The Aging Person
A Holistic Perspective

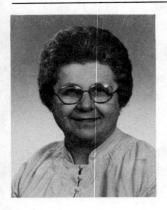

Lucille D. Gress, R.N., M.A., is an Associate Professor in the University of Kansas College of Health Sciences, School of Nursing. She has taught gerontological nursing intermittently for a number of years and since 1977 has taught gerontological nursing. She has also been involved in a number of research projects related to gerontological nursing.

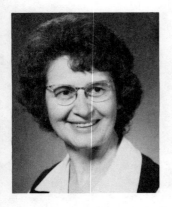

Sister Rose Therese Bahr, A.S.C., R.N., Ph.D., F.A.A.N., is a Professor of Nursing in the Department of Community Health Nursing and Program Director of the Gerontological Nursing Program preparing gerontological clinical nurse specialists in the Master of Nursing Program at the University of Kansas College of Health Sciences, School of Nursing. She has taught nursing process and the nursing and behavioral theories of aging in graduate nursing education and has conducted research related to sleep patterns and disorders, health beliefs and practices, and blood pressure, pulse, and temperature norms in aging subjects. Her current activities include participation in a national research study investigating curricular and practice issues of nurse administrators in long-term care facilities as well as clinical practice with ambulatory elderly Hispanic clients.

The Aging Person
A Holistic Perspective

LUCILLE D. GRESS, R.N., M.A.

Associate Professor, Department of Medical-Surgical Nursing,
Co-Program Director, Gerontological Nursing Program for
Graduate Students in Nursing, The University of Kansas,
College of Health Sciences, School of Nursing,
Kansas City, Kansas

Sister ROSE THERESE BAHR, A.S.C., R.N., Ph.D., F.A.A.N.

Professor of Nursing, Department of Community Health Nursing,
Program Director, Gerontological Nursing Program for
Graduate Students in Nursing, The University of Kansas,
College of Health Sciences, School of Nursing,
Kansas City, Kansas

Illustrated

The C. V. Mosby Company

ST. LOUIS   TORONTO   1984

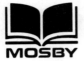

MOSBY

A TRADITION OF PUBLISHING EXCELLENCE

Editor: Julie Cardamon
Assistant editor: Bess Arends
Manuscript editor: Stephen Dierkes
Design: Suzanne Oberholtzer
Production: Carol O'Leary, Teresa Breckwoldt, Judy England

The C.V. Mosby Company
11830 Westline Industrial Drive, St. Louis, Missouri 63146

Library of Congress Cataloging in Publication Data

Gress, Lucille D.

The aging person.

  Bibliography: p.
  Includes index.
  1. Geriatric nursing. I. Bahr, Rose Therese.
II. Title. [DNLM: 1. Aging—Nursing texts. 2. Geriatrics—
Nursing texts. 3. Holistic health—Nursing texts.
WY 152 G832a]
RC954.G73   1984   362.6'042   83-8209
ISBN 0-8016-2032-5

AC/VH/VH 9 8 7 6 5 4 3 2 1   01/D/015

To our grandparents, parents, other family members, and friends,
who in many ways contributed toward the philosophy
of life and aging inherent in this work.
They contributed to an appreciation
of older persons' humanness and
value in leavening the wholeness of life;
the energizing life force and the caring concern
expressed by these people is inspirational to and
supportive of others along the life continuum.
Life at the end of a long journey is as valued as at its beginning.

Foreword

Holism emphasizes the wholeness of the older person and his or her self-agency. This wholeness encompasses the concepts of body, mind, and spirit and interactions with the environment; it promotes respect for human beings, their unique needs, and their right to continue development of personhood across the life span. Ultimately, the older person is worthy of respect and dignity whatever his or her status may be. This view projects life as a continuum from birth to death, calling attention to the wholeness of life as well as to the wholeness of the older person.

Because the needs of older persons are complex, individuals from many disciplines are needed to promote health and wellness in each dimension of the person: physical, psychological, sociological, and spiritual. The personhood of the older individual is the primary focus of this book; its content has implications for individuals of various professional orientations and for lay persons concerned with their own older family members.

What is caring for the older person all about? Answers found in this book can facilitate an understanding of the person experiencing the universal process of aging, and of the role that nursing and other related disciplines play in making the transition from one developmental stage to the other easier. This book is aptly titled, for it reflects all the dimensions of the older person.

During the past decade there has been a marked increase in literature concerning care of the older adult. From my perspective as a nurse, I see that nurses with expertise in caring for the aged are slowly but surely helping to correct misconceptions about the care of older adults.

In the newly emerging specialty of gerontological nursing, the challenge of fulfilling basic human needs is being met by nurses who recognize the necessity of preparation in the area of human development and aging and of acquisition of the requisite skills. Gerontological nursing is complex in nature and experimental by design, and requires continuing education. As more nurse scholars, such as the authors of this volume, share their knowledge of caring for the aged, nurses will have an opportunity to develop consensual yet creative methodologies for the provision of high-quality holistic care to older adults.

Attempts have already been made to define care of the older person from a holistic perspective. These authors, by placing emphasis on the spiritual dimension, have helped to close a gap in the literature. Attending to the spiritual dimension of the older person is an acknowledgment of the continuing development of the interior self characteristic of older persons. Enhancement of the spirit promotes health and wellness in the older individual.

The authors of this book are highly energized individuals who inspire others to view older persons holistically. They demonstrate a deep sensitivity for students and older clients alike. As scholars they are ever searching for the truth about and beauty of older persons. I have had the distinct pleasure of working with Sr. Rose Therese Bahr and Lucille Gress for approximately 5 years as they implemented an innovative grant aimed at the preparation of gerontological clinical nurse specialists. This book is a natural result of their philosophy and lives. I feel honored and privileged to introduce their book. The holistic perspective in this book should help its readers to have more of an understanding of themselves as older persons, of nursing as a dynamic, unique profession with a logical methodology called nursing process, and of the beautiful, inspiring, and awesome challenge that is gerontological nursing. Readers should sense the authors' enthusiasm as they draw nurses and others into a congruent, humanistic, holistic, and truly professional perspective of older persons—our present and future selves.

Delores M. Alford, M.S.N., R.N., F.A.A.N.
Gerontological Nursing Consultant
Dallas, Texas

Preface

Writing this book came about because of our interest in older persons and our concern for the increasing need to understand them as fully human persons. In view of their increasing longevity, demographics, and basic needs and rights, attention should be given to a holistic approach to persons in the later years of life. Although many books on gerontology and the aging process have been written, few focus on the continuing development of older adults from a holistic perspective.

The emphasis of this book is on the older person having the right to self-determination through the exercise of self-agency and self-care. Learning to exercise self-determination is a part of the developmental process that enables the person to become whatever he or she is capable of becoming. From a holistic perspective, this developmental process is achieved through the dynamic interchange of the whole person—mind, body, and spirit—with his or her total environment. If dependency needs arise and assistance is required, helping persons should respect and protect the integrity and the rights of the older person.

During aging, the person becomes increasingly differentiated and unique, and often more introspective. Self-understanding, the relationship of the self to the environment, and the question of the purpose of life often become a greater challenge to the person in later years than was the case in earlier years. Appreciation of this challenge is important to those who are interacting with and helping the older individual to maintain integrity.

Our intent is to explore within a holistic framework various factors influencing the continuing development of the older person. Although many variables contribute to the complexity of the human being, the thrust of the life force is toward a unified whole. We contend that, having received the gift of life, the older person no less than the younger person should experience the affirmation of being and share in the joys and celebration of life as a fully human being.

This book is intended for use as a textbook by graduate and undergraduate nursing students, and as a reference book for nurses working with older persons in various settings and individuals from other disciplines, such as social workers, pharmacists, nutritionists, clergymen, and occupational and physical therapists. The primary focus is on the humanness of older persons and their right to continue developing their potential as thinking, feeling, loving, and acting human beings. The book is aimed at promoting understanding and appreciation of older persons who continue striving toward personhood during their later years. Hence it has implications for anyone concerned with the well-being of older individuals.

In Chapter 1 an overview of the older person in the later years of development is offered within a holistic framework. A brief description of aging and an exploration of concepts related to holistic health and health care are presented.

Chapter 2 provides an overview of health and wellness applicable to the older person. Individual, community, and national perspectives are offered as a foundation for understanding the importance of health and wellness in the life of each person who is aging.

The terms *person, personhood,* and *personality* are analyzed in Chapter 3. This discussion encompasses philosophical, psychological, and sociological consideration of the essence of human nature as it matures over a life span and culminates in the beauty of character expressed in the personhood of the older individual.

Chapter 4 considers the older person from a developmental perspective. Attention is given to the concepts of development, various definitions and types of aging, growth and development in the later years, developmental orientations and theories, and other related topics.

The changes of aging—biological, psychological, sociological, and spiritual—and the challenges these changes pose for older persons are explored in Chapter 5. In addition, the challenges that these changes hold for care givers are examined.

The focus of Chapter 6 is on the concepts of motivation and high-level wellness as they relate to the older person. The concept of motivation and selected theories of motivation and personality development are discussed. Developmental aspects of motivation and models of aging are presented with a final commentary on the relevance of motivation to high-level wellness.

A discussion of those theories of self-care related to continued betterment of the older adult is presented in Chapter 7. The use of theories and theory-building in health care and nursing practice is described as an essential component in the care of older individuals. The self-care movement as a societal trend is analyzed; Orem's self-care agency theory and Kinlein's theory of care are used in demonstrating the importance of developing the self-care agency of older adults for the promotion of health, wellness, and independence.

Chapter 8 presents the promotion of personhood of aging individuals, using for analysis the components of life satisfaction, health, and the celebration of life as demonstrated through a variety of coping and adapting processes (e.g., relationships, communication techniques, zest for living, and achievement of life's goals). Two case histories of older adults who celebrate life daily are presented as examples for all older individuals.

In Chapter 9, an overview of the historical development of gerontological nursing is presented, based on Nightingale's formulation of nursing and the societal forces that created current issues and dilemmas faced by health professionals.

Chapter 10 deals with the older person and the nursing process. It includes a historical perspective of the nursing process and components of a philosophy of nursing. Four phases of the nursing process are defined and elaborated on with respect to the older person.

The older person and support system networks are discussed in Chapter 11. Systems theory, the concept of support, and support systems are briefly described. In addition, the concept of networks and types of support system networks are presented. Models of informal support systems and changing relationships in the informal support systems network are examined with consideration of strengthening the support systems. A review of support systems networks as they pertain to the rural elderly is also included. Finally, examples of support systems and the services they provide in support of the self-agency and strengths of older persons are given.

The Epilogue deals with perspectives of aging, past, present, and future. Aging is viewed within the context of social change. This concept of aging and continuing societal developments is explored and includes the concomitant development of the nursing profession in the field of aging. The perspectives of the future and challenges of aging are also explored. The potential for a bright future and the concept of a new world of brotherhood based on the worth and dignity of human beings are presented. Issues are raised regarding human values and rights with respect to the quality of life of each person in terms of humanness and in view of scientific advancements. The importance of helping each person realize a greater quality of life (as a priority over quantity of life) is pointed out. Meeting the challenge of this priority would, in turn, contribute to the well-being of society and the attainment of world brotherhood.

Our approach to the subject of this book is an outgrowth of our early experience within family constellations where a respect for and appreciation of older persons was a natural part of family relationships and interactions. Our philosophy of aging has continued to be expressed to students of gerontological nursing, numerous older persons, their adult children, and professional colleagues. In addition, our research efforts and presentations at workshops on national, regional, and local levels have reflected a continuing appreciation of the worth of older persons engaged in the pursuit of personhood. Attendance at various international and national meetings related to gerontology and gerontological nursing has expanded the breadth and scope of our knowledge. We have acquired expertise in direct interactions with older persons in various settings. Our convictions about older persons and their care have been reinforced by an ongoing review of the literature and by the response of older persons, family members, and professional colleagues.

Lucille D. Gress
Sister Rose Therese Bahr

Acknowledgments

We are grateful to the many persons who contributed to the development of this book including the older persons who graciously and freely gave of themselves and in so doing enhanced the quality and authenticity of this work.

We appreciate the cooperation and contribution of the administration and older persons at Mid-City Towers, Kansas City, Missouri, a high-rise primarily for the black elderly; St. Joseph Home, Kansas City, Kansas, a health care center for older adults; and El Centro, Kansas City, Kansas, a social center for Hispanic elderly. These individuals contributed toward the cultural diversity found in this book and demonstrated the enrichment that can occur with the celebration of life in later years.

In addition, we wish to acknowledge the Department of Audio-Visual Services at the University of Kansas College of Health Sciences and Hospital for the illustrations and photographs.

We also wish to express appreciation for the encouragement, support, and guidance provided by members of the staff of The C.V. Mosby Company. Their prompt, courteous response to numerous questions facilitated the writing process and helped make it a valuable learning experience for us.

Our grateful appreciation is extended to the reviewers who carefully read and critiqued the rough drafts of the manuscript. Feedback from these "invisible" persons influenced the quality of the final manuscript and their comments and interest afforded support to us.

Special thanks is extended to members of the staff and older adult participants at the Shepherd's Center, Kansas City, Missouri, a multipurpose center with programs designed by and for older adults in the metropolitan area. The interest in and support of gerontological nursing at the University of Kansas College of Health Sciences, School of Nursing, continues to be a source of strength to us.

Finally, we wish to express our heartfelt thanks to Jan Black, who shared a personal interest in the development of the manuscript and painstakingly typed beautiful copy from the almost illegible rough drafts. Her unfailing interest in and enthusiasm for the project helped us stay the course and meet the deadline for submission of the completed manuscript. Jan's loyalty and perseverance is commendable and deeply appreciated.

Contents

Chapter 1   A Holistic Perspective: an Overview

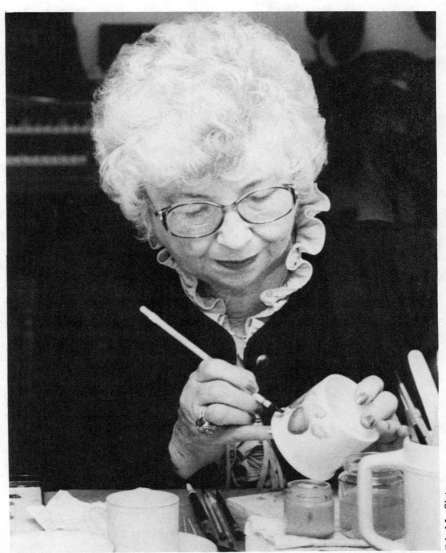

From a holistic perspective, the older person may be viewed as a human being striving toward unity and wholeness throughout the life span. This striving takes place within the context of an ever-changing environment, internal and external. Through a dynamic, interdependent relationship with these environments, the individual is influenced by and influences the sociocultural milieu that contributes toward personhood and wholeness. This chapter describes the older person in later years and that individual's right to be a self-determining, contributing member of society.

Holistic theory, according to Smuts (1926), is based on the concept of man responding in a unique manner as an individual and as a total being. Man consists of millions of particles, such as cells, which are subsets of larger, more complex parts, such as organs. These particles function in such a way as to support the parts, and the parts, in turn, support the whole person. Mind and body are viewed as inseparable; whatever happens in one part affects the whole being.

The holistic perspective is based on a concept of wholeness that may be examined by studying the structure and functions of human beings (Levine, 1971) and the dynamics of their relationships with their environment. Whatever changes occur, the whole person responds (Bower, 1982) and attempts to reestablish a dynamic balance among the interdependent variables of person and environment.

An illustration that may be used in depicting a holistic perspective was developed by Byrne and Thompson (1978) (Fig. 1-1). Concentric rings were used for portraying the individual's subordinate systems (cell, organ, organ systems) and superordinate systems (family, community, society). We

Fig. 1-1. **Levels of behavioral organization.**

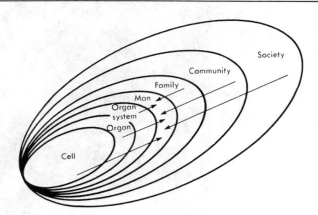

From Byrne, M.L., and Thompson, L.F.: Key concepts for the study and practice of nursing, ed. 2, St. Louis, 1978, The C.V. Mosby Co.

suggest use of this diagram for conceptualizing the older adult holistically. This perspective may be further developed by studying the dynamics of human behavior and relationships within the sociocultural milieu. This is in keeping with the assertion of Byrne and Thompson that a person cannot be understood apart from his or her environment.

Whitehead (1964), in turn, asserted that the body is inseparable from the natural world—that the brain and the body are actually continuous with the rest of the world. This concept of wholeness is illustrated in the work of those studying therapeutic touch. Krieger (1979), for example, speaks of an energy field that extends beyond the physical boundary of the skin of the body and of therapeutic touch as a mode of human interaction. She refers to a space between persons that can be perceived as a natural extension of the self and that may be used both to increase self-understanding and, because of this understanding, to promote the well-being of others. The concept of the transfer of energy from one person to another relates to the concept of wholeness defined previously and to the systems theory that will be discussed later.

A Holistic View of Aging

A holistic view of aging calls for a philosophy of aging. This philosophy should encompass beliefs about the nature of the human being, the world in which he or she lives, and the aging process. The human being is an active, changing individual who becomes increasingly differentiated and unique over time. The older person, in turn, develops within and adapts to a continually changing, sociocultural, physical, psychological, and spiritual environment. In the holistic view, the older person is expected to share in a give-and-take relationship with his or her environment. This means that the older person should have the opportunity to contribute to and benefit from resources that better the human condition.

Aging has been defined in various ways in the holistic perspective; it may best be viewed as the total of life experiences occurring in time. This broad definition encompasses changes in the person-environment context whatever the source or direction. Aging may be viewed as more than an either-or phenomenon of decremental or incremental nature; it can be viewed as a developmental process wherein constant change is multidimensional and multidirectional. The older person can learn new ways of relating to the self, to others, and to the world. He or she can continue to develop and to experience the joy that arises from relationships with others and the giving and receiving of affection.

A holistic philosophy of aging can be useful in combating "ageism," the tendency to discriminate against people on the basis of chronological age alone (Butler, 1969). Perhaps an indication of change in this attitude is evidenced in the election of Ronald Reagan to the presidency of the United States at the age of 69 and the implantation of a mechanical heart in 61-year-old Barney Clark, a retired dentist. Furthermore, the effect of elderly buyers on the market has recently been acknowledged ("Elderly buyers . . .," 1982). According to this report, 17.7 million family units have people 65 years of age or older as head. The elderly have already been acknowledged as an important segment of the voting population (approximately 16%), since they turn out to vote. Thus, there is some evidence of a developing attitude toward aging that takes into account the contribution older persons can make for the benefit of themselves and society.

A Holistic View of the Older Adult

A holistic view of the older adult may be achieved, in part, by giving attention to the dimensions of the individual. These dimensions—the physical, the psychological, the sociological, and the spiritual—will be examined further throughout the text. It is important that these dimensions be recognized as integral components of the whole person-environment milieu. If the older person reaches the point of needing assistance, helping persons should be mindful of the individual's right and responsibility to participate in problem-solving, decision-making processes in keeping with his or her state of well-being. Exercising the right of self-determination is essential to the person's sense of control over his or her destiny; it is also crucial to discharging social responsibility. No one lives in isolation; therefore individual and societal needs are important considerations within the holistic perspective.

Holistic Health

Demographics indicate that the oldest segment of society, people 80 years of age and above (Maddox, 1982), is the most rapidly increasing segment of the population throughout the world. These demographics reflect the increasing longevity, which in the United States is now 74 years. Since this older segment of the population is at risk for changes in health status, attention to the health needs of this population should be a priority within the holistic perspective.

Holistic health is a concept used to refer to the natural tendency toward self-healing (Jaffe, 1980). This integration of body, mind, and spirit (McKay, 1980) is achieved primarily by establishing a life-style that tends to promote a higher level of wellness (Ardell, 1977). Thus the locus of control for health is within the person who, in turn, is responsible to a great extent for his or her own state of well-being.

Benefits from a change in life-style can be experienced by older adults just as by younger persons. Achieving harmony among the various components of the individual necessitates attending to spiritual needs as well as physical, psychological, and sociological needs. Defining a philosophy and purpose in life is essential to achieving the state of well-being wherein the affirmation of the person can be realized (Brallier, 1978).

Holistic Health Care

Holistic health care emerged as a popular ideology in the 1970s. People began to turn to preventive health care programs such as the Kaiser-Permanente in California and to implement personal behaviors, such as exercise, weight control, and the giving up of smoking, as a means of regaining a measure of control over their well-being. This shift of emphasis from illness care to preventive health care and health promotion seemed to stem from the realization that the medical system affects only about 10% of the indices used for health measurement (Wildavsky, 1977; McKeown, 1978). The other 90% are determined by factors such as individual life-style, social conditions, and the physical environment, which are more subject to the control of individuals and groups of individuals involved in policy-making activities.

Various approaches to holistic health care have been developed, including stress management, biofeedback, muscle relaxation, meditation, visualization or use of guided imagery, and positive thinking (Brallier, 1978). Whatever the method, the goal is to help the person achieve a greater degree of harmony between himself or herself and the natural world (Jaffe, 1980). The emphasis is on health promotion and self-care. Although research is needed to provide a scientific basis for holistic health methods, many people, older adults included, are learning to use and apparently benefit from various methods and techniques for promoting wellness and increasing their zest for life.

Holistic Nursing and the Older Adult

Holism encompasses a multidisciplinary approach because of the many dimensions and needs of the human being. Holistic nursing is based on the concept of the person as a developing individual who is constantly involved in the process of change (Schrock, 1980). The older adult is recognized as a survivor of many life changes, positive and negative. These events have influenced his or her perception of and response to the experiences of daily life. Thus, determining the person's perceptions is of primary importance in the holistic nursing of older adults.

Achieving and maintaining wholeness may be as much a goal of the older person as of the younger person (Jaffe, 1980). It is coming to be recognized as one of the major challenges for older persons. Whereas younger persons tend to experience their bodies intensely, older persons may become intensely interested in learning about their bodies and how to take care of them. Older adults may be highly motivated toward self-care, since they generally value independence and desire to maintain mastery over their lives.

The integrated approach to health care of older adults calls for a comprehensive approach and a respect for their health beliefs and practices. The nurse and other health care providers have a responsibility to help older persons maintain their integrity. Evidence of the individual's ability to identify and deal with factors interfering with wellness is available in the report of Cousins (1979) and the findings of researchers Krieger (1979) and Rahe (1973). Holistic nursing is person centered and emphasizes the educational process; the older individual often needs to learn about the physiology of his or her body and about variables that affect its state of wellness.

An example of holistic nursing is practiced by Dolores M. Alford, who initiated the first independent gerontological nursing practice in the United States in April 1974 (Alford, 1982). Alford has promoted holism by assisting older persons to exercise their self-care agency and self-care management abilities and to use their strengths to achieve a high or higher level of wellness.

When Alford's practice expanded beyond what one nurse could handle, she recruited a partner; continuing expansion has since led to the addition of an associate. The agency they established is known as Nursing Associates. These nurses have incorporated principles of holistic nursing in their practice; they continue assessing health needs and screening for health problems and potential problems. They are involved in teaching clients how to acquire positive health habits so they can be healthy in body, mind, and spirit. Spiritual problems, for example, may arise when older persons are uprooted from their homes, which are often located in smaller towns or rural areas, and moved to larger metropolitan areas. These nurses practice nursing by promoting the self-care agency of their clients in a therapeutic relationship.

Services provided by the Nursing Associates include taking a wellness inventory, assessing the stress level of older adults, performing a physical examination, providing health counseling services and health education programs, and assisting the client with developing a comprehensive plan for the promotion of wellness.

Health promotion services of the Nursing Associates (1982) are offered at their office or at satellite locations such as day care centers, business offices, senior centers, schools, and apartment complexes. Nursing actions with older adults include contacting guardians regarding client needs, such as that for eyeglasses; prescribing a day at a beauty salon for comprehensive services, such as care of the hair, a manicure, and a pedicure; assisting the client with obtaining legal advice about financial affairs; teaching physical exercises; and providing health education.

Holistic nursing, as practiced by Alford and her associates, is comprehensive and includes attention to person-environment factors and the dynamics of interpersonal relationships. The approach is organized within the framework of the nursing process and guided by the American Nurses' Association's Standards of Gerontological Nursing Practice (ANA, 1976). A person-centered approach is used with an emphasis on wellness and health promotion.

Summary

A holistic perspective of the older person encompasses the whole person and his or her self-agency and life experiences. Whether the source of changes is physiological, psychological, sociological, or spiritual, the whole person experiences and responds to the changes. A holistic perspective is essential to understanding the older person and appreciating his or her unique needs as a thinking, feeling, acting human being. Throughout the book, the older person in the later years will be viewed holistically: as a person who has the potential for continuing development, experiencing affirmation and zest in daily living, and sharing with others in the celebration of life.

References

Alford, D.M.: Personal communication, Dec 27, 1982.

American Nurses' Association: Standards of gerontological nursing practice, Kansas City, Mo. 1976, A.N.A., Division of Gerontological Nursing.

Ardell, D.: High-level wellness: an alternative to doctors, drugs, and disease, Emmaus, Pa., 1977, Rodale Press, Inc.

Bower, F.L.: The process of planning nursing care: nursing practice models, ed. 3, St. Louis, 1982, The C.V. Mosby Co.

Brallier, L.W.: The nurse as a holistic health practitioner: expanding the role again, Nurs. Clin. North Am. 13(4):643-655, 1978.

Butler, R.N.: The effects of medical and health progress on the social and economic aspects of the life cycle, Industrial Gerontology 1:1-9, 1969.

Byrne, M.L., and Thompson, L.F.: Key concepts for the study and practice of nursing, ed. 2, St. Louis, 1978, The C.V. Mosby Co.

Cousins, N.: Anatomy of an illness as perceived by the patient: reflections on healing and regeneration, New York, 1979, Bantam Books, Inc.

Elderly buyers affect market, The Kansas City Star, December 19, 1982, 4B, Kansas City, Mo.

Jaffe, D.T.: Healing from within: how to gain greater control over your own health, New York, 1980, Bantam Books, Inc.

Krieger, D.: The therapeutic touch: how to use your hands to help or to heal, Englewood Cliffs, N.J., 1979, Prentice-Hall, Inc.

Levine, M.E.: Holistic nursing, Nurs. Clin. North Am. 6(2):253-264, 1971.

Maddox, G.L.: Aging people and aging population: a framework for decision making. In Thomas, H., and Maddox, G.L., editors: New perspectives on old age: a message to decision makers, New York, 1982, Springer Publishing Co.

McKay, S.: Wholistic health care: challenge to health providers, J. Allied Health 9(3):194-201, 1980.

McKeown, T.: The determinants of health, Hum. Nature 1(4):60-67, 1978.

Nursing Associates (brochure), Dallas, 1982.

Rahe, R.H.: Subjects' recent life changes and their near future life reports, Ann. Clin. Res. 4:1-16, 1973.

Schrock, M.M.: Holistic assessment of the healthy aged, New York, 1980, John Wiley & Sons, Inc.

Smuts, J.C.: Holism and evolution, New York, 1926, Macmillan Inc.

Whitehead, A.N.: Adventure of ideas, New York, 1964, Mentor Press.

Wildavsky, A.: Doing better and feeling worse: the protective pathology of health policy, Daedalus 106(1):105-123, 1977.

Chapter 2 Perspectives on Health and Wellness

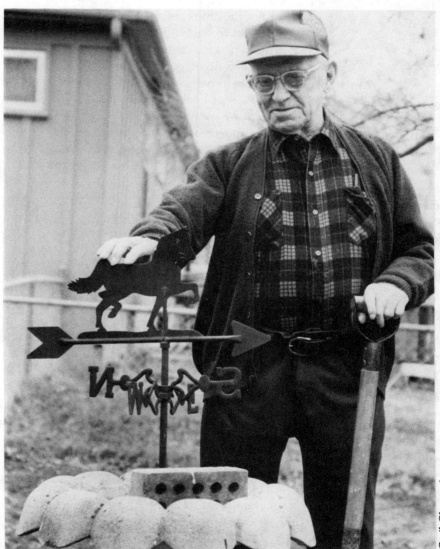

An individual wishing to fully enjoy life appreciates the need for health as a goal in his or her life. Attainment of health, resulting in satisfaction with one's life, requires developing the necessary inner resources. Life satisfaction touches many aspects of the individual including personal circumstances, work situation, and any social interaction. Achievement of health necessarily encompasses the four dimensions of the human person: the physiological, psychological, sociological, and spiritual realms. A positive life experience is expected when each dimension is fulfilled to its fullest potential throughout the life span.

For the older person health is a more urgent goal. Levels of wellness are expected to evolve into a greater measure of good health. Through wellness, self-actualization of the person is facilitated. Self-actualization is the achievement of potential reflected in the emergence of the individual's creative, dynamic personality.

Issues of health and wellness have been evident throughout the literature for a number of years. Controversies regarding the nature of health and wellness abound. These terms are defined in a variety of ways, depending on the perspective from which they are seen. Each of these terms is discussed in the following paragraphs.

Health and Wellness: Definitions

Health, according to Keller (1981) may be perceived as a state (Parsons, 1958; Dubos, 1965; King, 1971; Knight, 1974; Twaddle, 1974; Terris, 1975; Callahan, 1977; Duval, 1977; McDermott, 1977); a process (Greifinger, 1977; Hoke, 1968); a diagnosis (Twaddle, 1974; Sebag, 1979); a task (Illich, 1976); a response (Murray and Zentner, 1975); or a goal (Goodrich, 1932; Dubl, 1976; Wan and Livieratos, 1978). A definition of health that is generally accepted by most health professionals is the statement promulgated by the World Health Organization (1947) defining health as "a state of complete physical, mental, and social well-being and not merely the absence of disease and infirmity."*

Although this definition stresses health's various dimensions, in today's society illness or sickness continues as the basis of present provision of health care. When illness is the primary societal orientation, not having illness is considered to be health. Health is thus couched in negative terms. That sickness remains the major focus today is evidenced by the large number of institutions providing acute care. Money contributed from state and federal funding resources supports the sickness model to a much greater extent than the preventive health care model.

*From World Health Organization: Constitution of the World Health Organization, Chronicle World Health Organization, 1(1-2):29-43, 1947.

When health is perceived more positively, that is, as well-being in the physical, mental, and social domains suggested by the World Health Organization, emphasis is placed on measures of wellness that contribute to a desirable state of health. Health measures include sufficient nutrition, fluids, recreation, sleep, diversity of activities, work, solitude, social relationships, and spiritual development. When these measures are practiced, the individual is nurtured and enjoys a higher level of wellness and health.

Wellness, as opposed to health, is seen as an integrating force energizing each dimension of the human personality: physical, psychological, sociological, and spiritual. Dunn (1961) notes that wellness produces the capability within the individual to perform at an optimum level of functioning; that is, so that any task can be undertaken and completed in a zestful manner that is satisfying to the individual. Jourard (1971) speaks of wellness as comprising several components that result in a personality promoting physical health. With this personality people are concerned about diet, rest, and solitude. They are informed about principles of general hygiene; they are motivated to care for their teeth, sleep sufficiently to restore their energy, exercise to keep fit, and maintain a level of morale or "spirit" that produces a challenging and satisfying life. Bruhn and co-workers (1977) note that the wellness process is composed of the following:

1. Personal growth
2. Internal control
3. Knowledge about health-related activities and habits

Wellness, then, is perceived as a growth and development process throughout life.

Wellness for the individual is constantly developing; it never remains at a static stage. Because wellness is perceived as a process, wellness tasks need to be identified and implemented throughout life. Numerous models of wellness that identify wellness tasks are given in the literature. One such model, presented by Havighurst (1972), is based on Erikson's eight developmental stages (Erikson, 1963). In this model the tasks of wellness for those in middle adulthood (generativity vs. stagnation) include the following:

1. Accepting aging of self and others
2. Coping with pressures of social and occupational responsibilities and mobility
3. Recognizing the importance of good health habits and practices
4. Completing a periodic personal reassessment of life goals

For those in Erikson's last stage of maturity (ego integrity vs. despair) wellness tasks include the following:

1. Becoming aware of risks to health, and adjusting life-style and habits to cope with risks

2. Adjusting to loss of job, income, and family and friends through death
3. Redefining self-concept
4. Adjusting to changes in personal time and new physical environment
5. Adjusting previous health habits to current physical and mental capacities*

Through use of a wellness model, the level of wellness attained by an individual is readily identified and assessed.

Jahoda (1958) projected a model of wellness pertaining to positive mental health. This model suggests six approaches or categories of the concept of mental health for the purpose of assessment. Wellness tasks projected for mental health include:

1. Attitudes of an individual toward his own self
2. The individual's style and degree of growth development or self-actualization as expressions of mental health
3. Integration of all aspects of the personality
4. Autonomy describing degrees of independence
5. Perception of reality
6. Environmental mastery†

Through use of Jahoda's model, the wellness modality for the mental health of older persons may be assessed. Using the models projected by Havighurst and Jahoda, it is possible to grasp the essence of wellness as it relates to good health.

Older persons are capable of achieving and maintaining high-level wellness throughout their life spans. The health professional can aid in this attainment by:

1. Understanding the aging process as well as the health behaviors and belief systems of the older person
2. Providing instruction and anticipatory guidance about the functioning of the human body, mind, and spirit, and how these three components are an integral part of a healthy personality

When the developmental tasks of each phase of the life span are completed, when there is an absence of clinical disease, and when there is integration of the person within the social environment, the threshold for wellness and self-actualization is cleared for the older person. Thus, the older person is capable of enjoying a higher level of wellness any time, regardless of risks, injuries, and temporary delays in the approach to health experienced in his or her lifetime.

A National Perspective

Larson (1983) recently reported that Americans spend 287 billion dollars on health care annually and that this amount increases each year. Health

*From Bruhn, J.G., and others: The wellness process, J. Community Health **2**(3):209-211, 1977.
†From Jahoda, M.: Current concepts of positive mental health, New York, Copyright © 1958, Basic Books, Inc., Publishers.

care is the largest industry in the United States; 10% of the gross national product is spent in pursuit of wellness. He noted that more hospital beds, more drugs, and improved technology have demonstrated very little return on the health dollar.

Heart disease, stroke, and cancer continue to account for 70% of all deaths. However, only a small fraction of the national health budget is aimed at preventing and detecting these diseases. Larson suggests that people in the United States are literally killing themselves because of careless health habits, environmental pollution, and stressful social conditions that result in illness rather than wellness. To a degree, the life-styles of many Americans indicate a national orientation toward nonwellness rather than a positive orientation toward wellness.

Literature suggests, however, that a national revolution of health may be taking place. Realization that health practices are essential to the maintenance of good health and wellness is becoming more prevalent in the minds of individuals promoting self-care agency. Many more individuals are becoming nonsmokers, reducing high-level sodium content in foods, obtaining better rest and sleep, using relaxation techniques, and working toward improvement in mental health status. However, many individuals still do not subscribe to programs in weight control, exercise, and social activity essential to a well-balanced positive life-style.

Realization that the pursuit of health involves personal responsibilities must become more widespread; health is not merely a privilege or a gift. When citizens of various ages subscribe to health and wellness as a goal, the sickness model may turn into a wellness modality. When this occurs, health care dollars at the national level will be channeled into wellness promotion and prevention of illness rather than used primarily for treatment of after-the-fact acute and chronic illnesses.

A Community Perspective

A community comprises various ethnic and cultural groups who perceive health from their own perspectives. Individuals within each cultural group appreciate their relationship to the group and its beliefs and subscribed ritualistic health practices. For example, the orthodox Jewish community has a religious overtone in preparation of their food, using certain utensils and a prescribed number of washings of those utensils to promote health and well-being. Other groups also demonstrate cultural, ethnic, or religious differences that have an impact on health and wellness. The beauty and uniqueness of these variations may be appreciated.

Urban Dwellers

Citizens living in the urban community are exposed to various environmental factors impinging on their health and wellness: a high noise level from airplanes flying overhead, air pollution caused by automobile exhaust fumes and industrial waste, fat content of food purchased at fast-food chain stores, and interruptions of sleep by street cleaning equipment or jackhammers at nearby construction sites. Urban dwellers have a unique set of barriers to good health and wellness; these barriers must be evaluated and strategies planned and implemented to promote wellness. For example, a drive to a park outside the city for tranquil communing with nature may be a wellness task promoting balance in one's life. Another example is a working mother preparing food over the weekend for family meals in the coming week, rather than relying on doughnuts with high fat content or hamburgers for a quick but less healthful meal or snack.

Concern for the health of the urban dweller accompanies concern for the aged, for whom a fixed income and other factors result in less than adequately nutritious meals. The older person needs adequate nutrition as well as the younger person.

Rural Dwellers

Another component of the community is rural residents. In the rural setting, health programs, funded by state and national organizations, are often minimal or nonexistent. This problem leads to health practices initiated by the self-reliant rural dweller. For example, the rural dweller may join with other rural dwellers to butcher an animal for protein content in their meals during the cold winter months. A variety of community-based initiatives promoting health and wellness show the motivation and initiative of those who may not have access to health professionals or to a systematic provision of health care. The community's health and wellness depends on commonly held goals.

Many rural dwellers are older individuals (Kersten, 1979). They maintain a long, arduous workday tilling the soil. They seldom retire from farming because they lack financial resources to support such a retirement. Health practices for them continue to be time-tested remedies handed down through generations, such as garlic soup and mustard plasters for combating chest colds and congestion, or a mixture of chamomile tea and honey heated thoroughly and sipped slowly to combat gastrointestinal disorders. This self-reliant approach has resulted in more than merely physical survival. A large group of healthy, long-lived farmers are happy with their life-style and goal of independent living. Group effort has led to the building of a strong rural America.

An Individual Perspective

Each individual defines, to a great extent, his or her own status of health or illness. This personal definition is a primary factor stimulating health behavior. The individual is, of necessity, responsible for placing a value on health and then taking action to attain and maintain it. Attaining health requires choosing foods; determining amounts of rest, exercise, social relaxing, and privacy; and seeking ways to fulfill certain basic human needs. All these activities comprise the essence of self-care and self-responsibility for health; the individual can assess his or her self-care measures in these areas.

In assessing the health of the elderly individual, assessment of functional ability becomes imperative. Functional ability significantly determines the older person's life-style and appreciation for life. The health professional uses the assessment of functional ability to aid the elderly person with reviewing his or her life-style practices and health beliefs. It may bring to light deficiencies creating difficulties. Therefore, it is important that the individual subscribe to the value of health in his or her life. The wellness components of the physiological, psychological, sociological, and spiritual dimensions are encompassed within the total life-style of the older person. It is the older person who is ultimately responsible for his or her own health and wellness.

Summary

Health and wellness are goals of the older person. Through an appreciation of what health and wellness means, and through the establishment of healthy life-style practices, the older person aids in the maintenance of optimum functioning in whatever the setting. The beauty of body, mind, and spirit are maintained through health and wellness and can be constantly developed to bring joy and zest for living.

References

Bruhn, J.G., and others: The wellness process, J. Community Health 2(3):209-211, 1977.

Callahan, D.: Health and society: some ethical imperatives. In Knowles, J.H., editor: Doing better and feeling worse—health in the United States, New York, 1977, W.W. Norton & Co., Inc.

Dubos, R.: Man adapting, New Haven, Conn., 1965, Yale University Press.

Dubl, L.J.: The health planner: planning and dreaming for health and wellness, Am. J. Health Planning 1(2):7-14, 1976.

Dunn, H.L.: High-level wellness, Arlington, Va., 1961, Beatty, Ltd.

Duval, M.K.: The provider, the government, and the consumer. In Knowles, J.H., editor: Doing better and feeling worse—health in the United States, New York, 1977, W.W. Norton & Co., Inc.

Erikson, E.: Childhood and society, ed. 2, New York, 1963, W.W. Norton & Co., Inc.

Goodrich, A.W.: The social and ethical significance of nursing, New York, 1932, Macmillan Inc.

Greifinger, R.B., and Grossman, R.L.: Towards a language of health: achieving high-level wellness, Health Values 1:207-209, 1977.

Havighurst, R.J.: Developmental tasks and education, ed. 3, New York, 1972, Longman, Inc.

Hoke, B.: Promotive medicine and the phenomena of health, Arch. Environ. Health 16:269-278, 1968.

Illich, I.: Medical nemesis—the expropriation of health, New York, 1976, Bantam Books, Inc.

Jahoda, M.: Current concepts of positive mental health, New York, 1958, Basic Books, Inc., Publishers.

Jourard, S.: The transparent self, New York, 1971, Van Nostrand Reinhold Co.

Keller, M.J.: Toward a definition of health, Adv. Nurs. Sci. 41(1):43-52, 1981.

Kersten, J.: Attitudes of the rural elderly toward health and their use of available community health resources, unpublished master's thesis, Kansas City, 1979, The University of Kansas.

King, I.M.: Toward a theory for nursing—general concepts of human behavior, New York, 1971, John Wiley & Sons, Inc.

Knight, J.A.: Spiritual psychology and self-regulation. In Godlway, E.M., editor: Inner balance—the power of inner healing, Englewood Cliffs, N.J., 1974, Prentice-Hall, Inc.

Larson, P.: Health strategy faltering: Americans told prevention best disease fighter, The Kansas City Star, Jan. 2, 1983, Kansas City, Mo.

McDermott, W.: Evaluating the physician and his technology. In Knowles, J.H.: Doing better and feeling worse—health in the United States, New York, 1977, W.W. Norton & Co., Inc.

Murray, R., and Zentner, J.: Nursing concepts for health promotion, Englewood Cliffs, N.J., 1975, Prentice-Hall, Inc.

Parsons, T.: Definitions of health and illness in light of American values and social structures. In Jaco, E.G., editor: Patients, physicians, and illness, New York, 1958, The Free Press.

Sebag, J.: The diagnosis of health, Prev. Med. 8(1):76-88, 1979.

Terris, M.: Approaches to an epidemiology of health, Am. J. Public Health 65:1037-1045, 1975.

Twaddle, A.C.: The concept of health status, Soc. Sci. Med. 8(1):29-38, 1974.

Wan, T.T.H., and Livieratos, B.: Interpreting a general index of subjective well-being, Milbank Mem. Fund. Q. 56:531-556, 1978.

World Health Organization: Constitution of the World Health Organization, Chronicle World Health Organization 1(1-2):29-43, 1947.

Chapter 3 The Older Person and Personhood

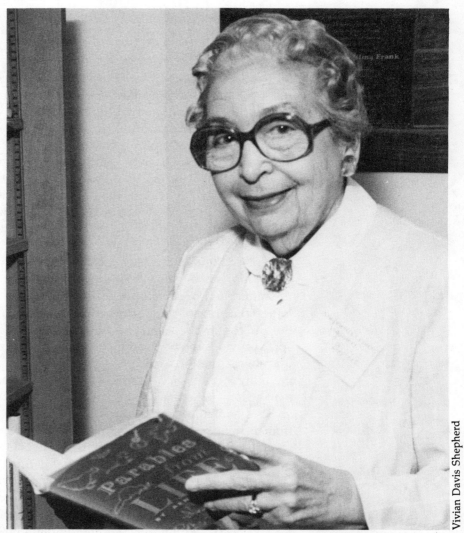

Vivian Davis Shepherd

Within the heart of every individual lies the most desired of needs—to be recognized as a person. This desire is so powerful that it remains a goal for a lifetime; personal identity is sought time and again in a variety of circumstances and life-styles. This desire continues throughout the life span but may become especially indomitable as an individual's age increases. What is this force that is so compelling? This phenomenon is the focus of this chapter—the meaning of personhood. In analyzing this phenomenon, the definitions of person, personality, and personhood and the varying components contributing to the development of the personality (cultural, biological, sociological, psychological, historical, and spiritual) are discussed. Particular emphasis is placed on the older adult and the goal of becoming a self-actualized person throughout the aging process.

The Human Person
Definition of Person

Because of the complexity of the human person, there is difficulty defining a human person in any specific way. Numerous philosophers, theologians, sociologists, and psychologists have given definitions of the human being with insight into the totality of the components. Theologians stress the essence of a nature created by God, in the Supreme Being's own image and likeness. In that regard, the human person, in physical actions and mental capacity, reflects the goodness, truth, and beauty of the person's Creator. In this belief, the human person is defined as mirroring the Creator's attributes, and thus having an intent always to do good to others, who also are created by God. What truly constitutes an action as human is the free will choosing that action (Strecker, 1981).

Philosophers often view the human person as a composite of body, mind, and spirit (soul, life principle). In this perspective, holism reflects the interaction of all components of the human person, giving rise to the importance of each component in the appreciation of human nature. In the philosopher's belief, the human person is a network for which the spirit provides the permeating life principle for growth of mind and body. It is always the three interacting components that determine the action of the human. Philosophers, then, are often interested in the essence of human action, sometimes taking into account the theological orientation that ascribes human nature to a Creator. Theologically and philosophically, the human person is one who is able to think, love, act, and become freely responsible for actions because the interconnecting network of body, mind, and spirit reflects God's spiritual nature. The human person, then, chooses freely to take responsibility for actions regarding moral laws, civil laws, and community regulations. These human actions differ from animal acts, which only accord to the animal nature (Strecker, 1981).

The classic definition is that the human person is a rational animal. In this view, the human person has a nature similar in its physical needs to that of an animal, and the only attribute unique to that person is rationality—the ability to reason and think through any situation calling for responsible action. This particular definition was promulgated by many classical and medieval philosophers, including Socrates, Plato, Aristotle, Thomas Aquinas, and others. This definition still holds true for contemporary human beings; the main tenet in considering humanness continues to be rationality.

A psychologist views the human being not as a static entity but as a system of dynamic and everchanging needs (Maslow, 1970). In this orientation, Maslow contends, many of the same elements needed by animals are also needed by humans, but humans express their needs in a unique way. Not only do humans know their needs, but they also have the capacity of understanding why the need exists. Consequently, humans may devise particular ways of meeting their needs. Often the human person is identified as a biopsychosocial, spiritual, and sexual human being, thus including the various dimensions of humanity—the inner world of human nature.

The sociologist views the human person from an interactional model. Since the human person is a social being, interaction between the person and others—family, neighborhood, community, and society—is as essential to living as the interaction with environment. Byrne and Thompson (1972) note that the intermingling of the person's inner environment and vast external environment brings about harmonious relationships.

Defining the human person from theological, philosophical, psychological, and sociological perspectives, then, helps to view and gain understanding of the myriad components and behaviors commonly attributed to a human being. Thus the complexity or development of an individual can be more deeply appreciated, and so can the fact that no life is without worth and dignity, because of its sacred origins and potential for improving society. Another concept to be explored is personhood, the object of lifetime pursuit. This concept is essential to understanding the human person's development.

Definition of Personhood   For Ashley and O'Rourke (1978), the embodied intelligent freedom highlighting the faculties of intelligence and free will are the two main projections in defining the human person. The intellect, with its capacity for receiving information from the five senses, can place these elements of information into an orderly and logical presentation for synthesis, interpretation, and evaluation. It is this reflective capacity of the human mind that allows an individual to make choices and to act responsibly in demanding situations. Ashley and O'Rourke note that to be a fully developed person means to live an intelligent freedom. This opportunity is given only to humans and allows for living fully. To be fully human means to express personhood uniquely in a relationship with every individual. In other words, personhood is a relational component of humanness (Happel, 1974). As a social being, a person is not able to be independent to the degree of isolation. Consequently, each person develops in relationship to others. Through this orientation socially accepted behavior is learned and awareness of the uniqueness of each life is deepened.

The task for attaining personhood begins with the question, "Who am I?" and, as answers are sought from others—mother, father, friends— another question arises: "Why am I?" One's existence—being born and through life attempting to achieve meaningful goals—becomes both a gift and a task (Happel, 1974). This growth process aids in understanding one's origin, sexuality, and ability to adapt to change and risk; in continually viewing life as a means to an end; in becoming the multidimensional person that one is capable of becoming; and in meeting in a meaningful way the needs of others. This purposeful approach to living brings about the fullness of personhood. It is a lifelong pursuit.

In other words, personhood is a process rather than a product. It is understood, then, that the terms *person, personhood,* and *personality* are not identical. *Person* describes the essence of human nature incorporated in the body, mind, and spirit of an individual. *Personhood* describes the continued development of one's total being in the physical, psychological, sociological, and spiritual dimensions toward self-actualization. *Personality* is the expression of personhood through the freely intelligent manner of acting, thinking, and loving.

Development of Personality

The development of the human personality begins at the moment of birth when the infant finally perceives an environment outside of the mother's womb. The individuals with whom this new, unique human being interacts have a profound impact on his or her personality development. This human being, with no life history other than gestation, is open for stimulation from a variety of sources. These sources greatly influence the immediate shaping of this human being into a human person. The infant's attention, through the biological development of the central nervous system, becomes attracted to elements in the environment. These elements take on symbolic meaning: certain messages that will have importance in life. For example, if the infant becomes attuned to a certain style of music in the home, this stimulation begins to convey the personalities of the mother and father and to evoke responses from the child.

It is very important that the newborn child be stimulated in many ways so that the senses of smell, taste, touch, sight, and hearing can help intellectual development keep up with biological development. Ashley and O'Rourke (1978) note that the human person is corporeal as well as intelligent, a unique body-person entity in constant interaction with the environment. The body's needs are totally integrated with the mind and spirit so that a holistic frame of reference emerges.

Numerous theories that attempt to interpret the personality and its development have been proposed. A brief overview of the major theories of personality aids in the identification of important concepts explaining personality and its evolution.

Theories of Personality

Freud, the father of psychoanalysis, was the first scientist to propound a theory regarding the development of human behavior. Primarily, the tenets of his theory include that a human being has an unconscious mind (id), ego, superego, and drives that are divided into sexual aggressions and unconscious conflicts. Little of the supernatural exists in his understanding of human functioning; nor is the will of the human person ever free. Freud has little appreciation for a person's belief in God; he suggests that such a religious belief is a person's mental projection to aid in everyday life (Gill, 1981). Freud's psychotherapy probes deeply ingrained conflicts in an effort to resolve existing pathological behavior. His theory of personality was a bold attempt to explain personality development and formed the foundation for subsequent theories.

Rogers (1951), who promotes client-centered therapy, proposes a theory that personality development occurs in the here-and-now; he does not emphasize past experiences as much as Freud did. Rogers states one fundamental need for personality development: to actualize all facets of the individual for growth. In this orientation, Rogers believes that the individual is capable of becoming everything he or she can be while moving toward self-actualization, the process of becoming oneself. Rogers notes that a healthy personality is a process, not a state of being, and that the process of self-actualization is ongoing. He suggests further that self-actualized persons live lives that are full of meaning, challenge, and enrichment, and that they are truly themselves. For Rogers, the fully functioning person is capable of experiencing a wide range of positive and negative emotions and lives every moment fully with a spontaneous and free orientation, on the level of feeling more than reason. This approach to personality development for Rogers was a breakthrough in personality development and aided a positive approach to perceiving oneself and an openness to all experiences in life (Gill, 1981).

Maslow, another psychologist, postulates that all human beings possess an innate tendency to become self-actualizing but that they move through a hierarchy of needs that must be satisfied if their development is to be complete. These basic needs relate to the physical or physiological aspects, to safety and security, feelings of belonging, love and esteem and, finally, self-actualization (Maslow, 1954, 1970). It is through the process of self-actualization that Maslow believes full humanness is achieved. A self-actualized person comes into close contact with the true self, the essence of being, and even with God (Gill, 1981).

May (1953) stresses the importance of the concept of becoming and the process of self-development (fulfilling one's potential). Making deliberate choices to attain self-fulfillment, the individual is able to create his own essence by transcending the natural level to full self-development. Through these decisions, the human potential is brought to mature fulfillment (Gill, 1981).

Erikson (1963) influenced theories of personality development by viewing the various stages of the life cycle as a series of phases or crises. These phases, according to Erikson, demand that all the earlier life tasks that serve as prerequisites for further human growth be accomplished before moving to the next task. Erikson identifies these particular stages in the life cycle as requiring qualities such as (1) a capacity for trusting, (2) autonomy, (3) initiative, (4) a sense of personal identity, and (5) an ability to relate to others with intimacy, that is, with a deep sharing of mind and heart. Specifically, Erikson identifies each phase or crisis as demanding the qualities portrayed in each of these six developmental cycles:

1. *Infancy and early childhood.* The quality to be developed is basic trust; and the crisis is mistrust.
2. *Middle childhood.* The quality to be developed is industry; and the crisis is fantasy.
3. *Adolescence.* The quality to be developed is identity; the crisis is nonidentity or identity confusion.
4. *Early adulthood.* Intimacy is the next stage of development; the crisis is isolation.
5. *Middle age.* Generativity is the quality to be developed; and the crisis is stagnation or self-absorption.
6. *Old age.* Ego integrity is the task/goal of this stage; and the crisis is distrust or despair.*

These categories provide the basis for evaluating and analyzing the personality as it develops. The personality, then, has dimensions that must be realized throughout life. The dimensions of personality identified by Ashley and O'Rourke include the following four levels of need.†

1. *The biological dimension* (Maslow's physiological needs). Human persons share with all living organisms the need to maintain themselves homeostatically in a dynamic relation with their environment, to grow and mature to full biological development as individuals, and to continue the species through reproduction. This is the level usually dealt with by biologists and physicians.

*From Erikson, E.: Childhood and society, New York, 1963, W.W. Norton & Co., Inc., pp. 247-284.
†From Ashley, B.M., and O'Rourke, K.S.: The right to be fully human. In health care ethics: a theological analysis, St. Louis, 1978, The Catholic Hospital Association.

2. *The psychological dimension* (Maslow's safety needs and also his belongingness and love needs in their more emotional aspects). We are psychic organisms which sense, imagine, and feel. This is the level of need generally dealt with by experimental psychologists and psychotherapists.
3. *The ethical dimension* (Maslow's esteem needs as well as the belongingness and love needs in their more developed aspects). This is the level of human free choice within the limits of an existing culture. It comprises the need of the individual both for self-control and social relations beyond those determined by the family. This is the level dealt with by lawyers, political leaders and clergy acting as moral counselors.
4. *The spiritual dimension* (Maslow's need for self-actualization including needs to know and understand, to contemplate and to create). This is the level of commitment, creativity, and transcendence at which we not only live within a culture, but criticize it, transcend it, and contribute to it. It includes all activity with a creative element in art or science or political innovation and, furthermore, religious activity as it extends to ultimate, cosmic meaning. This is the level dealt with by the inspiring teacher and spiritual guide.

These dimensions, essential to personality development, constitute the foundation for further analysis of growth. They suggest specific tasks to be accomplished within determined time frames in life's continuum. These tasks are dynamic and assist in the appreciation of the "who" and "why" of each individual.

Personality Development During the Life Span: the Fully Functioning Individual

Since personality development is considered a lifetime process, it is well to review specific developmental tasks occurring in the various phases (time frames) of the life span that assist the individual in continual positive development of the personality. The five stages of personality development, as formulated by Buscaglia (1978) include (1) infant and child, (2) adolescent, (3) mature adult, (4) intimate adult, and (5) old person. Each of these stages merits discussion to fully appreciate their importance to incremental enrichment of the personality.

1. *Infant and child.* Buscaglia indicates that the search for self is achieved through imitation of those placed in authority over the child, that is, parents or guardians. It is through this outward authority that the child begins to learn about the immediate world and the self. Through a variety of behaviors including play, the child explores this world, which becomes an entirely new arena for enjoyment, experiencing new events, and encountering other individuals. Havighurst (1972) discusses developmental tasks crucial for personality development in the periods from birth to 6 years and from 6 to 12 years. These developmental tasks are essential for promotion of that basic trust in the initial stages of life for a child given by Erikson, as well as of the basic human needs promoted by Maslow. The tasks for the first 6 years of life include the following:

a. Learning to walk
b. Learning to take solid foods
c. Learning to talk

    d. Learning to control the elimination of body wastes
    e. Learning sex differences and sexual modesty
    f. Forming concepts and learning language to describe social and physical reality
    g. Getting ready to read
    h. Learning to distinguish right and wrong and beginning to develop a conscience*

In middle childhood, from 6 to 12 years of age, Havighurst (1972) notes the following tasks to be accomplished:

    a. Learning physical skills necessary for ordinary games
    b. Building a wholesome attitude toward oneself as a growing organism
    c. Learning to get along with age-mates
    d. Learning an appropriate masculine or feminine social role
    e. Developing fundamental skill in reading, writing, and calculating
    f. Developing concepts necessary for everyday living
    g. Developing conscience, morality, and a scale of values
    h. Achieving personal independence
    i. Developing attitudes toward social groups and institutions

These tasks, when accomplished within childhood, form a foundation for strong personality development throughout the life span.

    2. *Adolescent.* The next stage of personality development is adolescence. Buscaglia notes that adolescence can be extremely joyful and filled with misery at the same time. During this stage the adolescent begins to perceive the self in a unique way and attempts to become more independent, moving further and further away from those responsible for child-rearing. This stage of development needs careful nurturing by parents or guardians to help the delicate balance of dependence and independence to achieve its full potential. In this stage all previous learning is questioned and placed in doubt until the adolescent can come to grips with true beliefs and make commitments about lifetime guiding forces. Choosing these directions aids in setting a course of action that brings satisfaction in both the personal and career life-styles. Havighurst (1972) gives the following developmental tasks for the adolescent 12 to 18 years of age. These developmental tasks include the following:

    a. Achieving new and more mature relations with age-mates of both sexes
    b. Achieving a masculine or feminine social role
    c. Accepting one's physique and using the body effectively
    d. Achieving emotional independence of parents and other adults
    e. Preparing for marriage and family life
    f. Preparing for an economic career
    g. Acquiring a set of values and an ethical system as a guide to behavior—developing an ideology
    h. Desiring and achieving socially responsible behavior

3. *Mature and intimate adult.* The mature adult's personality is constantly changing, constantly growing. Each day brings a new challenge and an opportunity to become more the person he or she has the potential to be. Each day, new experiences, such as encounters with unknown persons and new jobs to be accomplished in the household or at work bring opportunities for growth. All of these events help shape the behavior of the individual as he or she becomes more mature. Maturity is a lifelong process of growth. Life, then, includes the goal of actualization of all a human person's potential. Buscaglia (1978) notes that a person who is mature enjoys relationships: relationships with self, with others, with nature, and with his or her God. These spiritual elements become more and more ingrained in the mature person who finds that life is a wondrous thing to behold and is to be enjoyed fully at each moment. Buscaglia notes further that the mature person welcomes challenges to the potentiality of the self, so that the mastery of life may be appreciated fully. In maturity the person becomes fully functioning and, in Maslow's term, self-actualized. The self-actualized individual enjoys giving and receiving love and appreciates the uniqueness of others. The mature individual is an initiator and self-motivator, is creative, enjoys a sense of humor, and is comfortable in any situation because self-love is present. (The ability to touch others in love flows from self-love.) The mature person ascribes the wisdom that comes with loving as the guidepost for living life fully.

Havighurst (1972) notes that the developmental stage for the mature adult may be divided into two phases: early adulthood, 18 to 35 years of age and middle age, 36 to 64 years of age. Each phase has its own developmental tasks that are to be completed successfully as a foundation for further living. Havighurst (1972) identifies these developmental tasks for early adulthood:

a. Selecting a mate
b. Learning to live with a marriage partner
c. Starting a family
d. Rearing children
e. Managing a home
f. Getting started in an occupation
g. Taking on civic responsibility
h. Finding a congenial social group

Havighurst suggests these developmental tasks for middle age:

a. Assisting teenage children to become responsible and happy adults
b. Achieving adult social and civic responsibility
c. Reaching and maintaining satisfactory performance in one's occupational career
d. Developing adult leisure-time activities
e. Relating oneself to one's spouse as a person
f. To accept and adjust to the physiological changes of middle life
g. Adjusting to aging parents

A most noteworthy developmental task for the mature adult is intimacy. Intimacy is defined as a capability for enjoying close, warm, dynamic, comforting relationships with other persons. It is through intimacy that the adult person gains self-knowledge, wisdom, compassion, love, forgiveness, and the opportunity to touch another person deeply. Through intimacy and love, the person can be helped to grow and become who he or she really is. With intimacy, whether with a close friend or a spouse, each person is fulfilled. Togetherness helps in overcoming feelings of rejection, isolation, and loneliness, in experiencing life in all dimensions. This is not to say that intimacy is free of pain; but it does offer the opportunity to rise above selfish concern for oneself and to meet the needs for belongingness, love, self-esteem, security, and safety. It is a movement toward self-actualization (Buscaglia, 1978).

4. *The older person.* The healthy older person, 60 years of age or over, is a fully functioning human being with the wisdom of years and opportunities for self-actualization. Such opportunities are afforded by a dynamic family life, socializing, intimate relationships, a profession or occupation, and creativity in music, art, and literature. The older person develops and actualizes an inherent potentiality to the point where the true self emerges. It is true that many physical changes occur: wrinkles, weight loss, shortening of stature, difficulty hearing and seeing. But it is the human spirit, the world of inner resources, that the older person exhibits in such a beautiful way. It has been said that as the physical changes become more prominent in the older person, the inner world becomes more finely attuned to the environment. An older person has time to enjoy the beautiful and simple things: a leaf on a tree in autumn, the dew on rose petals, the greenness of grass, and the blueness of sky. By enjoying these things, the world becomes more beautiful. The companionship of both peers and younger people is sought and thoroughly enjoyed. The older person continues developing, growing and changing each day. As Erikson (1963) noted, it is in this stage of development that ego integrity occurs; that is, the older person, in perceiving the uniqueness of life, realizes that it was a good life regardless of the hardships, disappointments, and rejections that may have been a part of that life. In this stage, the main desire expressed by the older person is recognition of the dignity of his or her personhood. Through the respect of others, the older adult can continue to appreciate the beauty and worth of his or her own being.

Havighurst (1972) describes these developmental tasks for later maturity (60 years of age and older):

a. Adjusting to decreasing physical strength and health
b. Adjustment to retirement and reduced income
c. Adjusting to death of spouse

d. Establishing an explicit affiliation with one's age group
e. Adopting and adapting social roles in a flexible way
f. Establishing satisfactory physical living arrangements

Another task of the older person is acceptance of and preparation for death. This realism allows the older person to appreciate the finiteness of existence, the accomplishment of purpose, and the meaningfulness of life. Through this realistic orientation all aspects of life are placed in perspective for the older person and may suggest that there is an afterlife following death as well as life before death.

The Older Person: a Lifelong Goal of Personhood

The older person has overcome many obstacles to arrive at old age. Old age is an accumulation of experiences making an individual unique and precious as a resource for wisdom and insight, and for the understanding of events from a historical perspective. The aging person has lived through many events and changes in society. For example, within the United States, a 60-year-old or older person has moved from the horse and buggy to cars, planes, rockets, and missiles. What a tremendous monument to adaptability! To appreciate these changes is to appreciate the beautiful potential within each older person. They are survivors and thus outstanding examples of each older person's potential. With their perspective, his-

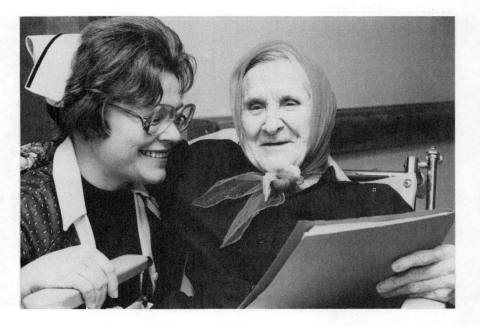

Fig. 3-1. **Dorothy Van Booven, R.N., Associate Administrator and Director of Nurses, and Isabelle Roches, a 92-year-old Irish resident at St. Joseph's Home, Kansas City, Kansas.**

tory may be appreciated as a story of people. They are members of the generation who had the intelligence, wisdom, and creativity that influenced the phenomenal progress prevalent in society today.

Society's attitude that the older person is unproductive and unwanted is an injustice. Gadow (1979) and Rayner (1979) suggest that the old should be assured of respect in society. However, the prevailing attitude in the United States is that the old are a burden rather than a resource for the present generation. Older persons are forced to retire from the work world even though their physical and mental capabilities are still very strong. They are forced into living at poverty level as a result of fixed incomes and inability to continue living in their own homes. Because of inadequate nutrition and limited social activities they are rejected by society and forced into isolation. Older adults have the same basic needs as other individuals. They have a right to expect from society that these needs will be filled in a spirit of justice and respect because they are persons, our brothers and sisters, who have aided in the development of the society we enjoy.

Gadow also notes that older persons should be afforded the privilege of being the essential carriers of culture. Culture embraces beliefs, practices, and traditions belonging to groups of people with a unique perspective and living within a particular geographical region or societal tradition.

Fig. 3-2. **Sister Rose Therese Bahr and group of Hispanic elderly at El Centro de Servicios para Hispanos, Kansas City, Kansas.**

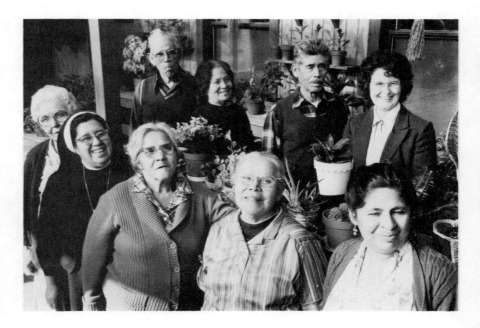

Culture is extremely important in giving us the subtle coloring and unique dimensions of people. Contemporary America is a multiethnic and pluralistic society (Nichols, 1983). An awareness that pluralism and ethnic diversity are important to the very fabric of society is emerging, just as the concept of the melting pot, so prevalent in earlier decades, is being given less credence (Simic, 1983). The multiethnic dimension of society is revealed in the many creative art forms produced by various cultural groups, such as special cuisines (Mexican, German, Chinese, Italian); music and dance (Greek, Irish, black); and family life patterns (American Indian, Hispanic, black, Asian). Each cultural group brings a delightful perspective on life to our world. These cultures are heritages that must be preserved. The older person is the bearer of a unique heritage and life-style. The older person comes from a specific cultural milieu and works to preserve many traditional practices. These aid in announcing to the world that older people are unique, important, and beautiful people (Figs. 3-2 and 3-3).

Another factor contributing to personhood of the older person is the value system embraced during life. Value systems have been the fundamental guides for most older persons and often include the values on

Fig. 3-3. **Lucille Gress and Cora Moore, a 93-year-old black woman residing in Mid-City Towers, Kansas City, Missouri.**

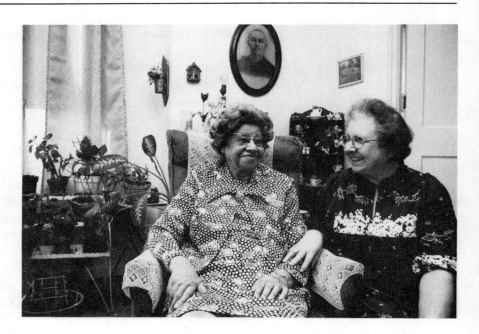

which this nation was founded: the pursuit of life, liberty, and happiness. These values provide an opportunity for the majority of older persons to creatively develop their own life-styles in the home and at work. These values—embracing love, justice, peace, liberty, compassion, harmony, and happiness—have molded the aging person's approach to life. For the aging person trustworthiness and honor are main principles in relationships with others. When they see these values betrayed (for instance, when robbed or cheated) the older person is confused simply because his or her world view does not subscribe to behaviors injuring others. A value system based on humanitarianism and on the respect accorded to another person is to some degree in opposition to much of the selfishness of the present era. In many cases, material possessions are far less important to the older person than those great qualities. Understanding this helps the caregiver to plumb the depths of the older person's world and to appreciate it for its strength.

Finally, education, both formal and informal, contributes much to the personhood of the aging individual. Many of today's older persons have not been formally educated in schools or institutions. Most of their education came from living. Thus they have developed a deep insight into the importance of intellectual stimulation, the value of the wisdom brought about by trial and error, and the ability to place importance on the essentials and less stress on the nonessentials. For the older person, life lived to its fullest is the essential mark of the truly educated person. Self-determination provides a purpose to life through understanding frustration and pain, intimacy and love, doubt and certainty, and a sense of connectedness to every human being (Buscaglia, 1978). Through self-education they appreciate the role of communication: to share what is in their environment so that others can continue to live with dignity and to have a spirit of friendliness and helpfulness. The golden rule, "Do unto others what you would have them do unto you," is a maxim guiding the lives of most older persons. There is no place for selfishness in their world. Much of their education is based on their relationship to nature, to others, and to their God. Education for many older persons took the form of reading the Bible with family members, so that faith was a factor inherent in their spiritual development. Faith continues to be strong in most older persons whether it is verbalized or not. It is through this type of education that the older person became aware of the dignity of all people. This education laid a strong foundation for living.

It is, then, the historical perspective, the culture, the value system, and the education that mold the personhood of the older individual. These factors help one to understand who the older person is in terms of thought process, life-style, and philosophy of life. The beauty of the aging person becomes apparent when one talks with them and sees aspects of life from their perspective. It is unfortunate that within the present century, as the aging population increases, society is less than eager to consider the older individual a treasured resource. To counter this attitude one must bring about an awareness of the various life-styles of older persons and the importance of these life-styles to the present. Each older individual has a right to be included within society. They have earned a right to be here, to live life fully through being contributing citizens. They have a right to live holistically, that is, with mind, body, and spirit. They wish to be allowed to give themselves to the world, to better it. They have personal ties that show their uniqueness and willingness to live fully, not merely to exist. The attitude of society must change. The older person must be allowed to pursue these elements of personhood:

1. Seeing life as the most precious gift from God
2. Continuing to think, love, and act responsibly
3. Exercising free will and maintaining spontaneity, flexibility, and receptivity
4. Being sensitive, stable, and strong
5. Exercising rights and assuming responsibility
6. Putting into practice their own value system

When these elements of personhood are understood and respected, the older person is given his or her rightful value within the home, the community, and society.

Summary

The older person is a composite of many aspects of living. Inherent in the personhood of the older person is the potential given by God to be actualized throughout the life span. The older person is capable of becoming a fully functioning person in every stage of life, from infancy through old age. The aging person should be given respect as a contributing member of society, whether employed or not. It is through the older person that many cultural traditions are preserved and many values interpreted. We all want to be fully functioning, loved, and respected. In this relational context, Buber's concept of I-thou emerges to promote the personhood of each of us (Buber, 1958). Buscaglia describes what he considers the essentials of living.* They include the following:

1. Right knowledge to supply you with the tools necessary for your voyage
2. Wisdom to assure you that you are using the accumulated knowledge of the past in the manner that would best serve the discovery of your presence here and now

*From Buscaglia, L.F.: Living, loving, and learning, Thorofare, N.J., 1978, Charles B. Slack, Inc., pp. 82-83.

3. Compassion to help you accept others whose ways may be different from yours with gentleness and understanding as you move with them or through them or around them on your own way
4. Harmony to be able to accept the natural flow of life
5. Creativity to help you to realize and recognize new alternatives and unchartered paths along the way
6. Strength to stand up against fear and move forward in spite of uncertainty without guarantee or payment
7. Peace to keep you centered
8. Joy to keep you songful and laughing and dancing all along the way
9. Love to be your continual guide toward the highest level of consciousness of which man is capable
10. Unity which brings us back to where we started, the place where we are at one with ourselves and with all things.

It is through these avenues of personhood that the beauty of the individual shines forth. As the older person ages, the beauty of personhood also deepens.

References

Ashley, B.M., and O'Rourke, K.S.: The right to be fully human. In health care ethics: a theological analysis, St. Louis, 1978, The Catholic Hospital Association.

Buber, M.: I and thou, ed. 2, New York, 1958, Charles Scribner's Sons. (Translated by R.G. Smith.)

Buscaglia, L.F.: Personhood: the art of being fully human, Thorofare, N.J., 1978, Charles B. Slack, Inc.

Buscaglia, L.F.: Living, loving, and learning, Thorofare, N.J., 1982, Charles B. Slack, Inc.

Byrne, M.L., and Thompson, L.F.: Key concepts for the study and practice of nursing, ed. 2, St. Louis, 1978, The C.V. Mosby Co.

Erikson, E.: Childhood and society, New York, 1963, W.W. Norton & Co., Inc.

Freud, S.: The ego and the id. In Standard edition of the complete psychological works of Freud, vol. 19, London, 1961, Hogarth Press.

Gadow, S.: Advocacy nursing and new meanings of aging, Nurs. Clin. North Am. **14**(1):81-91, 1979.

Gill, J.: The development of persons, Hum. Dev. 2(1):31, 1981.

Happel, S.P.: Personhood, liberty and justice for all: a discussion guide, Washington, D.C., 1974, National Conference of Catholic Bishops.

Havighurst, R.J.: Developmental tasks and education, ed. 3, New York, 1972, Longman Inc.

Maslow, A.: Motivation and personality, New York, 1954, Harper & Row, Inc.

Maslow, A.: Motivation and personality, ed. 2, New York, 1970, Harper & Row, Inc.

May, R.: Man's search for himself, New York, 1953, W.W. Norton & Co., Inc.

Nichols, E.J.: The influence of culture and heritage on the aging process. Paper presented at the Regional Forum on Aging, Kansas City, Mo., May 26, 1983.

Rayner, E.: Human development: an introduction to the psychodynamics of growth, maturity, and ageing, ed. 2, London, 1979, Allen & Unwin.

Rogers, C.: Client-centered therapy, Boston, 1951, Houghton Mifflin Co.

Simic, A.: Ethnicity and aging: an anthropological overview. Paper presented at the Regional Forum on Aging, Kansas City, Mo., May 26, 1983.

Strecker, I.J.: Proper vision of human sexuality enriches person, society, family, The Leaven 2(28):3, 1981.

Chapter 4 A Developmental Perspective

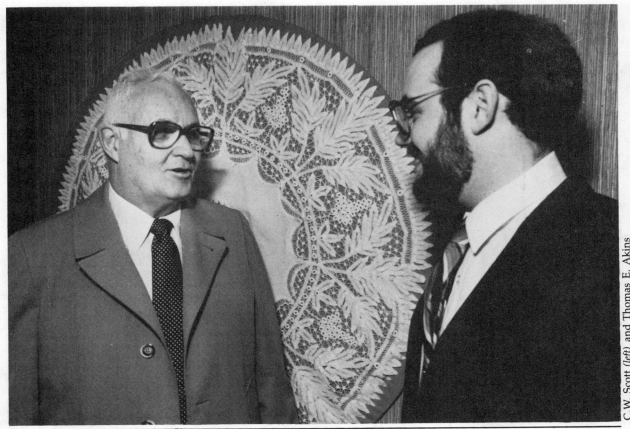

C.W. Scott (*left*) and Thomas E. Akins

The older person has experienced many changes, which may be viewed from a developmental perspective. These are evolutionary changes, which reflect a progression from a simple to a more complex, highly organized state of being (Schuster and Ashburn, 1980). The individual continues adapting to a continually changing internal and external environment and striving toward personhood.

In this chapter, attention is directed toward various aspects of development as they pertain to the older person. Implications of development for the well-being of the older adult are discussed holistically.

The Concept of Development

Development is defined in terms such as *growth* and *maturation*. These terms represent biological ideas and are used in reference to living beings and structures. *Development* refers to continuing processes of change over time. These processes of change tend to be progressive and irreversible; they may be molecular, cellular, physiological, or behavioral. They are reflected in the structure and functioning of the older person (Prechtl and Connolly, 1981).

Growth is commonly defined as a change in size. When used in association with development, however, it refers to a change in behavior and mental functions. Mental changes cannot be measured with the same precision as changes in size (Prechtl and Connolly, 1981). Growth in the developmental context indicates an increase in competence.

Maturation often refers to physical maturity. Generally, it implies a genetic control of development (Prechtl and Connolly, 1981). Precision requires that maturity be used with respect to particular properties or functions: for example, the maturation of red blood cells and their capacity to carry oxygen, and the maturation of kidney nephrons and their capacity to maintain the fluid and electrolyte balance of the body. According to Prechtl and Connolly, if maturity is used in the general sense, rather than the particular, it becomes merely a synonym for development.

The ideal development, according to Deci (1975), contributes to individualism. It encourages the expression of biological, psychological, and sociological needs by the individual. Rogers (1961) theorizes that human beings have intrinsic psychological needs, which become more specific with experience. These needs seem to give rise to motivations toward goals such as self-fulfillment, self-reliance, and achievement. Reaching these goals, however, depends on development of the whole person.

Self-development occurs in a cultural environment shared with other persons. Psychological needs are important, but they occur within a biological organism. Sociological and spiritual needs also arise from the whole

person. From a developmental point of view, the self is constantly changing and interacting with a constantly changing environment; therefore a
holistic approach is needed.

The holistic approach takes into account the dynamics of the ever-
changing individual interacting with everchanging internal and external
environments (Riegel and Meacham, 1976). The internal environment is
the structure of the person's whole being. The external environment includes family and society. The developmental concept can be used with
respect to the individual, the family, and society; thus it is useful in the
holistic approach.

Little attention used to be paid to human development in the later
years. Development tended to be viewed essentially as ending with the
attainment of physical maturity, whereas aging tended to be viewed as
following the physical growth and maturity of the individual. Decremental
aspects of aging were emphasized, and incremental aspects were minimized. Although physical capacities and functions decline in old age, it has
been found that mental and social capacities tend to increase in the last half
of life (Peck, 1956). Today, recognition of the human being's various dimensions and the varying rates, degrees, and directions of the process of
aging has resulted in changing the earlier concepts about aging. The realization that development occurs throughout the life span has contributed
toward a more comprehensive view of human aging and of holism itself.
Human development in the later years has become a recognized area for
study.

According to Peck (1975), there are three reasons for looking at human
aging from a developmental perspective. The first is to comprehend past
development as a means of exploring its influence on persons currently;
the second is to explore developmental aspects of the later life cycle, such
as increases in mental ability and social competence; and the third is to
identify the drive to expand life experience. Peck indicates that mental and
physical abilities do not necessarily show parallel decline. Knowledge of
the differing rates and varying degrees of changes in the biological, psychological, sociological, and spiritual dimensions of the individual may be
organized by using the developmental framework. This framework may be
useful to health care personnel concerned with helping older adults continue to develop.

Gaps in knowledge of human development and aging exist, and the
rapidly increasing number of older adults calls for closing them. In spite of
those gaps, strengths of older persons can be supported to a great extent.
Prevention of premature decline of capacities and abilities is essential if
older adults are to realize their potential.

Definitions of Aging

Further consideration of developmental aspects of aging needs a definition of aging. Biologists, psychologists, sociologists, clergy, and others have attempted to define it. Biologists seek to explain aging by describing changes at the molecular and cellular level (Finch, 1976, 1977; Hayflick, 1975, 1977). Developmental psychologists speak of changes before physical maturity as differentiation of the individual and changes after physical maturity as aging (Birren and Renner, 1977). Sociologists describe the aging process in terms of changes in roles and role functions (Neugarten and Hagestad, 1976). Spiritual aging, according to those concerned with it, encompasses changes in the inner being: the continuing unfolding of a philosophy of life and changing motivations (Moberg, 1971). Spiritual aging is not as clearly defined as the other dimensions of aging, probably because of its intangibility. Nevertheless, we consider the spiritual dimension important and its definition essential in the holistic approach to older adults.

Aging has been described as the total of time-related changes experienced by individuals. Gerontologists, on the other hand, have agreed that aging encompasses changes regularly experienced in mature, genetically representative individuals who live under representative conditions (Birren and Renner, 1977). These definitions of aging are not exhaustive, but they provide a way of viewing the aging process. A single definition is obviously insufficient for explaining the complex changes of aging.

Types of Aging

In addition to citing definitions, further examination of aging may be accomplished by looking at its various types. These types are commonly described as biological, psychological, functional, and sociological. The spiritual aspect of aging, although not as frequently referred to in the literature as are the other types, is included. There is some overlap with these types, but a consideration of them may enhance understanding of aging and the developmental concept.

Biological aging refers to changes in structure and functions of the body that occur over the life span (Zarit, 1980). Some of these changes in body organs and systems are hidden or occur very gradually. Other changes, such as graying hair and wrinkling skin, decreasing visual and auditory acuity, decreasing stature and change in posture, slower response time, and increasing susceptibility to disease, are more apparent. Biological aging is influenced by genetic inheritance and internal and external environmental factors. However, although a person may be physically declining in the later years, there may be growth in the other dimensions—for instance, the psychological and sociological dimensions (Birren and Renner,

1977). The interrelation of the various dimensions and the differences in direction of changes help alleviate the impact of biological aging.

Psychological aging refers to behavioral changes, changes in self-perception, and reaction to the biological changes. Psychological age is influenced by the condition of the body, such as of the cardiovascular and renal systems. It is also influenced by changes in the brain that affect memory, learning, motivation, and emotions (Birren and Renner, 1977).

Functional aging is closely related to psychological aging; it refers to the capacities of individuals for functioning in society, as compared to that of others of the same age (Birren and Renner, 1977). Attempts are being made to develop standards of functional ability (which involves adaptive capacity, revealing the close connection between psychological and functional aging).

Sociological aging refers to the roles and social habits of individuals in society (Birren and Renner, 1977). For older persons it includes changes in norms, expectations, social status, and social roles. Sociological aging is evaluated largely on the basis of norms in social behavior. Norms are the expected kinds of behaviors and beliefs established by the group. Age-graded expectations of behavior are influenced by the culture and by the person's biological and psychological characteristics (Hall, 1980). Social age differs in a sense from biological and psychological age, since it refers to social competence (related to the external environment) rather than to physical status or adaptive capacity (related to the internal environment).

Spiritual aging refers to changes of self and perceptions of self, of the relationships of self to others, of the place of self in the world, and of the self's world view (Stallwood and Stoll, 1975). Introspection increases in the older person, according to Jung (1933). The person's value system changes (Moberg, 1971). Interpersonal relationships tend to take priority over concerns with such matters as status in the working world and acquisition of material objects. Developing a philosophy of life in keeping with the changes of aging is a part of spiritual aging. The spiritual self, like the social self, is defined partly through interaction with others. It is also defined in the later years through introspection and contemplation—development of the inner self.

Growth and Development in the Later Years

The process of growth and development begins with fertilization of the ovum and the formation of the embryo. From the time of conception, growth and development of the organism proceed in a continuous and orderly process during the prenatal and postnatal periods (Timiras, 1972). Alternating slow and accelerated cycles are typical of physical and mental maturation. Gradually the infant begins the process of self-discovery and differentiation from others. The infant enters the stage of childhood and starts to assume various social roles and functions. During adolescence, self-identity becomes a priority in the continuing process of the individual's growth and development. Soon responsibilities of the young adult are assumed, and the person moves on toward the next developmental stage—the middle years. Once the reproductive capability is over, the person often struggles with a sense of meaninglessness. Shortly thereafter retirement from work adds to the question about the purpose of life. Adapting to these changes requires decision-making, and problem-solving—new approaches to life that challenge the capacities of the aging person. Thus it is apparent that growth and development continue throughout what is commonly perceived to be the downward side of life.

The concept of growth is often used as an indication of change in a positive direction rather than simply as an indicator of an increase in size. Development, on the other hand, refers to a differentiation or an unfolding of the person over time.

Jourard (1964) speaks of growth in terms of change in a desired direction. This concept of growth is a change in the definition from an earlier period. Growth in a positive direction in the physical and in other dimensions of the person may occur simultaneously. Growth in the psychosocial and spiritual dimensions, on the other hand, may occur long after physical maturity has been achieved. There are differences in the rate, type, and duration of growth. Different criteria than those commonly used to measure physical growth are needed to measure growth in these other dimensions. According to Jourard's definition, there is no time-related limit for the growth process; it can occur throughout the life span.

Development, on the other hand, is used in reference to an increase in size or to the form and function of the person. It corresponds with the chronological age of the individual to some extent (Birren and Renner, 1977). Development of capacities, such as the acquisition of wisdom and judgment, are the expected direction of change in the aging adult. Development is a concept that refers to processes that are genetically inherent within the person, and to those processes influenced by the external environment over time.

The concepts of growth and development are most often used to refer to persons in the childhood and adolescent stages preceding physical maturity. Consideration of the growth and developmental potential of older adults is important, however, if they are to become all they are capable of becoming. Older adults should not be deprived of the opportunity to continue their pursuit of personhood simply because of their age. With minimal assistance many older adults can achieve worthwhile personal goals and contribute to the well-being of others.

Two dominant orientations have evolved and been clearly differentiated: the organismic and the mechanistic. Both orientations have human nature as the basic premise, yet the human being is viewed differently in each case. The dialectical orientation is another view. These orientations provide a basis for the exploration of the developmental aspects of individuals of various ages, including later maturity.

The Organismic Orientation

The organismic orientation is based on the concept of organic wholeness. Development, according to this model, usually requires an organized system with a definite structure. Sequential changes occur that consequently affect the structure and function of the system. In this model the human being is viewed as actively initiating action rather than passively waiting to be acted on by an external force. Discovery of principles of organization is important in this model, since synthesis (rather than analysis) of basic elements is the major mode of inquiry. Attention is directed toward explaining the relationship between the parts and wholes and between structure and function, rather than analyzing those basic elements (Reece and Overton, 1970). Qualitative, discontinuous change occurs that is not considered reducible to simple elements of behavior. The term development is viewed by those formulating the organismic model as theoretical; it is used in explanations of observed behavior changes (Reece and Overton, 1970). Evidence of the organismic model can be seen in the work of Bühler (1953), Erikson (1950, 1963), and Havighurst (1953, 1972). These will be reviewed later.

The Mechanistic Orientation

The mechanistic orientation is based on the machine. The world is conceptualized as a machine with many parts moving through space according to basic laws (Hultsch and Plemons, 1979). In this view the individual is considered passive, or reactive; activity is believed to occur as a reaction to an external force (Reece and Overton, 1970). Quantitative changes occur; complex changes are considered reducible to simple elements. Analysis is the mode of inquiry, and the goal of analysis is to discover causal relations that can explain the behavioral change. Development is viewed as behavioral change that is predictable from antecedents; it is viewed as a descriptive term, which labels phenomena to be explained (Reece and Overton, 1970). The works of Selye (1956) and Holmes and Rahe (1967) show use of this model. These works will not be reviewed here, since they are readily available. Furthermore, this orientation has not gained widespread acceptance as a developmental model, since it does not reflect the internal motivation of human beings to be active participants in determining their lives.

The Dialectical Orientation

The dialectical orientation is a more recently formulated orientation; it requires working out a conceptual compromise between the organismic and the mechanistic models. Although the organismic and the mechanistic models are described as clearly differentiated and therefore irreconcilable, the dialectical process of thesis, antithesis, and synthesis allows for another view of development to be derived from their opposition. The dialectical model is also labeled the relational (Looft, 1973) and the dynamic interactive (Lerner, 1978).

According to Riegel's (1975) dialectical orientation, development occurs simultaneously within at least four dimensions: the inner-biological, the individual-psychological, the cultural-sociological, and the outer-physical. The process of development or unfolding proceeds through the stages of thesis, antithesis, and synthesis. This process is marked by dynamic tension, conflict, and interrelation of the parts. Contradictions between events occurring in the progressions of the inner and outer dimensions bring about developmental changes, and lack of harmony among the dimensions creates disequilibrium, providing the basis for further development. This development may be in either a positive or negative direction. In the dialectical orientation acceptance of contradiction is encouraged, since it is in the resolution of contradictions that further development is achieved. The dynamic interplay between the individual and the environment may be unidirectional or bidirectional. That is, change may be initiated by either internal or external forces or a combination of the two. The dialectical model is another way of viewing development by focusing on the ever-changing individual interacting with an everchanging environment.

The Family Development Orientation

The family development orientation is another widely used way of viewing development, although the family is not a biological organism and the concept of development cannot be used in the same manner as with the individual. However, the family is a unit of interacting biological individuals; hence, some developmental ideas apply.

According to Hill and Mattessich (1979) family development involves continuing structural differentiation throughout the family history and family members' changing roles as they attempt to carry out functions essential for survival and adapt to life changes. This model is developmental in character, since research has shown variations in family organization to be predictable.

Although these orientations are not exhaustive, they point out that older individuals experience developmental processes over time as individuals and as members of family units. Although there are other ways of viewing aging, the focus of this chapter is on developmental aspects within a holistic framework. In the next few paragraphs, human development and the dimensions of older persons—biological, psychological, sociological, and spiritual—are holistically explored.

Biological Development

Biological development is usually given priority over the other developmental orientations, since the biological being provides the locus for the other dimensions. Perhaps the best way to approach the biological aspects of development is to examine selected biological theories of aging.

Biological theories of aging have come about through the efforts of researchers who have focused attention on the aging processes and directed their efforts toward answering questions about how aging occurs and what physiological changes take place. The intent is to determine the basis of decremental changes of aging as a step toward preventing or staving off such changes for a longer period of time. Lack of definitive research findings has been a limiting factor, but continuing research efforts are ameliorating this situation. One of the difficulties has been distinguishing between aging changes and changes caused by disease (Finch, 1976; Rossman, 1977). For example, memory loss for recent events and decreased intellectual function were previously believed to be part of the normal aging process. However, research has shown that these changes tend to occur in persons suffering from high blood pressure (Wilkie and Eisdorfer, 1971), depression (Gurland, 1976), or other deteriorative diseases (Barnes and others, 1981). Capacity for sexual activity was previously thought to be lost with aging; this belief also has been invalidated (Kinsey and others, 1948; Masters and Johnson, 1966). Further investigation of the biology and physiology of aging is needed to show more clearly the difference between normal changes of aging and those arising from a pathological process.

Biologic theories of aging arise from two basic views: (1) the view of aging as a universal, involuntary process based on genetic factors and (2) the view of aging as a response to multiple external environmental factors. The sequential and consequential relationships among the variables of biological aging contribute toward their classification as developmental theories. A brief review of selected theories representative of these basic views is presented in the following paragraphs.

An example of the genetically programmed theory of biological aging is the theory of the biological clock. This theory is based on the idea that a genetically determined program controls the aging and dying process and the rate of the process (Kent, 1982). Researchers have thought that it may be possible to locate the biological clock and learn about the mechanism involved, thereby being able to interfere with this mechanism and ward off the changes of aging.

Hayflick's (1975) experiments with human embryo fibroblasts support the biological clock theory. These fibroblasts are capable of doubling an average of 50 times in vitro before showing evidence of deterioration. Hayflick proposes that the cell nucleus is the locus of the biological clock of aging. The limited capacity of the fibroblasts for doubling seems to indicate a genetically programmed life span of human fibroblasts and a biological clock that influences the aging process.

The free radical theory is another of the theories directed toward answering the question of why we grow old (Harmon, 1971). Free radicals are described as intermediate chemicals having an odd number of electrons. Because of their structure, free radicals readily react with other compounds, resulting in rapid change. Free radicals may be found in chemicals in food, smoke, air, and water. These free radicals are believed to react with unsaturated fatty acids and form nonfunctional peroxide molecules, causing intracellular disruption and cellular death (Kent, 1976). Since these free radicals readily react with other compounds, the likelihood of the random process and cell loss occurring is increased. Because of the random process and the cumulative effects involved, this theory is often classified as stochastic. Aging, according to this theory, results from an increasing number of events and their cumulative effects within the cell (Busse and Pfieffer, 1969).

Biological theories of aging tend to deal with changes at the cellular or tissue level. Biological theories, while necessary, are insufficient to explain the aging process holistically. The biological aspects of aging are important, but it is the whole person who acknowledges the changes of aging and responds to them. If the person has marked strengths in the other dimensions, biological changes of aging may not be too troublesome. This does not deny the need for further research and development of biological theories of aging, the value of current theories explaining aspects of the aging process, or the worth of the historical development of these theories. They can be useful for those working with aging persons. They provide a basis for understanding some of the changes occurring over time and the influence of these changes on functional abilities and interpersonal relationships. Biological theories of aging are in a process of development, and one needs to be informed of the status of this development and alert to new developments.

Psychological Development

Psychological development can be explored within the historical context of (1) the mechanistic, or Anglo-American orientation; (2) the mentalistic, or continental European orientation; and (3) the dialectical orientation (Riegel and Meacham, 1972).

The mechanistic, or Anglo-American, orientation may be partially understood by gaining appreciation of the darwinian philosophy of evolution and the struggle for survival (Darwin, 1900). Mental organization and social order are lacking in this approach. Neither the individual nor the environment are emphasized. Rather than being judged on their own merits, individuals are evaluated against a standard of success established by young adult white males. Those failing to meet the standards are labeled with such negative terms as deficient, retarded, or deviant. Intellectual excellence is judged according to the amount of information accumulated in keeping with the lockean concept of the mind. In this case, the mind is a tabula rasa, or clean slate, dependent on external contingencies for its development (Riegel, 1979). The mechanistic orientation to psychological development stresses the passive nature of the individual.

According to Riegel (1979), integration of a philosophy of man and society with psychology is largely the result of the efforts of Sir Francis Galton (1822-1911). Galton is also recognized as the originator of a psychology dealing with individual and developmental differences, including those related to adulthood and the aging process. Galton's orientation led to the development of the field of eugenics. He tried to justify his position by asking why races best suited to play their roles in life should be crowded out by those who were less competent, sick, or dependent.

The mechanistic Anglo-American orientation to psychological gerontology dates back several centuries. Early societies valued competition, and individuals were judged against a standard set by their most successful competitors. Individuals in this environment counted for little; they struggled against great odds for survival.

The mentalistic, or continental European, orientation represents a social philosophy wherein young people are evaluated against independent multiage, multigenerational, and multicultural standards rather than against those established by the most successful young adults. In this view, competition with others is minimized. Rousseau sums up this position by saying that a child more accurately reflects the harmony of the human being than does an acculturated adult (Riegel, 1979). Civilization, in this case, is viewed as generating injustice and social differences from which innocent children should be shielded as long as possible.

Rousseau's social philosophy began to have impact on educational institutions on the European continent (Riegel, 1979), and simultaneously age stratification, with the assignment of specific roles to various age groups, came into practice. The most recent expression of the European movement is said to be Piaget's work (Flavell, 1963; Furth, 1969). Piaget's psychology is based on a stepwise progression of development. Each developmental stage is evaluated against its own standards and is incompatible with other levels of behavior (Riegel, 1979).

The mentalistic model developed in societies whose landed aristocracies supported identifiable social stratification. Competition in this social structure occurs within rather than between classes. Political and economic decisions come from the top; duties are greater for the less privileged. Nevertheless, the educational philosophy reveals sensitivity to differences between ages and social groups in the assignment of appropriate roles (Riegel, 1979).

Personality theories, in addition to Piaget's theory of cognitive development, are representative of the continental European orientation. Early theories, however, such as Freud's psychoanalytical theory, focus on dynamics occurring within the individual. Advancement in theory development, leading to study of adults in later life, occurred with consideration of social conditions surrounding these individuals. Examples of attention to adult development include the work of Bühler (1953), Erikson (1963), Jung (1933), and Riegel (1979).

In spite of advancements, the mentalistic model continued to focus on the individual within whom development occurred and who faced the world alone. Although individual interaction with the social world occurred, development was acknowledged solely as the outcome of the activities of the individual. Dynamic interaction of the individual with the social environment was denied in this approach (Riegel, 1977). Failure to take the environment sufficiently into account gave rise to a third view: the dialectical orientation.

The dialectical orientation focuses on the developmental interdependence of the person and the environment (Riegel, 1979). In contrast to the mentalistic and mechanistic orientations, the dialectical orientation views individuals as active participants in interactions that are dialectical in character. These interactions depend on both inner-individual and outer-cultural development. In the ongoing developmental process individuals change nature, and the changing nature of the environment changes individuals. Development of language and invention of tools, and the changing social and physical conditions under which these processes took place, are examples of the dialectical process and developmental change (Riegel, 1979).

Riegel (1979) cites the individual in the process of retiring as an example of the dialectical orientation. Discord and conflict arise out of this change in life-style. Loss of interpersonal relationships and loss of job, with the consequent decrease in income and increase in leisure time, stimulate change in the individual. A reassessment process usually occurs, and the individual establishes new goals and looks for new ways of achieving them. Once this situation is under control, however, tension among the dimensions of the individual increases, and the dialectical process is initiated again. Change occurs as the result of disharmony; therefore equilibrium is not a goal of the dialectical orientation.

With this review of the mechanistic, mentalistic, and dialectical orientations, it is easier to understand differences in approaches of general and developmental psychologists. These differences may become fuzzy when interpreted by those outside the field of psychology who use content from the field in their own work. Their work gives rise to an interdisciplinary concept of development.

Sociological Development   The sociological orientation focuses on social development and aging. It is based on the question of how the process of aging and the position of the aged change over the course of time. Individuals organize their life courses and interpret life experiences on the basis of age and societal change. Chronological age is converted to social age as individuals take their place in work roles, family roles, and roles assumed in retirement. Neugarten (Hall, 1980) states that chronological age is becoming increasingly less predictive of the life-style of older individuals. She predicts that the involvement of adults with various educational programs will become a powerful force in changing patterns of life. During this period of rapid social change flexibility of older persons may be as important as economic fluidity in the ongoing process of development.

The sociological orientation is based on information gathered from a variety of sources. Three major sources of historical information on aging are (1) continuing records of vital statistics (births, marriages, and deaths), (2) census documents of a statistical nature and censuslike documents of an earlier period, and (3) literary and other materials (Laslett, 1976).

From continuing records of vital statistics fairly reliable estimates can be obtained on mortality rates; life expectancy rates from several countries, such as Japan and England, are available in addition to those from the United States. Earlier censuslike documents can be used to obtain additional data on personal and family situations of older persons throughout history. Examination of any social developments actually changing the position of the aged can be made if data are available from before and after the significant change. Literary and other materials cover a greater time span (some 3000 years), but this is considered a short period of time from which to make assertions about human development. As time goes on and record keeping improves, more precise data will become available for the before and after assessment of significant changes in the position of the aged.

The paucity of formal theory on societal development and aging is thought to be caused by the primitive state of historical gerontology and the only recent development of gerontology itself (Laslett, 1976). The sociological orientation, therefore, is based on propositions believed to underlie sociological development.

Laslett cites historical events as of major importance in the subject of aging. A "before" and "after" in the study of aging is evident in the record of transitions from one uniform situation to another. These transitions accompany developments such as industrialization; there is question, however, as to where the line dividing the "before" and "after" of these social developments should be drawn. Nevertheless, the assertion remains that aging in the past was different from what it has become.

Laslett (1976) presents four sets of propositions to represent the body of informal theory on aging: (1) historical propositions, (2) normative propositions, (3) functional propositions, and (4) domestic propositions.

Historical propositions are complicated, according to Laslett, by the tendency to equate the historical distinction of a given society when, for instance, industrialization was present and absent with contemporary industrial and nonindustrial societies. As in other areas of study, care should be taken not to reach conclusions based on inaccuracies.

Normative propositions indicate that in the "before," aging was accepted, and the aged were entitled to universally accorded respect. In the "after," aging has been rejected as unworthy of recognition: the aged are not accorded prestige, and society tends to act as if they do not exist. This depersonalization and rejection has created problems for many older persons, especially those who have survived their families and peers.

Functional propositions maintain that in the "before" the aged had specific, valued economic and emotional roles that were indispensable in the multigenerational household. In the "after," aged persons do not have obvious functions. This situation creates a sense of purposelessness in some older people.

Domestic propositions assert that in the "before" the constitution of the domestic group was specified by universally accepted social assumptions. The group was expected to allot membership to all senior persons within the kin network. In the "after," a family consists of a man, his wife, and their dependent children. Any responsibility for caring for aged persons is fulfilled by economic assistance or by visiting, not by changing the specified shape of the family group. While there may be exceptions, these are the general patterns that seem to be supported by existing data.

Social development in the later years may be considered in terms of the direction of change in social roles and functions. Older persons occupy roles such as spouse, parent, grandparent, great-grandparent, church member, golfer, and seamstress—and function accordingly. Social roles are based on an interpersonal process between two or more individuals. This concept is in contrast to the psychological view that an individual acts alone (Kaplan, 1979). The sociological view supports the notion of a cultural system that influences social roles and interaction among the elderly.

In the sociological orientation, the person fulfills ascribed roles involving definite rights and responsibilities. The function of the person depends on the needs of the group. Examples of rights and privileges given to the person concern bodily existence, material or economic rewards, and social standing. These rights and privileges bestow status and prestige on the person.

Certain regularities in behavior occur because individuals behave according to established, age-appropriate behavioral norms (Neugarten and Hagestad, 1968). These norms vary and may be formal or informal; but they are changing, and society is becoming less rigid (Hall, 1980). "May-December marriages" are becoming more acceptable, and older persons are not necessarily expected to retire and avail themselves of Social Security benefits when they become eligible, as they once were. Behavioral norms permit a much wider range of behaviors than the former age-graded norms of behavior did.

A number of sociological theories of aging exist, but perhaps those most frequently mentioned are the *disengagement theory* (Cumming and Henry, 1961) and the *activity theory*.

Essentially, Cumming and Henry concluded from their study of adult life that role activity decreased as part of the normal and successful aging process of older persons. According to the disengagement theory, at the same time these persons are disengaging from society, society is disengaging from them. Mandatory retirement is evidence of this situation. Although this theory is no longer supported because of its lack of universality, it is noteworthy for its heuristic value. It was a major effort to identify factors pertinent to normal aging and has stimulated a great deal of research on successful aging.

The activity theory (Havighurst, 1963), on the other hand, suggests that to age successfully, individuals should continue the roles carried out in the middle years to the fullest extent possible. This theory also has stimulated a great deal of research on successful aging and has encouraged programming of activities to keep older persons involved.

Neither the disengagement theory nor the activity theory has gained acceptance as the single theory explaining social aging. Another theory, the developmental, or continuity, theory (Neugarten and Hagestad, 1964), has been proposed. It is uncertain whether the developmental theory will gain a wider acceptance than the other two theories.

The developmental theory states that by identifying patterns of behavior of individuals in their earlier years, predictions about their patterns of adaptation can be made. Factors that influence social aging may vary over time, but there seems to be a common thread, a continuity, in the individual's development.

Although sociological theory is undeveloped at this time, the attempted development of theory is valuable. With new knowledge, a clearer picture of aging's social aspects is beginning to emerge. Undoubtedly further studies will help develop sociological theory and moreover serve to point out the interdisciplinary nature of studies of developmental aspects of aging. Because of the complex nature of aging human beings, it is difficult to envision the likelihood of a single theory that would explain aging.

Spiritual Development

The orientation to spiritual development is less clearly defined than the orientations to other dimensions of the person—which is not to say that the spiritual dimension is less important. Older persons often emphasize the spiritual aspects of life, whether they are rooted in a formal religion or not.

Spiritual aging, like aging in the other dimensions, occurs over time as individuals continue to develop a philosophy of life. It involves getting to know the interpersonal relationships defining self in give-and-take situations and coming to an appreciation of one's relationship to the universe. Coming to accept one's experience, both pleasant and unpleasant, is part of spiritual development. In distilling the experiences of life, most individuals come to the realization that all of life's experiences are transitory. Joy can be realized after mastering difficult life events, such as the death of a loved one. Drawing on an inner strength, the person may be able to endure adversity and to increase self-esteem. Sharing experiences with others helps to develop inner strength and establishes the human bond, love, which is a source of support. If aging is seen as the unfolding of human potential, the development and use of inner resources comprise the spiritual growth and development of older persons.

The term *spiritual* is defined in various ways; it does not necessarily mean religious in the formal sense. *Spiritual* and *philosophical* may be used interchangeably to describe spiritual development. According to Bayly (1969), spiritual refers to the invisible inner aspect of the human being, which is considered immortal. Montagu (1966), an anthropologist and social biologist, speaks of a progression in goodness, which might be considered spiritual development. Montagu defines goodness in terms of the ability to love, experience, and respond to the environment with sensitivity. He describes the person as a problem searching for a solution. In any case, the person is viewed as a spiritual being.

Spiritual development in the later years involves achieving a more mature outlook on life and religious beliefs. Being a good listener and tolerating others' differing beliefs is part of the process. Striving to understand the ideas of and the relationship to other persons and to the universe contributes toward developing humanness and personhood. As beliefs change, evidence of the pervasiveness of the spirit in the development of older people's personalities becomes visible in their interpersonal relationships and views of the universe.

According to Ebersole (1979), spiritual development probably encompasses numerous qualities, such as wisdom, compassion, morality, and ethics. Jung (1933) speaks of the development of the inner self of people in the last half of their lives. Erikson (1968, 1975) also supports the concept of spiritual development in describing the last stage of life as ego integrity versus despair: ego integrity reflects a love and respect of self giving rise to a sense of the spiritual dimension of the person. Peck (1968) elaborates on Erikson's theory of psychological development and raises issues about spiritual development in the later years. For example, the question is raised as to whether a person is worthwhile only for doing full-time work, or whether the person can be worthwhile for being and performing in roles other than work roles. Another example is the idea that persons may choose to leave a legacy that would contribute toward a better world. This kind of concern is one of the ways in which older persons can transcend the physical self and find meaning in life. Spiritual development is not clearly defined, but evidence of its occurrence does exist.

Although the holistic approach is supported by many, the spiritual dimension of older persons probably receives the least consideration of the dimensions. This is especially true with respect to research, which should undergird approaches to spiritual needs and problems just as it does the needs and problems in the person's other dimensions. It is probably equally true with respect to clinical application of empirically established principles of spiritual well-being (Bahr, 1982). Because the spirit is intangible, it is more difficult to define and study; theories of spiritual development are more notable by their absence than their presence. Attention to spiritual needs and problems of older adults is imperative if a holistic approach to the elderly is to be used by health care workers to improve their care.

In summary, various orientations to development have been presented. The four dimensions of the aging person—biological, psychological, sociological, and spiritual—have provided the basis for further consideration of developmental concepts. It is not illogical to think that development might proceed at different rates in the different dimensions. This possibility makes it necessary to consider the effect of these variations on the development of personhood of the older individual. Although development is an ongoing process of change, the direction of that change may be incremental or decremental. Change, whatever the direction, helps shape the personality of older people as they make choices and act on their perceptions of events and the world around them. Development, then, can be viewed as a dynamic, continuous process involving growth, decline, and reorganization throughout the life span; it should be viewed from an interdisciplinary point of view (Kimmel, 1980).

Developmental Theories

In the next few pages, developmental theories with a life span orientation are reviewed. More specifically, attention is directed toward selected theories dealing with the later stage of the life cycle. Major developmental theories to be presented include those of Jung (1933), Bühler (1953), Erikson (1959), and Havighurst (1948). These theorists did early work in adult development and illustrate emergence of the concept of developmental tasks.

Jung's Theory of Individuation

Jung (1933) was one of the first theorists to take exception to the prevailing psychoanalytic view that the sense of identity established in adolescence produces consistency in behavior thereafter (Neugarten, 1973). Jung described stages of development in adulthood, noting an increase in introversion and reorganization of value systems in middle and later life.

According to Jung, the personality is composed of three separate interacting systems: the ego, the personal unconscious, and the collective unconscious. The ego is the mind that encompasses all of the perceptions, meanings, and feelings coming into the individual's awareness at any time. In view of constant sensory bombardment, the mind must be selective in its perceptions. The two attitudes that influence perception of and reaction to the world are introversion and extroversion. These opposite orientations of consciousness and personality may change over time; for instance, the nondominant personality may increase in strength. The personal unconscious is viewed as a storehouse for material that is no longer at the conscious level, but which is easily returned to consciousness. Memories and thoughts that are threatening or relatively unimportant comprise the material in the storehouse. The conscious, or ego, must recall needed material when the occasion demands. Complexes are a part of the personal unconscious. These complexes (such as inferiority complexes) are clusters of emotions, memories, and thoughts organized around a common theme. They are a small part of the total personality but have a great deal of influence on the person's behavior. Since complexes are in the personal unconscious, the individual is unaware of the control they exert. Perceptions, values, interests, and motivations are determined largely by these complexes.

Psychological functions include the rational (thinking and feeling) and the nonrational (sensing and intuiting). Each of these sets are opposing functions and require energy from the individual for determining the action to take. Only one part of the functions can be dominant at one time, according to Jung's theory.

Experiences of the collective unconscious are manifest as archetypes or universal patterns. Examples of archetypes, according to Schultz (1977), are birth, death, God, and the earth mother. Of the archetypes possible, apparently only a few are of significance in our lives. Selected archetypes are treated as separate systems within the personality. These are identified as the persona, the anima and the animus, the shadow, and the self.

Persona is the mask the individual may use to present the self differently from the real self. Individuals play many roles in life, using many masks.

Jung believed the persona useful in helping individuals cope with various events of life. Often at midlife, individuals become aware that they have not been expressing their true selves and have neglected the development of some aspects of their personalities. The healthy personality seeks to decrease the power of the persona and increase development of other parts of the personality.

The anima and the animus are related, in that each individual has biological and psychological characteristics of the opposite sex. A man's personality has some feminine components (the anima) and the woman's personality has some masculine components (the animus). Repression of these masculine and feminine characteristics undermines psychological health; all aspects of the personality must be developed in harmony, according to Jung.

The shadow houses the animal instincts, vestiges of prehuman ancestry. It is also the locus of the wellspring of spontaneity and deep emotion, which is essential to full humanness. Again, there is evidence of opposites that must be blended or balanced to achieve the harmony Jung speaks of in a healthy personality. The dark side of the personality is part of the shadow, but without expression of the whole shadow, the vigorous and emotional part of the personality is lacking.

Most important is the self. The self is the ultimate goal of life. Since the goal of life is achieved through the striving toward wholeness of the personality, it is understandable that Jung places importance on the last half of life. Personality, according to Jung's theory, can hardly achieve integration and unity without the life experiences of the last half of life.

Jung was the first theorist who took issue with the idea that personality is determined during infancy and childhood. He indicated instead that personality continues to develop throughout a person's life and that it undergoes a crucial transformation between the ages of 35 and 50. According to Jung, personality develops over four stages: childhood, youth and young adulthood, middle age, and old age. At midlife, when the meaning of life is questioned by many individuals, Jung reminds us that effort must be devoted to development of the subjective world. In this phase, interest must shift from the physical and material to the religious and philosophical aspects of life. This is essential for the process of self-realization—the final stage of personality growth. The person must accept the inevitability of death. Successful integration of the unconscious with the conscious and with the experience of the inner being places individuals in a position of psychological health, a condition Jung refers to as individuation.

The individuated person, by achieving harmony between the various aspects of the personality, becomes similar to other individuated persons, according to Jung. Individuals achieving individuation achieve final release from the influences of childhood. In this respect, they are more alike than different.

Jung attempted to explain personality development in terms of the dynamics of the intrapsychic process, minimizing the external environment. He indicated that individuals are born with an inherited capacity to form symbols; this capacity is the collective unconscious. Jung focused on the individual's own capacity to try to make sense of his world and to change his behavior by changing his perspective. This process, by which integration of personality takes place, is individuation, or self-realization; it is a natural process.

Bühler's Theory of the Course of Human Life

Bühler (1953) became interested in looking at development in the later years partly to learn about effects of childhood and youth on personality development. Bühler identifies some of the fundamental changes in personality during the life span.

Bühler is one of the early theorists on development in the adult years. She conducted empirical studies in an effort to identify general principles that underlie change throughout the life span and shifts in motivations and needs that might be considered typical of persons in the various phases of adulthood. Investigating biological and psychological aspects of development, records of production and performance, and autobiographies and biographies, Bühler described a progression of life phases based on changes in events, attitudes, and achievements.

The phases of life, according to Bühler (1961) include (1) childhood and youth, or the beginning of life, (2) the period between 45 and 65 years, a time of assessing the outcomes of previously set goals, and (3) the period beginning at age 65, when the individual becomes aware of a sense of fulfillment or failure (Brunner and Suddarth, 1980). Bühler concluded from her studies that this realization of achievement or failure is crucial to adjustment in old age.

Erikson's Theory of Ego Identity

Erikson (1963) presents a psychosocial theory of ego development and ego identity, which is among the first to deal with personality development throughout the life span. Development, according to Erikson, is a two-dimensional process wherein eight stages of social development parallel the eight stages of individual development. The psychological stages of Erikson's theory are "(1) basic trust versus mistrust, (2) autonomy versus shame and doubt, (3) initiative versus guilt, (4) industry versus inferiority, (5) identity versus role confusion, (6) intimacy versus isolation, (7) generativity versus stagnation, and (8) ego integrity versus despair."* The sociohistorical stages of this theory are not as clearly identified as the psychological stages, however. Erikson indicates that the person and so-

*From Erikson, E.H.: Childhood and society, ed. 2, New York, 1963, W.W. Norton & Co., Inc.

ciety evolve simultaneously, and he views society as basically supportive.

At each stage of development, according to Erikson's theory, the individual experiences conflict and a subsequent crisis or turning point. The crisis has positive and negative components. If the conflict is resolved in a positive direction, the individual proceeds to the next stage in a healthy manner; if the conflict is unresolved, it interferes with further development. Resolution or nonresolution of a psychological conflict at any stage of ego development affects subsequent stages. For example, ego identity is a major concern during adolescence; it is a concern in adulthood and in old age as well. If conflict arises with ego integrity, adequate resolution of the conflict is necessary before the individual can successfully progress toward the next developmental stage and adaptation contributing toward a healthy state of being.

The later stages of Erikson's theory are not as well developed as stages relating to childhood. Peck (1968) elaborated on Erikson's theory by developing a more definitive description of the later developmental stages. For example, he examined the issue of ego differentiation versus work role preoccupation and the impact it often has on men in the sixth decade of life. He suggests a shift in value system whereby individuals facing retirement can reappraise and redefine their worth. The issue is whether persons can be worthwhile outside of working full time—worthwhile just for being the persons they are.

Peck (1968) also speaks of the issue of body transcendence versus body preoccupation. He indicates that although decreasing restorative capacity and increasing body aches and pains may be incapacitating to some older individuals, others seem less incapacitated by physical discomfort and appear to enjoy life in spite of their infirmities. Why some individuals have the power to avoid preoccupation with bodily conditions and to transcend their bodies and others cannot is an issue worth exploring.

Ways of looking at and accepting one's mortality are offered by both Peck and Erikson. This includes living in such a way that one's anticipation of personal death becomes less important than the knowledge of one's contributions that will extend beyond one's lifetime. Peck (1968) believes that this kind of living would not only indicate successful aging but probably be measurable as well.

Although criticism has been leveled at Erikson's theory of ego identity because of his failure to elaborate on the stages of adulthood, his theory is one of the first with a life-span orientation; it has provided a basis for further refinement. If one subscribes to the dialectical approach, dealing with differing ideas and theories of development may be viewed positively. Out of the ferment created by differences may come further refinement of developmental theories.

Other Developmental Theorists

More recently, Gould (1972, 1976, 1978) and Levinson (1977, 1979) have contributed to developmental theory. Gould focuses on the sequential nature of change in individuals over time. He indicates that around age 50, individuals realize that there are no magical powers by which the world can be subjected to their will—which frees them to develop another frame of reference. New perceptions may gradually allow freedom from pettiness, struggles over control, and competition. Gould refers to the inner direction that occurs in the transformation after midlife. This transformation reminds one of Jung's (1933) theory about development of the inner self in the last half of life. Gould views this change as part of the developmental process in which individuals reorient their internal world.

Levinson (1977, 1979) studied the development of life structure, which he defines as the pattern of a person's life at any given time. This life structure is composed of two aspects by which the individual's interaction with the world is evidenced: the external, that is, the individual's pattern with respect to roles, memberships, life-style, and long-term goals; and the internal, that is, the meaning of external events, inner identities, values, and so on. Levinson divides the life cycle into four eras of approximately 25 years each; they are (1) childhood and adolescence, (2) early adulthood, (3) middle adulthood; and (4) late adulthood. These eras are referred to as seasons of a person's life (Levinson, 1979). The eras are distinctive and unifying. Transitions occur when one era ends and another begins. Each period has identifiable developmental tasks and processes and is defined in terms of these tasks. Levinson's theory is concerned with development of all the components of an individual's life. In Levinson's view, evolution of the life structure is the essence of adult development.

The Developmental Task Theory

Havighurst (1953) is credited with much of the early formation of the developmental task theory, although he first heard the term *developmental task* from Frank in about 1935. This theory is based on the view of the individual as a learner who grows through learning. Learning occurs at differing rates and with varying degrees of intensity throughout the life cycle. An individual must learn developmental tasks that contribute toward individual happiness and success in life. Havighurst defines a developmental task as

. . . a task which arises at or about a certain period in the life of the individual, successful achievement of which leads to his happiness and to success with later tasks, while failure leads to unhappiness in the individual, disapproval by the society, and difficulty with later tasks.*

*From Havighurst, R.: Human development and education, New York, 1953, David McKay Co., Inc., p. 2.

Havighurst likens the sociopsychological tasks to the biological tasks of the body and cites examples of outcomes if the tasks are not successfully achieved.

According to Havighurst, developmental tasks arise from physical maturation, from cultural expectations of society, and from the individual's personal values and aspirations. The infant grows, learns to walk, and is expected to continue learning throughout life. This expectation includes learning to talk and read in preparation for contributing to society. As discussed previously, the interrelationship of the various dimensions within the individual is evident. In the holistic approach, development in the various dimensions occurs simultaneously, affecting the whole person.

Havighurst presents developmental tasks for each stage of life. These tasks reflect the biosocial development and the development of the mind. He indicates that the developmental tasks of later maturity differ from those of other stages in only one respect: the defensive strategy is aimed at holding on to life instead of reaching out for more life. Havighurst speculates, however, that boundaries of the spiritual dimension need not be narrowed but may instead be widened. This view alludes to the potential for incremental changes within the person even in late life. The concept of developmental tasks, promoted by Havighurst and others, continues to influence approaches to various stages of development. This influence is perhaps most notable on considerations of the later stage of maturity.

The Concept of Family Development

Family development is a process in which the family structure and functions change over time (Duvall, 1950, 1977). Traditionally, the family has been defined as nuclear, consisting of husband, wife, and children. The nuclear family continues to serve as the norm (Rakel, 1977). Modern forms of the family are emerging, such as individuals living in groups that function in a similar manner to nuclear or extended family groups (Rakel). Some basic functions of the family are to ensure physical survival and to promote the essential humanness of its members (Ackerman, 1958). Patterns of family development are, for the most part, consistent.

Previously, the family development perspective was based on the concept of the family as a closed system; the developmental dynamic was viewed as internal to the family (Hill and Mattessich, 1979). More recently, the perspective of the family has been based on the concept of the family as a partially open living system. Societal expectations and environmental changes influence the developmental process. Although external factors are a necessary part of the developmental process, they are believed to be insufficient by themselves to cause family development. The internal dynamics of the family, involving pressures such as those arising with changes of aging and changing roles, are still considered predominant in the development of the family.

In the dialectical perspective (Riegel, 1979) family development involves both continuity and discontinuity. The internal and external factors influencing the dynamics of family development are viewed as interactive and dependent. The family is in a pivotal position, on one hand looking at its individual members and their needs and on the other hand at the needs of society, which is also developing. Perhaps because of its semiopenness and the interdependence of the internal and external loci of the dynamic of development, the family stands as an example of developmental theory.

Summary

Aging is a universal process experienced not only by older adults but by those providing assistance to them. The developmental concept is one way of viewing the aging process; it provides a framework for organizing ideas and information and a means of increasing understanding of aging. Moreover, the developmental concept is versatile: it can be used at the individual and family levels of organization. The various orientations described previously also provide ways of looking at individuals.

A model for intervention by those providing care to older persons can be developed through knowledge of these orientations. Consideration of various orientations toward developmental patterns helps caregivers understand the older person. It involves exploring human nature philosophically. In the mechanistic orientation, based on knowledge of the individual's past behavior, the individual is passive and predictable. This individual would require specific directions regarding such things as life-style changes, exercises, and dietary modification. In the organismic orientation the individual would be expected to be more active in establishing goals and implementing plans for meeting them. In the dialectical orientation dynamic interaction, of the individual and the environment determines change. In this situation the care provider should be sensitive to these dynamics. The orientation one has toward human nature influences relationships with older persons. Most persons act on principles if they understand the rationale behind them. Both the caregiver and the older adult need an appreciation of the interchange dynamics, whatever the model of intervention.

References

Ackerman, N.W.: The psychodynamics of the family. In Ackerman, N.W., editor: The psychodynamics of family life, New York, 1958, Basic Books, Inc., Publishers.

Bahr, Sister R.T.: Holistic or wholistic health: a philosophy of practice in gerontological nursing? (editorial), J. Gerontol. Nurs. 8(5):262, 1982.

Barnes, R.F., and others: Problems of families caring for Alzheimer's patients: use of a support group, J. Am. Geriatr. Soc. 29(2):80, 1981.

Bayly, J.: View from a hearse, Elgin, Ill., 1969, David C. Cook Publishing Co.

Birren, J.E., and Renner, J.V.: Research on the psychology of aging: principles and experimentations. In Birren, J.E., and Schaie, K.W., editors: Handbook of the psychology of aging, New York, 1977, Van Nostrand Reinhold Co.

Brunner, L.D., and Suddarth, D.S.: Textbook of medical-surgical nursing, ed. 4, Philadelphia, 1980, J.B. Lippincott Co.

Bühler, C.: The curve of life as studies in biographies, J. Appl. Sci. 19:405, 1953.

Bühler, C.: Old age and fulfillment of life with consideration of the use of time in old age, Vita Humana 4(½):129, 1961.

Busse, E.W., and Pfieffer, E.: Behavior and adaptation in later life, Boston, 1969, Little, Brown & Co.

Cumming, E., and Henry, W.E.: Growing old: the process of disengagement, New York, 1961, Basic Books, Inc., Publishers.

Darwin, C.R.: Origin of the species, by means of natural selection, New York, 1900, P.F. Collier. (Originally published in 1859.)

Deci, E.L.: Intrinsic motivation, New York, 1975, Plenum Publishing Corp.

Duvall, E.M.: Changing roles in the family cycle, J. Home Econ. 43:435, 1950.

Duvall, E.M.: Marriage and family development, ed. 5, New York, 1977, J.B. Lippincott Co.

Ebersole, P.: The inherent strengths of middle-aged men and women. In Burnside, I.M., Ebersole, P., and Monea, H.E., editors: Psychosocial caring through the life span, New York, 1979, McGraw-Hill, Inc.

Erikson, E.H.: Childhood and society, New York, 1950, W.W. Norton Co., Inc.

Erikson, E.H.: Identity and the life cycle: psychological issues, New York, 1959, International Universities Press, Inc.

Erikson, E.H.: Childhood and society, ed. 2, New York, 1963, W.W. Norton Co., Inc.

Erikson, E.H.: Generativity and ego integrity. In Neugarten, B.L., editor: Middle age and aging: a reader in social psychology, Chicago, 1968, The University of Chicago Press.

Erikson, E.H.: Life history and the historical movement, New York, 1975, W.W. Norton & Co., Inc.

Finch, C.E.: The regulation of physiological changes during mammalism aging, Q. Rev. Biol. 51:49, 1976.

Finch, C.E.: Neuroendocrine and autonomic aspects of aging. In Finch, C.E., and Hayflick, E., editors: Handbook of biology of aging, New York, 1977, Van Nostrand Reinhold Co.

Flavell, J.H.: The developmental psychology of Jean Piaget, New York, 1963, Van Nostrand Reinhold Co.

Furth, H.G.: Piaget and knowledge, Englewood Cliffs, N.J., 1969, Prentice-Hall, Inc.

Gould, R.L.: The phases of adult life: a study in developmental psychology, Am. J. Psychiatry 129(5):521, 1972.

Gould, R.L.: Adult life stages: growth toward self-tolerance, Psychol. Today 8:74, 1976.

Gould, R.L.: The end of an era: beyond mid-life. In Gould, R.L., editor: Transformation: growth and change in adult life, New York, 1978, Simon & Schuster, Inc.

Gurland, B.J.: The comparative frequency of depression in various adult groups, J. Gerontol. 31:283, 1976.

Hall, E.: Acting one's age: new rules for the old, Psychol. Today 9(1):66, 1980.

Harmon, D.: Free radical theory of aging: effect of the amount and degree of unsaturation of dietary fat on mortality rate, J. Gerontol. 26(4):456, 1971.

Havighurst, R.: Developmental tasks and education, Chicago, 1948, Chicago University Press.

Havighurst, R.: Human development and education, New York, 1953, David McKay Co., Inc.

Havighurst, R.: Successful aging. In Williams, R.H., Tibbitts, C., and Donahue, W., editors: Processes of aging, New York, 1963, Atherton Press.

Havighurst, R.: Developmental tasks and education, New York, 1972, David McKay, Inc.

Hayflick, L.: Current theories on biological aging, Fed. Proc. 34(1):9, 1975.

Hayflick, L.: The cellular basis for biological aging. In Finch, C.E., and Hayflick, L., editors: Handbook of the biology of aging, New York, 1977, Van Nostrand Reinhold Co.

Hill, R., and Mattessich, P.: Family development theory and life-span development. In Baltes, P.B., and Brim, O.G., Jr., editors: Life-span development and behavior, vol. 2, New York, 1979, Academic Press, Inc.

Holmes, T., and Rahe, T.: The social readjustment rating scale, J. Psychosom. Res. 11(8):213, 1967.

Hultsch, D.F., and Plemons, J.K.: Life events and life span development. In Baltes, P.B., Jr., and Brim, O.G., Jr., editors: New York, 1979, Academic Press, Inc.

Jourard, S.M.: The transparent self: self disclosure and well-being, New York, 1964, Van Nostrand Co., Inc.

Jung, C.F.: Modern man in search of a soul, New York, 1933, Harcourt Brace Jovanovich, Inc.

Jung, C.F.: The portable Jung, New York, 1971, Penguin Books. (Translated by R.F.C. Hull; edited by J. Campbell.)

Kaplan, M.: The concept of social role. In Kaplan, M.: Leisure, lifestyle and lifespan: perspectives for gerontology, Philadelphia, 1979, W.B. Saunders Co.

Kent, S.: Why do we grow old? Geriatrics 31(2):135, 1976.

Kent, S.: The biologic aging clock, Geriatrics 37(7):95, 1982.

Kimmel, D.C.: Adulthood and aging: an interdisciplinary developmental view, ed. 2, New York, 1980, John Wiley & Sons, Inc.

Kinsey, A., and others: Sexual behavior in the human male, Philadelphia, 1948, W.B. Saunders Co.

Laslett, P.: Societal development and aging. In Binstock, R.H., and Shanas, E., editors: Handbook of aging and the social sciences, New York, 1976, Van Nostrand Reinhold Co.

Lerner, R.M.: Nature, nurture, and dynamic interactionism, Hum. Dev. 21:1, 1978.

Levinson, D.J.: The mid-life transition: a period in adult psychosocial development, Psychiatry 40:99, 1977.

Levinson, D.J., and others: Seasons of a man's life, New York, 1979, Alfred A. Knopf, Inc.

Looft, W.: Socialization and personality throughout the life-span: an examination of contemporary psychological approaches. In Baltes, P.B., and Schaie, K.W., editors: Life-span developmental psychology: personality and socialization, New York, 1973, Academic Press, Inc.

Masters, W.H., and Johnson, V.E.: Human sexual response, Boston, 1966, Little, Brown & Co.

Masters, W.H., and Johnson, V.E.: Human sexual inadequacy, Boston, 1970, Little, Brown & Co.

Moberg, D.O.: Spiritual well-being, Washington, D.C., 1971, U.S. Government Printing Office.

Montagu, A.: On being human, New York, 1966, Hawthorn Books, Inc.

Neugarten, B.L., and Hagestad, G.O.: A developmental view of adult personality. In Birren, J.E., editor: Relations of development and aging, Springfield, Ill., 1964, Charles C Thomas, Publisher.

Neugarten, B.L.: Adult personality: toward a psychology of the life cycle. In Neugarten, B.L., editor: Middle age and aging: a reader in social psychology, Chicago, 1968, The University of Chicago Press.

Neugarten, B.L.: Personality change in late life: a developmental perspective. In Eisdorfer, C., and Lawton, M.P., editors: The psychology of adult development and aging, Washington, D.C., 1973, American Psychological Association.

Neugarten, B.L., and Hagestad, G.O.: Age and the life course. In Binstock, R.H., and Shanas, E., editors: Handbook of aging and the social sciences, New York, 1976, Van Nostrand Reinhold Co.

Peck, R.: Psychological developments in the second half of life. In Anderson, J.E., editor: Psychological aspects of aging, Washington, D.C., 1956, American Psychological Association, Inc.

Peck, R.: Psychological developments in the second half of life. In Neugarten, B.L., editor: Middle age and aging: a reader in social psychology, Chicago, 1968, The University of Chicago Press.

Peck, R.: Physiological developments in the second half of life. In Sze, W.C., editor: Human life cycle, New York, 1975, Jason Aronson, Inc.

Prechtl, H.F.R., and Connolly, K.J.: Maturation and development: an introduction. In Connolly, K.J., and Prechtl, H.F.R., editors: Maturation and development: biological and psychological perspectives, Philadelphia, 1981, J.B. Lippincott Co.

Rakel, R.E.: Principles of family medicine, Philadelphia, 1977, W.B. Saunders Co.

Reece, H.W., and Overton, W.F.: Models of development and theories of development. In Goulet, L.R., and Baltes, P.B., editors: Life-span developmental psychology: research and theory, New York, 1970, Academic Press.

Riegel, K.F.: Adult life crisis: toward a didactic theory of development. In Datan, N., and Ginsberg, L.H., editors: Lifespan developmental psychology: normative life crises, New York, 1975, Academic Press, Inc.

Riegel, K.F.: History of psychological gerontology. In Birren, J.E., and Schaie, K.W., editors: Handbook of the psychology of aging, New York, 1977, Van Nostrand Reinhold Co.

Riegel, K.F.: Foundations of a dialectical psychology, New York, 1979, Academic Press, Inc.

Riegel, K.F., Meacham, J.A., and Riegel, R.M.: Development, drop and death, Dev. Psychol. 6:306, 1972.

Riegel, K.F., and Meacham, J.A., editors: The developing individual in a changing world, vol. 2, Social and environmental issues, Chicago, 1976, Bevesford Book Service.

Rogers, C.: On becoming a person: a therapist's view of psychotherapy, Boston, 1961, Houghton Mifflin Co.

Rossmann, I.: Anatomic and body composition changes with aging. In Finch, C.E., and Hayflick, K., editors: Handbook of the biology of aging, New York, 1977, Van Nostrand Reinhold Co.

Schultz, D.: Growth psychology: models of the healthy personality, New York, 1977, Van Nostrand Reinhold Co.

Schuster, C.S., and Ashburn, S.S.: The process of human development: a holistic approach, Boston, 1980, Little, Brown & Co.

Selye, H.: The stress of life, New York, 1956, McGraw-Hill, Inc.

Stallwood, J., and Stoll, R.: Spiritual dimensions of nursing practice. In Beland, I.L., and Passos, J.Y., editors: Clinical nursing, ed. 3, New York, 1975, Macmillan Inc.

Timiras, P.S.: Developmental physiology and aging, New York, 1972, Macmillan Inc.

Wilkie, F., and Eisdorfer, C.: Intelligence and blood pressure in the aged, Science 172:959, 1971.

Zarit, S.H.: Aging and mental disorders: psychological approaches and assessment and treatment, New York, 1980, The Free Press.

Chapter 5   Changes and Challenges

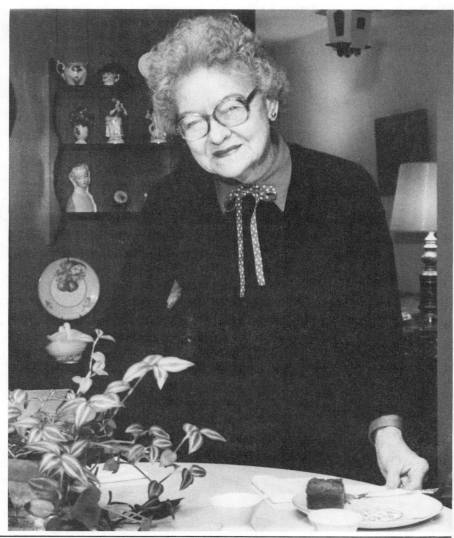

The older person faces many challenges imposed by aging. These changes occur gradually within the physical, psychological, sociological, and spiritual dimensions of the person. Whatever the changes, it is the whole person who responds—through the process of adaptation—to the challenges they present.

This chapter explores some of the normal changes of aging and the challenges they present to the older adult and the health care provider. Knowledge of these factors provides the basis for understanding and coping with the changing capacities of older persons.

Physiological Changes of Aging

The aging person may be viewed as an open system maintaining a steady state by continuing an exchange of energy and matter with the environment. The steady state of the individual depends in part on the ability of the biological system to maintain itself in a constantly changing environment. Integrity of the person is maintained partly by various physiological processes stimulated by alterations in the environment, such as changes in the blood glucose concentration (Groër and Shekleton, 1983). Knowledge of these alterations is important, since even minute changes may compromise the steady state of the older person.

Normal changes of physiological aging can be examined through various parameters, such as cardiac output, peripheral resistance, pulmonary function, and glomerular filtration rate. Although impairment measured by these parameters may not seriously interfere with the person's functional ability in a relatively stress-free environment, a fall or an infection can disrupt the steady state and may result in an inability to regain equilibrium (Groër and Shekleton, 1983).

General Physiological Changes

A brief presentation of selected general physical changes of aging follows. For example, the cardiac output (the amount of blood forced from the ventricle per minute) is significantly decreased in the older adult (Timiras, 1972). The average of 5 L/minute may be decreased 50% by the age of 80 (Forbes and Fitzsimons, 1981). In the elderly, exercise accelerates the cardiac rate and increases blood pressure, but these responses are insufficient to compensate for the decreased cardiac output. Inability to meet the needs of contracting muscles is a limiting factor in the elderly.

Changes in the lung also affect the adaptive response of the older person, since oxygenation of the blood is essential for muscular function. The rate of oxygen uptake in the older person is about 1.5 L/minute, compared with an average of approximately 4 L/minute in the young adult. To meet the need of contracting muscles, the older person must move approximately 50% more air than the younger person. The decrease in the absorption of oxygen is probably related partly to the decreased cardiac output, but the major difference is likely to be caused by changes in the lung tissue itself (Timiras, 1972). Shortness of breath has been identified as one of the first indicators of aging changes. In the words of one older person, "You can't fool a flight of stairs."

A decrease in mechanical efficiency of the lung is evident in the decreased turnover of air and the increased dead air space. The total volume of the lung is essentially unchanged, but the vital capacity decreases with age. This change is evident in the maximum breathing capacity of the older person; it shows a decrease of approximately 40% in individuals between 20 and 80 years of age (Timiras, 1972). This change in capacity occurs because of the inability to maintain a rapid respiratory rate. It is believed to reflect changes in neuromuscular ability. Given this change of aging, it is evident that the older person tends to have difficulty contending with stresses such as increased exercise or with conditions such as pneumonia or chronic obstructive lung disease.

The glomerular filtration rate also declines with age. A decline in the number of nephrons, the functional units of the kidney, occurs. Degenerative changes occur in the remaining nephrons, but under normal conditions the kidney is able to maintain the acid-base balance of the body. However, with the decrease in the general circulation, the renal filtration rate declines approximately 6% per decade. Arteriosclerotic constriction of the renal arteriole results in the blood being channeled to other parts of the body and contributes to the decline in the glomerular filtration rate (Forbes and Fitzsimons, 1981). Changes in the renal system have implications for the older person in such areas as fluid intake and ability to handle medications.

In addition to the generalized changes of aging just cited, a number of other changes occur, which are summarized in Table 1.

Specific Physiological Changes

More specific physiological changes affecting the elderly include sensory-motor changes, oral-digestive changes, and thermoregulatory changes.

Sensory-motor changes contribute toward limitations of varying degrees and affect the older person's response to the aging process. The tendency to focus on limitations rather than on the potential for adaptation hinders the adaptive process. Changes in visual acuity, for example, affect the individual's ability to manage the environment. Change in the lens of the eye eventually affects the ability to accommodate for near vision (presbyopia) (Fozard and others, 1977). Yellowing of the lens decreases the amount of light that can be transmitted to the retina. Yellowing of the lens also affects color discrimination, resulting in decreased sensitivity to the shorter wavelengths of the blue-green end of the spectrum. It becomes more difficult to differentiate the green traffic light against the blue sky. An opacity of the lens (cataract) may further compromise visual acuity. The

Table 1. **Normal Physical Assessment Findings in Older Persons**	**Cardiovascular changes**	
	Cardiac output	Heart loses elasticity; therefore heart contractility decreases in response to increased demands
	Arterial circulation	Decreased vessel compliance with increased peripheral resistance to blood flow occurs with general or localized arteriosclerosis
	Venous circulation	Does not exhibit change with aging in the absence of disease
	Blood pressure	Significant increase in the systolic, slight increase in the diastolic, increase in peripheral resistance and pulse pressure
	Heart	Dislocation of the apex is due to kyphoscoliosis; therefore diagnostic significance of location is lost
		Premature beats increase, but are rarely clinically important
	Murmurs	Over half the aged have diastolic murmurs; the most common are heard at the base of the heart due to sclerotic changes on the aortic valves
	Peripheral pulses	Easily palpated because of increased arterial wall narrowing and loss of connective tissue; vessels feel more tortuous and rigid
		Pedal pulses may be weaker due to arteriosclerotic changes; lower extremities are colder, especially at night; feet and hands may be cold and have mottled color
	Heart rate	No changes with age at normal rest
	Respiratory changes	
	Pulmonary blood flow and diffusion	Decreased blood flow to the pulmonary circulation; decreased diffusion
	Anatomic structure	Increased anterior-posterior diameter
	Respiratory accessory muscles	Degeneration and decreased strength; increased rigidity of chest wall
		Muscle atrophy of pharynx and larynx
	Internal pulmonic structure	Decreased pulmonary elasticity creates senile emphysema
		Shorter breaths taken with decreased maximum breathing capacity, vital capacity, residual volume, and functional capacity
		Airway resistance increases; there is less ventilation at the bases of the lung and more at the apex
	Integumentary changes	
	Texture	Skin loses elasticity; wrinkles, folding, sagging, dryness
	Color	Spotty pigmentation in areas exposed to sun; face paler, even in the absence of anemia
	Temperature	Extremities cooler; perspiration decreases
	Fat distribution	Less on extremities; more on trunk

From Ebersole, P., and Hess, P., editors: Toward healthy aging: human needs and nursing response, St. Louis, 1981, The C.V. Mosby Co.; based on data from Malasanos, L., and others: Health assessment, ed. 2, St. Louis, 1981, The C.V. Mosby Co.; Blake D.: Physiology and aging seminar for nurses, 1979, Napa, Calif.; and Wardell S., and others, editors: Acute interventions: nursing process throughout the life span, Reston, Va., 1979, reprinted with permission from Reston Publishing Co. a Prentice-Hall Co.

Continued.

Table 1. Normal Physical Assessment Findings in Older Persons—cont'd	**Integumentary changes—cont'd**	
	Hair color	Dull gray, white, yellow, or yellow-green
	Hair distribution	Thins on scalp, axilla, pubic area, upper and lower extremities; facial hair decreases in men; women may develop chin and upper lip hair
	Nails	Decreased growth rate
	Genitourinary and reproductive changes	
	Renal blood flow	Due to decreased cardiac output, reduction in filtration rate and renal efficiency; subsequent loss of protein from kidneys may occur
	Micturition	In men frequency may increase due to prostatic enlargement
		In women decrease in perineal muscle tone leads to urgency and stress incontinence
		Nocturia increases for both men and women
		Polyuria may be diabetes related
		Decreased volume of urine may relate to decrease in intake, but evaluation is needed
	Incontinence	Occurrence increases with age, specifically in those with organic brain disease
	Male reproduction	
	Testosterone production	Decreases; phases of intercourse slower, refractory time lengthens
	Frequency of intercourse	Changes in libido and sexual satisfaction should not occur, but frequency may decline to one or two times weekly
	Testes	Decreased size; sperm count decreases, and the viscosity of seminal fluid diminishes
	Female reproduction	
	Estrogen	Production decreases with menopause
	Breasts	Diminished breast tissue
	Uterus	Decreased size; mucous secretions cease; uterine prolapse may occur due to muscle weakness
	Vagina	Epithelial lining atrophies; canal narrows and shortens
	Vaginal secretions	Become more alkaline as glycogen content increases and acidity declines
	Gastrointestinal changes	
	Mastication	Impaired due to partial or total loss of teeth, malocclusive bite, and ill-fitting dentures
	Swallowing and carbohydrate digestion	Swallowing more difficult as salivary secretions diminish Reduced ptyalin production impairs starch digestion
	Esophagus	Decreased esophageal peristalsis Increased incidence of hiatus hernia with accompanying gaseous distention
	Digestive enzymes	Decreased production of hydrochloric acid, pepsin, and pancreatic enzymes
	Intestinal peristalsis	Reduced gastrointestinal motility Constipation due to decreased motility and roughage

Table 1. **Normal Physical Assessment Findings in Older Persons—cont'd**	**Musculoskeletal changes**	
	Muscle strength and function	Decrease with loss of muscle mass; bony prominences normal in aged, since muscle mass decreased
	Bone structure	Normal demineralization, more porous
		Shortening of the trunk due to intervertebral space narrowing
	Joints	Become less mobile; tightening and fixation occur
		Activity may maintain function longer
		Posture changes are normal; some kyphosis
		Range of motion limited
	Anatomic size and height	Total decrease in size as loss of body protein and body water occur in proportion to decrease in basal metabolic rate
		Body fat increases; diminishes in arms and legs, increases in trunk
		Height may decrease 1 to 4 inches from young adulthood
	Nervous system changes	
	Response to stimuli	All voluntary or automatic reflexes are slowed
		Decreased ability to respond to multiple stimuli
	Sleep patterns	Stage IV sleep reduced in comparison to younger adulthood; frequency of spontaneous awakening increases
		The elderly stay in bed longer but get less sleep; insomnia is a problem, which should be evaluated
	Reflexes	Deep tendon reflexes remain responsive in the healthy aged
	Ambulation	Kinesthetic sense less efficient; may demonstrate an extrapyramidal Parkinson-like gait
		Basal ganglions of the nervous system are affected by the vascular changes and decreased oxygen supply
	Voice	Range, duration, and intensity of voice diminish; may become higher pitched and monotonous
	Sensory changes	
	Vision	
	Peripheral vision	Decreases
	Lens accommodation	Decreases, requires corrective lenses
	Ciliary body	Atrophy in accommodation of lens focus
	Iris	Development of arcus senilis
	Choroid	Structure shows atrophy around disc
	Lens	May develop opacity, cataract formation; more light is needed to see
	Color	Fades or disappears
	Macula	Degeneration occurs
	Conjunctiva	Thins and looks yellow
	Tearing	Decreases; increased irritation and infection
	Pupil	May be different in size
	Cornea	Presence of arcus senilis
	Retina	Vascular changes can be observed
	Stimuli threshold	Threshold for light touch and pain increases
		Ischemic paresthesias in the extremities are common

Continued.

Table 1. **Normal Physical Assessment Findings in Older Persons—cont'd**	**Sensory changes—cont'd**	
	Hearing	High-frequency tones are less perceptible, hence language understanding is greatly impaired; promotes confusion and seems to create increased rigidity in thought processes
	Gustatory	Acuity decreases as taste buds atrophy; may increase the amount of seasoning on food

pupil of the eye becomes smaller, creating the need for higher intensity lighting. A longer period of time is needed to adapt to differences in light or dark environments. These changes in visual acuity not only affect the person's ability to negotiate the environment; they also affect the person's fatigue level and sense of psychological well-being.

Hearing acuity is another physical change of aging that challenges older adults and those in contact with them. Decreasing hearing acuity results from sensorineural changes referred to as presbycusis. Loss begins with the higher tones because of changes in the organ of Corti and the eighth cranial nerve. Discrimination of sound is impaired and the older person may comment, "I hear you talking, but I can't make out what you say." In this case, decreased auditory acuity interferes with verbal communication and with the ability to pick up environmental cues important to the individual's safety. The inability to hear songbirds and music further limits the individual's enjoyment of life. The psychological impact of this physical impairment is great; it often leads to withdrawal and social isolation.

Change also occurs in the older person's ability to perceive and respond to proprioceptive sensations, which may affect the person's mobility. Proprioceptive sensations include the pressure sensations from the soles of the feet and the sensation of balance or equilibrium (Guyton, 1977). Proprioceptive sensations are relayed through the spinal cord in the dorsal columns (Ganong, 1975); most of the proprioceptive input goes to the cerebellum, and some goes to the cortex. Change in the conduction time for relaying the proprioceptive input is not clearly understood, but researchers think it may be related to changes within the synaptic mechanisms (Finch, 1977). Whatever the contributory factors, changes affecting proprioception affect the older person's self-esteem and ability to walk.

Sensory-motor changes, including changes in muscle tone, coordination, and balance, often affect the mobility of older persons. Fat, for instance, in the quadriceps muscles of the thigh, tends to replace some of the muscle tissue and decreases functional ability. Older persons often have increasing difficulty getting out of a chair or the bathtub. Changes in coordination may result in jerky movements, clumsiness, and a tendency to drop things. Balance, in turn, may be affected by anatomical changes, as well as by sensory-motor changes. Flexion of the hips and knees and kyphosis, resulting in a shift of the center of gravity, require more effort to maintain equilibrium. Changes in the feet, such as splayfoot (a wide forefoot in relation to the heel) and bunions further compromise mobility. Assistive devices—such as canes, walkers, and chairs designed to help a person stand—and a supportive environment should offset changes affecting mobility.

Changes in mobility tend to have great impact, since the person with limited mobility is keenly aware of dependence on others. The person's life space tends to become increasingly diminished with locomotor changes; this situation poses a challenge to the older person psychologically as well as physically. Problems with mobility are not insurmountable, however; this is illustrated by Mrs. W., an 80-year-old lady who lives in a high-rise for the elderly, which is located on the corner of a busy, four-lane thoroughfare. Arthritis and decreasing visual acuity limit her mobility, but she negotiates the familiar environment of the high-rise without undue concern. Mrs. W. is anxious about crossing the street and uses a white cane; she is determined not to become housebound. She jokes about the cane and the screeching of brakes when drivers suddenly realize the white cane signifies visual impairment. Mrs. W.'s determination to remain active is supported by various modes of adaptation.

Changes in the oral-digestive system include decreased motility of food and secretion of digestive juices. The oral cavity is of special importance, since the mouth is the primary means by which the individual seeks to obtain satisfaction (Kutscher, 1972), and since its importance is often overlooked. The mouth is important not only in the digestive process, but in the communication process. Changes in the oral cavity affect the well-being of the older person, including the individual's self-concept and self-esteem.

One of the physical changes in the oral cavity is a decrease in the secretion of saliva resulting in xerostomia (dry mouth). Dry mouth affects the digestive and communication processes. Older persons often find it necessary to take sips of water to compensate for the decrease in saliva; they may also use hard candies as a means of stimulating salivation. When there is marked decrease in the secretion of saliva, the antibacterial effect of saliva may be altered, contributing to the development of sordes (accumulation of decaying organic material and bacteria), which must be removed by artificial means (Brobeck, 1979). Sordes interfere with digestion and communication. The dehydrating effects of tranquilizers and other drugs compound problems associated with the decrease of saliva.

The digestive function initiated in the mouth is affected by the decreased secretion of saliva and the decreased ptyalin content of saliva. The digestive process begins with chewing, which breaks food into smaller particles. These particles are then coated with saliva and mucus containing ptyalin (salivary α-amylase), a digestive enzyme that hydrolyzes starches (Guyton, 1977; Jensen, 1980). This digestive process is continued in the stomach. Although the decrease of ptyalin in saliva (Timiras, 1972) is not a major problem of older persons, it can affect the older person's state of well-being. Coupled with other changes in the gastrointestional tract, such as decreased secretion of digestive juices and decreased enzyme content, it necessitates increased attention to the process of adaptation.

Changes in the thermoregulatory system are another challenge to older persons. Production of heat is normally achieved through basal metabolism, mostly associated with digestion of food and muscular activity. Heat loss occurs mainly by radiation, convection, and evaporation of moisture from the surface of the skin. Changes in the neural, endocrine, metabolic, and mechanical components (Finch, 1977) affect the capacity of older persons to adapt to environmental changes in temperature. Loss of heat is regulated to a great extent by change in the blood flow to the skin, which is affected by the nervous system. Receptors sensitive to minute changes in the central core blood temperature are found in the hypothalamus of the brain (Shock, 1977). Receptors in the skin also provide input to the brain about peripheral body temperatures. An increase in core body temperature stimulates vasodilation, which brings more blood to the surface for the dissipation of heat. With a decrease in core body temperature, the converse occurs, and vasoconstriction of the vessels in the skin helps conserve heat. In addition to these mechanisms, when the temperature increases, sweat glands are stimulated; evaporation of sweat results in heat loss. With a decrease in temperature shivering usually occurs, a muscular activity promoting heat production. However, changes of aging affect the mechanisms of the thermoregulatory system and alter the ability of older persons to respond, such as by shivering, and adapt to environmental changes in temperature.

Body temperatures of the elderly at rest remain within the same range as those of young people (between 35° C and 37° C) (Shock, 1952). Shock (1977), however, reports studies showing that elderly survivors of accidental hypothermia demonstrate impaired temperature-regulating mechanisms, which may last as long as 3 years following the episode. Persons showing a drop in core body temperature on exposure to cold did not indicate that they felt cold. Evidence indicates that although older people generally maintain their resting body temperature, some older persons seem at risk for developing hypothermia. Evidence also shows that the response of older persons to high or low environmental temperatures is less effective than that of the young (Shock, 1977). It appears that older persons can increase heat production the same as the young, but their mechanisms for conserving heat are not as effective. Body temperature in the elderly, therefore, decreases in a cold environment.

An increase in environmental temperature and a subsequent increase in body temperature normally stimulate vasodilation of the cutaneous blood vessels and increase sweating, heart rate, and respiratory rate (Shock, 1977). These compensatory mechanisms promote loss of body heat. Studies have shown, however, that the adaptive responses to an increase in environmental temperature are not as effective in older people as in young people. One of the factors influencing response to high environmental temperatures is the older person's slower response of sweat glands (Hellon and Lind, 1956). The rate of evaporation of moisture from the skin is also decreased in the aged (Krag and Kountz, 1952). As in most cases, the adaptive response of older adults involves multiple mechanisms reflecting the intricacy of human physiology.

The death rate from heat stroke is known to increase markedly in persons above 60 years of age, and mortality rates in institutions for the elderly increase during prolonged periods of higher than normal environmental temperatures (Friedfield, 1949; Timiras, 1972). Those above 70 years of age are increasingly vulnerable to either extreme of temperature. Muscular contraction, one of the defense mechanisms against cold, is less effective in the elderly. Decreased contractility of muscle hinders the ability of the older individual to adapt to low environmental temperatures. According to Jensen (1980), physiological defenses against hyperthermia (temperature above 39.5° C) are more effective than those against hypothermia (core body temperature significantly below 37.5° C). Although the thermoregulatory system is inactive at very low temperatures, the body may be rewarmed by external heat. Knowledge about thermoregulation in the elderly is essential for planning care, whether by caregivers or by the older person involved in self-care.

The concept of thermostatic control of food intake affords another view of factors affecting the thermoregulatory control of older persons. This concept is about the effect environmental temperature has on food intake (Brobeck, 1979). Food intake, it is suggested, is increased in cold temperatures and decreased in warm temperatures as a means of regulating body temperature. The anterior hypothalamus apparently integrates temperature regulation and food intake (Hamilton, 1975). This concept has implications for older persons and caretakers who are concerned with the holistic promotion of wellness. Many older persons are in a dilemma because of the high cost of energy and may feel forced to choose between heating or eating. The effect of food intake on heat production in the body renders a decision to heat or eat untenable. Dealing with thermoregulatory factors affecting older persons requires attention to individual needs and to the external environment—including economic factors and housing.

Research has shown that the temperature of the head does not necessarily correlate with the core body temperature (Ganong, 1975). A great deal of body heat can be lost from the head because of the nature of blood circulation to the area. Reference to the wearing of a nightcap is often found in the literature, usually in a humorous vein. Although there is a scientific basis for covering the head to conserve body heat, this information is disregarded by many people.

Thermoregulation in older adults is affected by structural and functional changes in the skin such as atrophy, dryness, loss of elasticity, decrease in the number of capillaries and decrease in the capacity by vessels to dilate in the skin of older persons (Timiras, 1972). Also affecting thermoregulation are age changes occurring in the heart and skeletal muscles. Need for increased oxygen on exposure to a relatively cold temperature, for example, becomes a stressor because of the difficulty of increasing the heart rate in elderly persons. The heart requires more time for contraction and relaxation; a greater refractory period occurs during which the heart does not respond to a stimulus. Thus, although the need for oxygen may increase, the capacity of the heart to circulate blood needed for transporting oxygen is decreased (Shock, 1977). Change in the capacity of muscles to respond to stress affects the ability to adapt to the stress of cold. Decrease in muscular activity, a major source of heat energy, further compromises the older person's adaptive capacity. Although functional ability of older persons may be adequate under ordinary conditions, they are less able to cope with physiological stress. Adaptive ability is compromised even further by the multiple aging changes occurring simultaneously in other dimensions of the person. Knowledge of human development and aging afford a means whereby older persons and caregivers can learn to cope more effectively with challenges posed by the physiological changes of aging.

Psychological Changes of Aging

Psychological changes of aging may not be as apparent as physiological changes of aging, but they can have marked impact on older persons. They can affect interest in life and will to live. Psychological aspects of aging involve the individual's perceptions of the experiences of life and, in turn, the ability to adapt to aging changes.

Gradually, human beings learn about themselves through their sensory systems and feedback from their sociocultural environment. Consideration of body image and self-concept is a means of examining aspects of psychological development. Body image, the view of the self and feelings about the body, is acquired as the individual differentiates the self from the environment. Objects regularly used by the person, such as false teeth and jewelry, often become a part of the body image and should be treated accordingly (Hogan, 1980). Self-concept is the view of the self as perceived by the self. Development of self-concept is affected by the environment, physical and human. If feedback from others is positive or negative, the individual tends to view the self accordingly. In an attempt to maintain an acceptable self-concept, the person tries to live up to self-perceptions, which are influenced by feedback.

Self-concept is one index of wellness (Engel, 1980). Relationships with significant others are also used to examine the development of self-concept. Frankl (1963) reports that the individuals imprisoned in concentration camps who had the will to live were those who felt accepted as human beings by others. They continued to believe that there was something worth living for in spite of the crisis they were experiencing. Fromm (1962) speaks of the person's uniqueness, which arises out of the awareness of self as a separate entity having a limited life span and being unable to control his or her birth or death. Buber (1957) also refers to the ability of the human being to perceive and to be aware of this perceiving. He suggests that people seek relationships with those who see them on their own terms. Buber speaks of the process needed by individuals that will confirm them for what they are as well as for what they may become. This process should be reciprocal and needs to be dealt with consciously. According to Buber, the greatest potential for inner growth of the self is through the process of confirming others. Thus, self-concept is feelings about the self that depend not only on self-perceptions but on perceiving the respect of others in the sociocultural environment.

As physical maturity is achieved, body image becomes integrated with psyche. Body image is expanded to include the thinking, feeling, and acting self. Individuals generally begin to appreciate themselves as having personalities by taking into account how they measure up to peers and whether they are on time—in the social sense—in such areas as finding a place in the worlds of work and marriage (Neugarten, 1968). Thus mature individuals have certain expectations of themselves; their feeling of worth depends to a great extent on the degree to which they measure up to these expectations.

In the middle and later years individuals tend to become increasingly introspective (Jung, 1933) and concerned with the meaning of life experiences, past, present, and future. In addition to concern about self-concept and body image, the desire for mastery over their lives and a sense of purpose in life are evident. Other characteristics that affect continuing development also exist. These characteristics include awareness (or consciousness), intelligence, motivation, the capacity to appreciate life and its experiences, and the ability to respond to other persons. Although these characteristics are generally viewed as subjective aspects of the personality, certain characteristics, such as motivation and intelligence, may also be viewed as objective aspects. This dual nature of personality characteristics affects the individual's self-esteem.

Self-esteem is the person's self-evaluation, influenced by the evaluations of others, and consequent approval or disapproval based on aspirations and expectations of the self (Murray, Huelskoetter, and O'Driscoll, 1980). Older persons, like younger persons, depend on their own feelings and the feelings and responses of others for a sense of belonging and worth. These feelings and responses are influenced by attitudes toward the aged and by values held by older persons themselves and others with whom they are associated. Attention to self-esteem needs of older persons becomes increasingly important when limitation of mobility and loss of significant others occur. Positive self-esteem is realized, to a great extent, through interaction with others who value the worth of human beings regardless of age or social status.

Intellectual Capacity

A major factor influencing attitudes toward the aged is intellectual capacity. It has been assumed that a decline in intellectual capacity occurs with aging; this assumption is internalized by many older persons, who tend to act accordingly. Other persons have accepted the assumption as true and have based expectations of older persons on the assumption. Studies show, however, that decline in the various psychological functions related to intellectual capacity is minimal in healthy older persons. The most consistent finding is that there is a decline in speed. Since ideas of intellectual capacity have a major importance in the formation of attitudes toward the aged, they will be explored as an example of the psychological aspect of aging.

Intellectual capacity as used here includes perception, cognitive ability, memory, and learning. Describing and identifying age-related behavioral changes that occur in intellectual function is a task for those concerned with developmental psychology; it is also of interest to those working with older persons. Such changes should be examined within a progressive-regressive framework, since the direction of these changes may vary at different stages of development.

Perception

Perception, the capacity to interpret the environment, is crucial to appropriate interaction with the environment. This capacity depends to a great extent on those sensory systems normally sensitive to various stimuli in the environment. With aging, changes in the sensory systems, such as the visual and auditory systems, alter perceptual ability and that, in turn, alters the capacity of older persons to respond to their environment. Perceptual capacity may also be affected by changes in the central nervous system, which alter the processes of receiving, processing, and responding to stimuli. Knowledge of these age changes, the reasons they occur, and factors influencing motivation in the later years is essential to understanding the adaptive process of older people. Because of the nature and impact of these age changes, older people often need assistance from others. Their acknowledgment of dependence needs may, in turn, be affected by their perception of both aging itself and the attitude of others from whom they would seek assistance.

The concept of stimulus persistence is believed useful in considering differences in the response of older persons to visual stimuli compared with that of younger persons. It is theorized that the first stimulus must be cleared before a second stimulus input can be processed and given a separate response. The central nervous system is believed to be the channel for processing and clearing the stimulus response. In older persons, it is believed that a trace of the first stimulus remains over time and leaves the individual either refractory to a second stimulus or slower to respond to a second stimulus (Botwinick, 1978). Thus perceptual ability may be affected by the capacity of the central nervous system as well as by the capacity of the sensory systems themselves.

Studies of visual illusions support the idea of alteration in visual abilities with aging. Findings from the studies are inconclusive, but the data regarding possible qualitative changes in perception with age are provocative (Elias and others, 1977).

Findings from the Müller Lyer illusion and the Titchener Circles illusion tests showed inconsistencies in the age span studied (Elias and others, 1977). These tests are designed to test perception of relationships of part to whole. However, several factors beyond the central processing mechanisms of older individuals make interpretation of these tests difficult. Inconsistent test results concern the way older persons with changes in perceptual capacity may be perceived by people who interpret the test. Loss of central vision because of changes in the vascular system, for example, may give the impression that older persons are incapable of managing independently. Macular degeneration, however, primarily limits close work such as reading; individuals are unlikely to become blind because of this condition. Affected individuals can learn to negotiate their environment by using peripheral vision. As in other changes in the visual sensory system mentioned previously, visual perceptions require organization. This organization depends not only on the structure and function of the visual sensory system, but on such factors as a functioning central processing system, intelligence, and motivation (Elias and others, 1977). Judgment should always be exercised in interpreting tests; this is especially true when testing older adults. They are challenged not only by the changes in perceptual ability but by the reactions of others, who may misinterpret their altered behavior as a sign of declining mental faculties. For older persons, environmental changes, such as higher intensity lighting and the delineation of steps with a stripe of white paint or white tape, would help offset physical changes.

Still another change in the sensory systems affecting perception and challenging older adults is impaired hearing. Like visual impairment, it affects the perceptions of older adults and frequently brings about marked psychological reactions. Unlike some other changes of aging, hearing changes are invisible; other people often forget the older person's problem with hearing. Change in hearing acuity occurs so gradually and painlessly that it is almost imperceptible to older persons themselves. They tend to deny the problem and to think other people are just not speaking loudly enough. Perceptions of hearing-impaired persons are frequently distorted, giving rise to feelings of paranoia and the notion that others are laughing at them. These misperceptions often lead to withdrawal from social inter- action. Moreover, other people often withdraw from those with hearing problems because of the difficulty in communicating with them. Even worse, they often treat these individuals as if the older persons were also mindless. This situation tends to make hearing-impaired persons feel like nonpersons or social outcasts—a great psychological impact.

Several changes contribute to hearing loss caused by the aging process (presbycusis): (1) sensory, occurring with atrophy of cells at the base of the organ of Corti, which results in loss of ability to hear high-pitched tones; (2) neural, which results in loss of speech discrimination because of loss of neurons in the pathways from the ear to the auditory cortex; (3) metabolic, which involves atrophy of the stria vascularis and loss of ability to hear pure tone; and (4) mechanical, which results in decreased flexibility of the basilar membrane and loss of ability to hear high-frequency tones (Rupp, 1970). Change in just one of the sensory systems has many contributing factors, which increase the complexity of its effects.

The changes in hearing acuity may be identified in terms of conductive and sensorineural functions. Conductive losses occur in the transmission of sound from the outer through the middle ear via the ossicles, the malleus, the incus, and the stapes. In this case the loss of sound is usually one of amplitude and does not involve distortion of sound. Sensorineural loss, on the other hand, involves the functioning of the inner ear (cochlea), which facilitates transmission of electrical signals from the inner ear via the cochlear nerve to the brain. Loss of function in this situation can include loss in amplitude and distortion of sound, which interferes with speech discrimination.

Loss of speech discrimination has potential for the greatest personal and social impact. Speech perception requires both peripheral and central processing mechanisms. Changes in speech perception, therefore, are of great import; they tend to limit social interaction and the satisfaction derived from association with others.

Older persons often experience tinnitus, or a ringing in the ears, because of circulatory changes or the effects of certain medications. Ringing in the ears becomes especially disturbing at night when other sounds that might mitigate its effects are diminished. Turning the radio on and tuning it to a point between stations is a simple but effective means of counteracting tinnitus. The buzzing sound, referred to as white noise, counteracts the tinnitus and allows the older person to sleep. Ability to sleep undisturbed often results in marked improvement in mood and sense of well-being.

Although perceptual ability has a biological basis, visual and auditory impairment of the sensory systems affect the psychological development and well-being of older persons. Moreover, this type of impairment affects the sociological and spiritual dimensions of these individuals as well.

Closely related to perceptual ability is cognitive ability, which refers to the ability to know and which depends to a great extent on the nervous system. The older individual may intellectually acknowledge certain facts, such as impending retirement, but have difficulty dealing with the facts psychologically. For the person whose identity and sense of personal fulfillment and worth depends to a marked degree on the work role and related social aspects, the behavioral reaction to impending retirement appears to be denial of the event's reality. This problem demonstrates a separation of perceptual and cognitive ability; it is a problem in the conceptualization, not the perception, of concrete reality. Both of these components of intellectual capacity influence the older person's response and ability to adapt to changes of aging. Practically speaking, these components are inseparable.

One of the interesting observations related to intellectual capacity reported by Elias and others (1977) is that intellectual functioning may show little change or even a slight increase up to the seventh decade of life, depending on the definition of intelligence. If long-term memory and use of acquired skills are included in the definition, relatively little decline occurs in healthy persons. Skills in some areas can increase over time, compensating for decline in other areas.

On the other hand, some researchers have noted that a decline in cognitive functioning may precede death (Kleemeier, 1961; Lieberman, 1965); this phenomenon is labeled *terminal drop*. Terminal drop is defined as a decline in performance on tests occurring a few years before death, which may be related to physiological decline (Kaluger and Kaluger, 1979).

A number of cross-sectional studies (Schaie, 1958; Riegel and Riegel, 1972) and longitudinal studies (Wilkie and Eisdorfer, 1971; Siegler, 1975) have been done, but the question of whether terminal drop is a problem with measurement or changes in the brain function of a person nearing death remains unanswered.

One of the problems in studying intelligence in older persons is the sampling problem, which is related to the research methods (Botwinick, 1967). The methods influence the results, creating a dilemma not easily resolved. The cross-sectional research method may erroneously magnify age decline because of the study's limited view at a given point in time. The longitudinal method, on the other hand, may minimize age decline, since subjects may drop out, leaving the more able ones to provide an increasingly biased sample as their age increases. In addition to problems with research methodology, numerous factors such as health, types of tests used, motivation, fatigue level, and perceptual-motor and speed functions influence the testing of older adults. The definition of intelligence also affects the testing process. The emphasis may either be on capacity, which is inferred, or on ability, which measures what is happening at the time of the test. Differences in the definition of intelligence influence the interpretation of the tests, often leading to controversy rather than clarification of the findings.

Interpretation of the various tests of cognitive ability is a complex process. In some cases, what appears to be decreased cognitive ability may be related to factors such as cautiousness and motivation. Older persons tend to hesitate in responding to test items for fear of making a mistake. There is question regarding the role of the central nervous system in the slowed response time of older persons and the implications for higher functioning. Such factors as physical exercise and motivation seem to influence the response time to varying degrees. Individual differences also pose questions about the significance of slowed response time to cognitive abilities of older persons. Slowed response may have been a characteristic of some individuals earlier in life and have little bearing on cognitive ability.

Additional clues to cognitive ability are provided by studies of problem-solving ability. Many more older than younger persons seem to prefer dealing with concrete tasks; others can deal with abstract thought and solve difficult problems without evidence of age decline until late life. The greater the educational background, the more likely older persons are to prefer dealing with problems requiring abstract thought (Botwinick, 1978).

According to Botwinick, older persons often fail to obtain knowledge of the goal before seeking information essential to solve the problem. There is a tendency to approach the information gathering process in a disorganized manner with repeated inquiries for the same information. This redundancy is believed related to a difficulty in seeing meaning in the information and in remembering it.

A new trend in the study of age and problem solving is to focus on the areas in which older persons have difficulties (Botwinick, 1978). Findings from these studies support the concept of lifelong learning ability in older persons. Part of the findings' success is probably related to the fact that the studies were conducted outside of the typical laboratory setting. This approach increases the probability that the process has more meaning to the older participants and is more likely to elicit a positive response. Thus one of the major challenges of the older person may be the decline of motivation rather than of cognitive ability. Another challenge is posed by those who view older persons as incapable of remembering recent events and incapable of learning.

Memory

Memory is an important component of intellectual capacity and is closely related to learning. Although these processes arise from the same biological base, they are different parts of a common phenomenon. For that reason, memory and learning are considered separately.

Memory is a term used to indicate retention of information about specific events occurring within a certain time frame and at a given place (Craik, 1977). Learning, on the other hand, may be referred to as the formation of new associations evidenced by a change in behavior that persists over time. The learning process depends to a great extent on memory and information processing. Changes of aging may modify the approaches to these mental operations, but they do not necessarily alter basic intellectual capacity.

Some researchers have found that divided attention may interfere with memory tasks of older persons. This situation may be less of a problem, however, when the memory task is presented in the auditory mode (Craik, 1973; Anderson and Craik, 1974). Apparently, auditory inputs can be retained briefly, even if they are not attended to immediately. This contrasts with input in the visual mode, which requires immediate attention. Thus concern for achievement of memory tasks by older persons should involve careful consideration of the various modes used in presenting stimuli.

Memory is sometimes referred to as a memory trace (Best and Taylor, 1966). The precise nature of the process by which a memory trace is achieved is unknown, but once impulses travel certain pathways within the central nervous system, other stimuli seem to provide the means whereby that material can be recalled.

Several factors may influence the development of the memory trace. For example, disruptions may interfere with stage one, in which the memory trace is transient and easily disrupted (Brobeck, 1979). Disruptive conditions include hypothermia, anorexia, and hypoglycemia. Their effect on the circuitry of nerve conduction and the capacity for processing information is variable, since they may vary in intensity and occur intermittently over time. On the other hand, it is believed on the basis of animal studies that intracellular synthesis of protein, which involves ribonucleic acid, may play a role in long-term memory trace. Moreover, there is considerable support for the hypothesis that repeated stimulation of the neurons in a closed circuit system maintains memory until permanent changes for fixation have been accomplished (Best and Taylor, 1966). Since the processing of a memory trace may continue over a period of time varying from several minutes to several months, the potential effect of disruptive conditions and physiological alterations in cellular metabolism is evident. It is also evident that however memory is defined it is a complex process.

Another way of viewing memory is through the distinctions of short-term and long-term memory. Short-term memory is referred to as primary memory, when material is still in the mind and the focus of conscious attention. It is the control system for thinking and remembering (Atkinson and Shiffrin, 1971). Long-term, or secondary, memory is that part of the process involved when the immediate memory span is exceeded and recall of items necessitates retrieval. Qualitative differences between primary and secondary memory arise out of differences in processes rather than in time intervals or experimental designs.

Apparently age differences mean little to primary memory, as long as the items are adequately perceived and reorganization of material is not required. Age differences in secondary memory probably mean variance in acquisition or retrieval. Older persons have more difficulty when there are divided attention situations and when stored material requires manipulation or reorganization (Broadbent and Gregory, 1965; Talland, 1965). There seems to be a greater difference in recall than in recognition for older persons; they apparently fail to organize material for more effective recall levels (Craik, 1977).

The belief that memory of older persons for remote events is unimpaired is based on anecdotes rather than on controlled research studies. Valid comparisons between recent and remote memory should be based on equating the material to be remembered and the conditions affecting its acquisition, according to Craik (1977). Childhood events have been recalled many times; therefore the older person is remembering not necessarily from 50 years ago but, to an undetermined extent, from the last description of the event. The accuracy of the recall also is open to question.

Currently the discrete-stage models of memory, although of heuristic value in the past, appear to have outlived their usefulness. Memory, it is suggested, should be thought of as a continuum (Craik and Lockhart, 1972). Durability of the memory trace is believed to be simply a function of the kind of processing carried out on the stimulus. Greater depth of the memory trace can be achieved by more elaborate encoding through exercise of semantic or categorical judgment as to what a word represents or through rating a word for its meaning. A major source of memory deficit is probably caused by poor acquisition of materials in the secondary memory, resulting in a production deficiency. Analysis suggests that if older persons were given an appropriate task to perform, rather than just being asked to learn inconsequential material, their performance would be close to the memory performance of younger persons.

Learning

Concern for changes in older persons' ability to learn requires considering some of the same components involved in the memory process: acquisition, storage, and retrieval of information. Although there is no single definition of learning, Botwinick (1967)* defines learning as the "acquisition of information or skills" that can be measured by improvement in an overt response. Demonstration of learning usually requires more time for the older person. Age-related decrement in performance has been attributed to a problem with retrieval of information rather than with storage. Older individuals have demonstrated the need for more time to search for stored information and to produce the response. In addition, older persons need to know how to search for the necessary item to produce the desired response. Some evidence points out that supportive instructions improve the performance of older persons (Ross, 1968; Lair and Moon, 1972).

Organizational processes also facilitate learning; they determine the amount of information that can be stored and retrieved. Evidence suggests that organization helps with recall, but older persons are less apt to organize material than younger persons. Thus retrieval becomes a problem for many older persons, but there are ways to offset it—such as by providing cues.

There are acknowledged differences in learning and memory of older persons, but there is less agreement on some of the factors influencing the change, such as susceptibility of interference. Interference is defined as the effect of the learning of one task on the retention of another (Arenberg and Robertson-Tchabo, 1977). Methodological problems such as coordinating the different age groups with respect to the degree of original learning and the rate of learning (Arenberg and Robertson-Tchabo) make it difficult to evaluate the susceptibility of interference. Thus the question of the effects of interference remains controversial.

Omission errors made by older persons seem related to response in-

*From Botwinick, J.: Cognitive processes in maturity and old age, New York, 1967, Springer Publishing Co., p. 48.

hibition (related to anxiety) or arousal (psychophysiological). They tend not to respond, seemingly out of caution or fear of being wrong. This behavior creates a problem with learning, since learning is minimal when responses are not required. Leech and Witte (1971) conducted a study based on the tendency of older persons not to respond. Their teaching strategy is to reward learners for correct responses. These investigators, realizing that learning would be difficult if older persons did not respond, rewarded all responses by older learners. A greater reward was given for correct responses than for wrong responses. Data from the study suggested that what seemed like a learning deficit may simply be a problem of response, which limits the expression of learned material (Botwinick, 1978).

Psychological changes of aging involve a number of components, such as intellectual capacity, perception, cognitive ability, memory, and learning. Although a number of studies have been conducted regarding these components, there is no consensus about the cognitive ability and performance of older persons. Generally, many agree that, given enough time, older persons will respond to testing as accurately as younger people. Further investigation of factors such as motivation and meaningfulness of learning tasks is necessary in the attempt to resolve differences regarding previously drawn conclusions (Botwinick, 1978). Attention should be directed toward identifying the strengths of older persons and ways of assisting them to maximize their potential as thinking, feeling, acting human beings.

Sociological Changes of Aging

Sociological changes of aging include changing social roles and the social integration of older persons into the surrounding community. These sociological changes are affected by the capacity of older persons to function in social roles. They are also influenced by opportunity for participation in socially sanctioned roles. Thus sociological changes of aging arise out of the person-environment context of a given culture.

Cultural values determine to a great extent the social behavior of older persons. In many cultures older members of society are revered for their wisdom. In our culture the high value placed on productivity has created a dilemma: on one hand adults are expected to be productive, and on the other hand many older persons, although strongly committed to the "Protestant work ethic," have been denied the opportunity to participate in a satisfying and productive work role. Instead, they have been expected to yield to younger persons in the work place, with a subsequent decrease in their productivity and social roles. It looks now as if this dilemma might be resolved by the declining birth rate and increasing proportion of older persons in our society. Concern is being expressed over the declining size of the work force as compared with the growing number of dependents. This concern is reflected in the recent change in the mandatory retirement age; in many places it is now age 70 instead of the previous age of 65. Because of changes in the composition of society, productivity will again be shared in part by older adults.

Social roles of older persons are less clearly defined than those of younger persons; fewer roles tend to be identified for older adults. This situation has led to what is described as the "roleless role" of older persons. Moreover, there is little socialization of older persons. Older persons face the challenge of learning behavior appropriate for the various roles they may play, such as retired person, grandparent, widow. However these social roles are defined, they are closely related to the continuing biological, psychological, and spiritual development of the individual. Older persons struggling with the process of socialization into the roles and activities of late adulthood may be challenged by the lack of clearly defined roles.

Older persons, like younger persons, may be admonished to act their age, but there are few established norms regarding acceptable behavior for them. Among behaviors not socially approved are social withdrawal, idleness, and disregard for religion (Hobert and Ginsberg, 1979), but these behaviors are not formalized to the same extent as are behaviors for earlier developmental stages. This relative lack of social norms or expectations creates feelings of ambivalence that may lead to a state of anxiety for some older persons. Anxiety is likely to be increased for older individuals who rely on others' approval for guidance.

In some cases there is evidence that older persons are beginning to meet the challenge of the "roleless role" by identifying and legitimizing new roles for themselves. Roles such as legislator and consumer advocate are being assumed with an expectation of change. Many in Missouri, the first state in the United States to have a silver-haired legislature, at first considered it to be a mock legislature, that is, one in which the members were simply learning about the legislative process. However, these members soon realized that not only could they identify issues and the need for related legislation, but that they could find sponsors for proposed bills in the postlegislation period. Their success is evident in bills that have been passed, such as the inheritance tax bill and the property tax bill. In some cases the needs of younger persons are served by the legislature to a greater extent than those of older persons. This seems to be proof of the stage of generativity referred to by Erikson (1963) and the fact that older persons are not necessarily motivated to participate in civic activities merely for the purpose of serving their own needs.

In Kansas a concerned citizens' group has made a concerted effort to upgrade care in adult care homes. Another group, the Kansas Coalition for Aging, wants geriatrics and gerontology included in the curricula of state supported institutions of higher learning. They have been successful in gaining support from the legislature on this issue. Many older persons are volunteering for the first time for various activities to achieve goals relevant to them. These activities are examples of the way in which older individuals are achieving one of the developmental tasks of later maturity cited by Havighurst (1953)—civic responsibility.

Several factors undoubtedly contribute to these sociological changes of aging. Persons are living longer, and many are experiencing a high level of wellness. Education is opening up more work roles to many older people. Many older individuals have increasing leisure time for pursuing their interests, and they are becoming more politically astute. Rather than being defeated by what, at times, seems to be overpowering opposition, many older persons are rising to effect social change.

Spiritual Changes of Aging

Spiritual aging involves changes occurring with the passage of time, like aging in the other dimensions of the person. Since the spirit is described as an intangible quality emanating from within the inner person (Dunn, 1959; Bayly, 1969), consideration of the aging process of the spirit differs somewhat from that of the biopsychosocial dimensions of the person.

Definition of the Spirit

Sinnott (1955) indicates the spirit is a "mass of natural impulses, desires, and emotions that well up out of protoplasmic purposiveness, setting up in us goals and longings of all sorts, conscious or unconscious." These, he continues, "are the highest expressions of biological goal-seeking."* Protoplasmic purposiveness arises out of the biological thrust of cells toward ongoing development. Sinnott views the body, mind, and spirit as three aspects of goal-seeking, which is the distinctive feature of life at all levels. In this view the mind and spirit have a biological basis. The organizing principle, according to Sinnott, is the universal spirit of God.

Jourard (1964, p. 104), on the other hand, interprets the spirit as "goals or purposes for living."† People need a sense of purpose for life to have meaning. Meaning arises out of the perceptions of the individual, whether based on a personal relationship with God or an activating force unrelated to a belief in God (Ellis, 1980).

*From Sinnott, E.W.: The biology of the spirit, New York, Copyright © 1955 Edmund W. Sinnott, The Viking Press, pp. vii, 121.
†From The transparent self by Sidney Jourard,
Copyright © 1971 by Van Nostrand Reinhold Company, p. 104.
Reprinted by permission of the publisher.

In Biblical times the view was set forth that God created things spiritually prior to their physical sojourn on earth. In this view the life force has spatial and corporeal form at the time of conception or birth. The spirit leaves the dying body with the last breath; it is considered timeless and immortal (Jung, 1933). Although this concept has not been accepted by modern science, it continues to be held by those who adhere to traditional Judaeo-Christian religious beliefs and practices. Any attempt to discuss spiritual aging requires consideration of the definition of the spirit.

Spiritual aging refers to the process of developing a philosophy of life and coming to terms with oneself, one's place in the world, and one's relationship to others (Stallwood and Stoll, 1975). Since aging refers to differentiation over time, it seems logical to view spiritual aging as differentiation occurring in the individual's inner resources over time. These inner resources reflect the value system that guides the person's conduct (Moberg, 1971). Spiritual aging, less visible than some of the physical changes of aging, becomes apparent through the individual's verbal and nonverbal expression of feelings and reactions to life experiences.

Spiritual Development

A concept closely related to spiritual aging is spiritual development. According to Montagu (1966) "the term 'spiritual' means progress in the ability to love and experience. It involves exercise of the ability to express the deepening sensitivity to the world, rather than relying on someone else's interpretation."*

Murray and Zentner (1979) refer to the mature religious outlook of the individual who still strives to incorporate broadened views of theology and religious action into the thinking process. The mature individual is described as one who can contemplate fresh religious and philosophical views in trying to understand ideas he or she has missed or interpreted differently. This individual feels a sense of worth experiencing these views. This aspect of spiritual development is evident in the reference made to the ongoing changing of views of the life experience and to the changing philosophy of life resulting from these new views. Formal religious organizations are but one part of the spiritual outlet available to older adults.

According to Ebersole (1979, p. 294),† "True spiritual development probably incorporates those elusive qualities of wisdom, morality, ethics, compassion, and self-actualization. Spiritual development may be seen as an integrative view of psychiatry (inner self) and religion (external God)

*From Montagu, A.: On being human, New York, Copyright © 1977, E.P. Dutton, Inc. (A Hawthorne Book), p. 99.
†From The inherent strengths of middle-aged men and women, by P. Ebersole. In Burnside, I.M., Ebersole, P., and Monea, H.E., editors: Psychosocial caring throughout the life span. Copyright © 1979, McGraw-Hill Book Co. Used with the permission of McGraw-Hill Book Company.

that is bridged as the spirit matures. The external evidence is seen in the bridges between people, a communal exchange, and the presence of caring.''

Ebersole presents a table illustrating the phases of spiritual development. This table identifies developmental characteristics of the individual and the symbolic corollary in Biblical history. Such information can be used to increase understanding of the spiritual development of older individuals and to facilitate nursing assessment.

Spiritual aging and spiritual development are concepts that require careful consideration. The spiritual dimension of the aging person should receive attention equal to that of the other dimensions (Bahr, 1982). Some do not acknowledge the spiritual component as one of the dimensions of the individual, but view it as a quality that permeates the other dimensions and gives meaning to life (NICA, 1977). Older persons and caregivers should examine their philosophy about the spiritual aspects of life before determining a course of action. Otherwise, the plan is not holistic.

Concepts of the spiritual dimension that differentiate it from the biopsychosocial dimensions tend to be qualitative. The developmental approach can be used to establish its identifiable characteristics, which are comparable to those of the other dimensions of the older individual. These characteristics are here examined as changes occurring over time, regardless of the direction of the changes. For example, biological changes include loss of nonmitotic cells, such as neurons, and changes in muscle cells. Psychological changes include differences in the capacity for memory and mental speed. Sociological changes include changing roles and responsibilities, such as those occurring with retirement or widowhood. Spiritual changes include increasing feelings of inferiority and changing feelings and thoughts about the life experience. Although the spiritual dimension is usually viewed as qualitatively different from the other dimensions of the person, qualitatively similar characteristics have been identified, such as the spirit-titre and the tendency toward continuing development of a philosophy of life. Consideration of spiritual aspects and quality of life experience can have a great impact on the elderly.

Spiritual aging and development can be described as beginning with conception; others hold a view of the spirit as an eternal component of being that exists before conception and continues after death. Certain identifiable biological events occur with conception; but there is a less tangible component referred to as the spirit. At the moment of conception the vital life force or spirit is set in motion, signifying the beginning of another human being. Cells begin to divide, differentiate, and form organs and organ systems essential to life. The brain and nervous systems, which control physiological activity of the body, are formed. In addition to serving physiological activity, these systems contribute toward psychological and sociological growth and development. These functions become evident in the postnatal period. During this period cells mature and die, but the life force continues, providing the impetus for growth and development that continues throughout the life span of the human being.

In utero and at birth the infant is in close proximity with other human beings, although there is little indication of its awareness of the association. As the normal infant progresses through the various developmental stages, however, evidence of psychological, sociological, and spiritual growth and development becomes increasingly apparent. The infant begins to demonstrate an awareness of the self and of separateness from others. It responds to others, expressing a range of human emotions. In the process, interpersonal relationships take on different characteristics from those present at the time of birth. Thus the process of aging and development that will challenge the coping ability of the individual later in life gets under way.

The dynamic of spiritual development involves a search for answers to the basic questions of life. This search gives purpose and direction to life. The child begins the quest for identity by raising such questions as "Who am I?" and "Why am I?" These questions are indicative of spiritual development. In later maturity the emphasis is on "Why am I?" or "What is the meaning of my life?" The older person has achieved identity but sometimes is forced to struggle with the possibility of becoming a nobody in a world that has placed high value on productivity and materialism. This situation brings into sharp focus the question of purpose in life. Searching for answers to questions, however, may lead to a greater sense of being and self-identity. In the process of searching for answers about the essence of life the person usually works out a philosophy of life that gives direction to the individual's conduct (Moberg, 1971). Knowledge tends to become distilled into wisdom, providing the individual with inner resources with which to meet the positive and negative experiences of life. The dynamic process of spiritual development adds zest, joy, and meaning to life in the later years.

Jung speaks of the stages of life that support the developmental approach. He indicates that the normal child has no real problems; it is only when grown up that the individual can have self-doubts and struggle with inner conflicts. Jung also speaks about the lack of preparation for the second half of life. He indicates that the individual "cannot live the afternoon of life according to the programme of life's morning."* Moreover, he believes that older individuals should know that their lives are not un-

*From Jung, C.G.: Modern man in search of a soul, New York, 1933, Harcourt Brace Jovanovich, Inc. p. 119.

folding and expanding, but that contraction of life is being inexorably forced by an inner process. This view implies that learning is necessary for older individuals; learning would be more clearly identified as developmental tasks by developmental theorists.

Jung cites the tendency toward introspection that begins in the middle years. He views the person throughout the later years as interested in continuing the quest for meaning in life and for answers to other basic questions. Jung states that he is far from knowing what the spirit is; yet he speaks of ways to deal with the forces of inner life. He refers to spirit as the living body seen from within, and body is described as the external manifestation of the living spirit. In spite of his admitted lack of knowledge of what the spirit is, Jung writes, "There are no misunderstandings in nature; they are only to be found in the realms that man calls 'understanding'" (Jung, 1933).* Thus it seems that Jung believes that the tendency toward introspection is part of the process of spiritual development.

Jourard discusses the issue of spirit and the lack of acceptance of the spirit in the realms of science and metaphysics. As a means of developing an operational definition for it Jourard attempted to look at what is observable and describable when a person is said to be "spirited" or "broken in spirit." In trying to resolve the dualism between the mind (or spirit) and the body, he speculated on regarding the spirit as a "mode of organization and the mind as but another system—the perceptual cognitive system."† The spirit would be affected by other systems and would affect them in turn. This view supports the concept of the spiritual dimension as having identifiable characteristics similar to those of the biopsychosocial dimensions. He suggests further study of the spirit, inspiration, and the determinants involved. Jourard maintains that there is likely to be a factor that "highly loads such variables as: the value and purposes which a man affirms and pursues; degree of integration of the components of the self-structure; creativity and inspiration . . .."† Such a factor would probably reveal that "hope, purpose, meaning, and direction in life produce and maintain wellness, even in the face of stress."†

Although Jourard does not speak of spiritual development directly, he developed the concept of spirit-titre as a means of facilitating the assessment of a person's level of wellness. The spirit-titre is the person's mood or feeling tone. He devised a scale for measuring spirit-titre objectively. Wellness in the normal person, according to Jourard, tends to be an outgrowth of "such events as having one's individuality respected and acknowledged."† Jourard states that receiving love from another can be a highly

*From Jung, C.G.: Modern man in search of a soul, New York, 1933, Harcourt Brace Jovanovich, Inc. p. 119.
†From The transparent self by Sidney Jourard
Copyright © 1971 by Van Nostrand Reinhold Company, pp. 97, 107, 141, and 96.
Reprinted by permission of the publisher.

inspiriting experience. Study of these concepts requires working with people who experience varying levels of the spirit-titre over time. He cites the example of men whose spirit-titre has become conditioned to a life-style limited by the pursuit of money, status, or prestige, and the effect on them of mandatory retirement. The problem that arises is what they can do in retirement that is of personal value. This type of question revolves around the essence and purpose of life and relates directly to the spiritual dimension.

Sinnott (1955) describes the human being as an organism with being arising out of the physical matter from which the person is composed. All aspects of the person are related to the biological process of self-regulation. This view differs from views that the spirit permeates all the other dimensions. Sinnott describes the organism as developing from an egg and regulating its growth as it moves progressively toward maturity; life and the mind are considered essentially as one. A goal-seeking tendency, according to Sinnott, is evident in the activities of the body and the mind and is a basic characteristic of life. This view supports the developmental concept that the organism strives toward an end point of maturity. The spirit is seen as part of the basic unity of the person. Sinnott questions why the person is "drawn toward some things and repelled by others."* Motivation is a crucial issue, particularly in the later years. Sinnott goes on to say that whatever the belief may be regarding the nature of the universe and one's relation to it, human qualities such as "goals, dreams, and aspirations"* deserve more attention. These factors motivate everything the individual does; they are distinctive characteristics of the person. This position also implies an ongoing process of development, since achieving goals or realizing aspirations requires time. Thus Sinnott too alludes to spiritual aging and development.

Kas (1975), writing on the search for maturity, indicates it is because of internal integrity and harmony that the person has the "courage to be," to affirm his or her existence and the "basic human right to be a person." He indicates that self-love is the result of self-acceptance and internal integrity and harmony. The person has a legitimate basis for anger when this integrity is threatened, when basic human dignity is disregarded, and when the personality is mistreated. Although Kas does not directly speak of spiritual development, he speaks of aspects that may be generally thought spiritual. The search for maturity implies a developmental process in spiritual aging.

May (1953) describes the experience of becoming a person as a process of becoming aware of the self. Discovery of sources of inner strength and

*From Sinnott, E.W.: The biology of the spirit, New York, Copyright © 1955 Edmund W. Sinnott, The Viking Penguin, Inc. pp. 82, 89.

security is the reward of the activity. He speaks of the development that begins in infancy as a process continuing into adulthood, regardless of how old the person may be, and that is directed toward achieving an identity. May points out that the organizing function within the individual is the self. The self is a "thinking, intuiting, feeling, and acting unity."* He emphasizes that the self is more than the roles one plays; it includes the capacity by which one knows he or she plays the roles. May also indicates that development is chosen and affirmed by the person to some extent rather than existing as an automatic process. Joy, according to May, is the outcome of fulfilling human potential.

In summary, spiritual aging and spiritual development can be described as changes occurring over time that have antecedents and are visible in the goal-directed activities of older persons. All living things change and age, and, since people may be described as living souls, the spirit or soul can be described as a life force within developing biological human beings. Spiritual development means striving toward harmony in the relationships with the self, God, and others. Harmony is essential to the person's state of well-being; lack of harmony tends to reflect decremental changes. Finally, in spite of the importance of spiritual growth and development, it should be remembered that the spiritual dimension is only one of the dimensions of the human being. Thus consideration of spiritual aging and development must be kept in perspective by an acknowledgment of the interrelationships of the various dimensions essential to the framework of the holistic approach.

In the later years, perhaps as part of a changing philosophy of life, individuals often seek forgiveness for the unkind acts or neglect that have affected their relationship with others or with their God. This action is not necessarily religious; rather, it may be their need to express their spiritual needs as one human being to another. In the process of the life review, differences with others probably seem trivial in the overall experience of life. It seems as if there is a need to make amends for any imagined or real wrongdoing in preparation for the next developmental stage, the final stage of life. During the period preceding death, older individuals often experience illness and suffering. It appears in some situations as if the meaning of such experience is to afford a new perspective and opportunity to make peace with the self. Often, the experiences of life and the interaction with others seem to allow the transcendence of physical pain, bringing joy in spite of infirmities.

Thus spiritual development, like development in the other dimensions of the person, involves a progression of changes resulting in a more highly

*From May, R.: Man's search for himself, New York, 1953, W.W. Norton & Co., Inc., p. 79.

organized and differentiated individual. With aging the individual places greater emphasis on human relationships and development of the inner self, which contributes toward his or her continuity and integrity.

Challenges to the Older Person and Caregivers

Challenges to the older person arise out of changes in functional ability. Whether these challenges can be faced with equanimity by older persons depends to a great degree on their attitude toward aging and their coping ability. Society's—and older persons'—attitudes and coping abilities may interfere with their capacity to meet the challenges of aging.

In the previous sections of this chapter examples of age changes posing challenges to older persons were presented. These examples could be multiplied many times over but would basically be the same, differing only in degree. Although there are limitations related to age changes, perhaps the greatest limitation is the attitude of society and individuals.

Although biological changes of aging were presented first, the spiritual changes of aging were discussed in greater detail in this chapter because of the relative lack of attention in the literature to the spiritual dimension. In addition, our experience with older persons continues to uncover their increasing concern with spiritual development.

The sociological dimension of older persons is apparent in the roles they assume and in their interactions with others. The fact that this dimension is dealt with less than the other dimensions does not deny its importance in the holistic approach to older persons. This dimension, as well as the other dimensions of older persons, are further explored in the chapters on nursing process and supportive networks.

The challenge to caregivers is to develop a philosophy of life that encompasses the life span and enables them to assist the elderly in meeting their unique needs as fully human persons.

References

Anderson, C.M.B., and Craik, F.I.M.: The effect of a concurrent task on recall from primary memory, Journal Verbal Learning Verbal Behavior **13**:103-113, 1974.

Arenberg, E.A., and Robertson-Tchabo, E.A.: Learning and aging. In Birren, J.E., and Schaie, K.W., editors: Handbook of the psychology of aging, New York, 1977, Van Nostrand Reinhold Co.

Atkinson, R.C., and Shiffrin, R.M.: The control of short-term memory, Sci. Am. **224**:82-90, 1971.

Bahr, Sister R.T.: Holistic or wholistic health: a philosophy of practice in gerontological nursing? (editorial) J. Gerontol. Nurs. **8**(5):262, 1982.

Bayly, J.: View from a hearse, Elgin, Ill., 1969, David C. Cook Publishing Co.

Best, C., and Taylor, N.B., editors: The physiological basis of medical practice: a text in applied physiology, Baltimore, 1966, The Williams & Wilkins Co.

Botwinick, J.: Cognitive processes in maturity and old age, New York, 1967, Springer Publishing Co., Inc.

Botwinick, J.: Aging and behavior: a comprehensive integration of research findings, ed. 2, New York, 1978, Springer Publishing Co., Inc.

Broadbent, D.E., and Gregory, M.: Some confirmatory results on age differences in memory for simultaneous stimulation, Br. J. Psychol. **56**:77-80, 1965.

Brobeck, J.R., editor: Best and Taylor's physiological basis of medical practice, ed. 10, Baltimore, 1979, The Williams & Wilkins Co.

Buber, M.: Pointing the way: collected essays, New York, 1957, Harper & Row Publishers, Inc. (Translated and edited by M. Friedman.)

Craik, F.I.M.: Signal detection analysis of age differences in divided attention, Paper presented at the meeting of the American Psychological Society, 1973, Montreal.

Craik, F.I.M.: Age differences in human memory. In Birren, J.E., and Schaie, K.W., editors: Handbook of the psychology of aging, New York, 1977, Van Nostrand Reinhold Co.

Craik, F.I.M., and Lockhart, R.S.: Levels of processing and a framework for memory research, J. Verbal Learning Verbal Behavior **11**:671-684, 1972.

Dunn, H.L.: High-level wellness for man and society, Am. J. Public Health **49**:786-792, 1959.

Ebersole, P.: The inherent strengths of middle-aged men and women. In Burnside, I.M., Ebersole, P., and Monea, H.E., editors: Psychosocial caring throughout the life span, New York, 1979, McGraw-Hill Book Co.

Elias, M.F., Elias, P.K., and Elias, J.W.: Basic processes in adult developmental psychology, St. Louis, 1977, The C.V. Mosby Co.

Ellis, E.: Whatever happened to the spiritual dimension? Can. Nurse **76**(8):42-44, 1980.

Engel, G.L.: The clinical application of the biopsychosocial model, Am. J. Psychiatry **137**(5): 535-544, 1980.

Erikson, E.H.: Childhood and society, ed. 2, New York, 1963, W.W. Norton & Company, Inc.

Finch, E.C.: Neuroendocrine and autonomic aspects of aging. In Finch, C.E., and Hayflick, L., editors: Handbook of the biology of aging, New York, 1977, Van Nostrand Reinhold Co.

Forbes, E.J., and Fitszimons, V.M.: The older adult: a process for wellness, St. Louis, 1981, The C.V. Mosby Co.

Fozard, J.L., and others: Visual perception and communication. In Birren, J.E., and Schaie, K.W., editors: Handbook of the psychology of aging, New York, 1977, Van Nostrand Reinhold Co.

Frankl, V.E.: Man's search for meaning: an introduction to logotherapy, Boston, 1963, Beacon Press.

Frieldfield, L.: Heat reaction states in the aged, Geriatrics **4**:211-216, 1949.

Fromm, E.: The art of loving, New York, 1962, Harper & Row Publishers, Inc.

Ganong, W.F.: Review of medical physiology, ed. 7, Los Altos, Calif., 1975, Lange Medical Publications.

Groër, M.E., and Shekleton, M.E.: Basic pathophysiology: a conceptual approach, ed. 2, St. Louis, 1983, The C.V. Mosby Co.

Guyton, A.: Textbook of medical physiology, Philadelphia, 1956, W.B. Saunders Co.

Guyton, A.: Basic human physiology: Normal functions and mechanisms of disease, ed. 2, Philadelphia, 1977, W.B. Saunders Co.

Hamilton, C.L.: Feeding and temperature. In Mogenson, G.J., and Calareslu, F.R., editors: Neural integration of physiological mechanisms and behavior, Toronto, 1975, Toronto University Press.

Havighurst, R.J.: Human development and education, New York, 1953, David McKay Co., Inc.

Hellon, R.F., and Lind, A.R.: Observations on the activity of sweat glands with special reference to the influence of aging, J. Physiol. **113**:132-144, 1956.

Hobert, A.S., and Ginsberg, L.H.: Human services for older adults, Belmont, Calif., 1979, Wadsworth, Inc.

Hogan, R.: Human sexuality: a nursing perspective, New York, 1980, Appleton-Century-Crofts.

Jensen, D.: The principles of physiology, ed. 2, New York, 1980, Appleton-Century-Crofts.

Jourard, S.M.: The transparent self, Princeton, N.J., 1971, Van Nostrand Reinhold Co., Inc.

Jung, C.G.: Modern man in search of a soul, New York, 1933, Harcourt Brace Jovanovich, Inc.

Kaluger, G., and Kaluger, M.F.: Human development: the span of life, ed. 2, St. Louis, 1979, The C.V. Mosby Co.

Kas, C.C.L.: Search for maturity, Philadelphia, 1975, The Westminister Press.

Kleemeier, R.W.: Intellectual changes in the senium or in death and the IQ, Presidential address presented at the annual meeting of the American Psychological Association, Division of Maturity and Old Age, 1961, New York.

Krag, C.L., and Kountz, W.G.: Stability of body function in the aged. II. Exposure of the body to heat, J. Gerontol. **7:**61-70, 1952.

Kutscher, A.H.: The psychosocial aspects of the oral care of the dying patient. In Schoenberg, B., and others, editors: Psychosocial aspects of terminal care, New York, 1972, Columbia University Press.

Lair, C.V., and Moon, W.H.: The effects of praise and reproof on the performance of middle aged and older subjects, Aging Hum. Dev. **3:**279-284, 1972.

Leech, S., and Witte, K.L.: Paired associate learning in elderly adults as related to pacing and incentive conditions, Dev. Psychol. **5:**180, 1971.

Lieberman, M.A.: Psychological correlates of impending death: some preliminary observations, J. Gerontol. **20:**181-190, 1965.

May, R.: Man's search for himself, New York, 1953, W.W. Norton & Co., Inc.

Moberg, D.O.: Spiritual well-being: background and issues, White House Conference on Aging, Washington, D.C., 1971, U.S. Government Printing Office.

Montagu, A.: On being human, New York, 1966, E.P. Dutton.

Murray, R.B., Huelskoetter, M.M., and O'Driscoll, D.L.: The nursing process in later maturity, Englewood Cliffs, N.J., 1980, Prentice-Hall, Inc.

Murray, R.B., and Zentner, J.P.: Nursing assessment and health promotion throughout the lifespan, ed. 2, Englewood Cliffs, N.J., 1979, Prentice-Hall, Inc.

National Interfaith Coalition on Aging: Spiritual well-being: a definition, Athens, Ga., 1975, N.I.C.A.

Neugarten, B.L., editor: Middle age and aging: a reader in social psychology, Chicago, Ill., 1968, University of Chicago Press.

Riegel, K.F., and Riegel, R.M.: Development, drop, and death, Dev. Psychol. **6**(2):306-319, 1972.

Ross, E.: Effects of challenging and supportive instructions on verbal learning in older persons, J. Educ. Psychol. **59:**261-266, 1968.

Rupp, R.R.: Understanding the problem of presbycusis: an overview of hearing loss associated with aging, Geriatrics **25:**100, 1970.

Schaie, K.W.: Rigidity-flexibility and intelligence: a cross-sectional study of the adult life span from 20 to 70 years, Psychol. Monographs **72:**462, 1958.

Shock, N.W.: Aging of homeostatic mechanisms. In Lansing, A.I., editor: Cowdry's problems of aging, ed. 3, Baltimore, 1952, The Williams & Wilkins Co.

Shock, N.W.: Systems integration. In Finch, E.C., and Hayflick, L., editors: Handbook of the biology of aging, New York, 1977, Van Nostrand Reinhold Co.

Siegler, I.S.: The terminal drop hypothesis: fact or artifact? Exp. Aging Res. **1:**169-185, 1975.

Sinnott, E.W.: The biology of the spirit, New York, 1955, The Viking Press.

Stallwood, J., and Stoll, R.: Spiritual dimension of nursing practice. In Beland, I.L., and Passos, J.Y., editors: Clinical nursing, ed. 3, New York, 1975, Macmillan, Inc.

Talland, G.A.: Three estimates of the word span and their stability over the adult years, Q.J. Exp. Psychol. **17:**301-307, 1965.

Timiras, P.S.: Developmental physiology and aging, New York, 1972, Macmillan Inc.

Wilkie, F., and Eisdorfer, C.: Intelligence and blood pressure in the aged, Science **172**(38): 959-962, 1971.

Chapter 6 Motivation and High-level Wellness

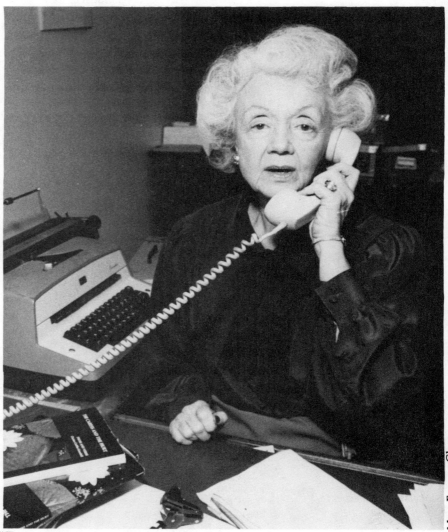

Mary Frances Glore

Motivation is critical for the older person's achievement of high-level wellness. Questions are raised as to why the individual makes certain choices, and what the effect of time is on these choices. Changes in motivation over time tend to influence the person's perception of wellness and inclination to maximize the potential for wellness. Consequently, these changes in motivation become a concern for health care providers.

This chapter focuses on various aspects of motivation as it pertains to older adults and their level of well-being. This focus is warranted by the rapidly increasing number of older persons, the current emphasis on personal choice and individual responsibility for self-care, and the limited health care resources.

The Concept of Motivation

Motivation is defined in various ways. Sometimes it is defined as an act or process of motivating; or it may be defined as a force, or drive, or as an incentive (Gove, 1971). The psychologist attempting to determine why individuals behave as they do speaks of goal-directed and need-satisfying behavior (Hilgard, 1957). Attempts to account for spontaneous and planned behavior arising from social motivation require consideration of internal and external influences. Whatever the source of motivation, a common denominator exists: a person who, for some reason, is moved to act.

Motivation is an abstract concept that refers to an inner response of the person to a stimulus or stimuli, which is based partly on emotion and partly on cognition (the way the person thinks). For example, a gray-haired gentleman who appeared to be in his 80s related how he stopped smoking. "I fell asleep watching TV, and when I opened my baby blue eyes, they were showing lungs and the effect of smoking on them. It wasn't a very pretty picture, so I stopped smoking." Regardless of the source, motivation has relevance for achieving a higher level of wellness among older people.

Dunn (1977) indicates that wellness is a direction rather than an optimum level. Wellness is a dynamic process of change in which the individual moves toward maximizing a state of well-being. Achieving better than the average level of wellness involves integration of the whole person, physical, psychological, sociological, and spiritual. At any time the individual can, if motivated, choose to move toward a higher level of wellness. The concept of high-level wellness is discussed more fully in Chapter 2.

Motivational Terms

Motivational terms are the tools with which to consider the concept of motivation as it relates to older persons. Definition of these terms is important, since confusion arises if they are used differently by various individuals. Elias, Elias, and Elias (1977) use *motivation* as a general term. They use more specific terms such as *incentive, drive,* and *need* to refine the definition of motivation. They acknowledge the difficulty of defining these terms and the disagreement among investigators regarding these definitions.

Drive, for example, may be defined as a state of restlessness that stimulates activity. Mobilization of energy occurs, satisfying needs, which in turn decreases the drive (Newcomb, 1963). This outcome of energy expenditure is called drive reduction. Examples of drives are the psychogenic drive to excel and the biogenic drive to quench thirst.

Elias and Elias (1977) further describe drive as a hypothetical state of energy activated by internal psychological or biological needs or by external stimulation that contributes toward an increased state of arousal. Drive, according to these psychologists, stimulates activity; the subsequent goal-directed behavior is guided by incentives. They also use the terms *push* and *activate* in describing the arousal effect of needs with respect to behavior.

Need, another motivational term, is defined in various ways. Maslow (1963) uses physiological needs as the point of departure for his theory of human motivation. He equates need with drive and cites hunger, thirst, and sex as examples of needs or drives. He describes drives as being hierarchical in nature, ranging from basic physiological needs such as oxygen, water, and food to the higher level need for self-actualization. Self-actualization, according to Maslow, requires a person to satisfy some of the needs that fall in the area of creative expression; self-actualization is more than physical survival. Moreover, according to Maslow, the desire to know and understand are basic needs of the personality, just as physiological needs are basic to the physical dimension. Satisfaction of basic needs in the various dimensions is essential to achieving wholeness in the human being. Schuster and Ashburn (1980) assert that one of the most basic motivational needs of an individual is to know that choices are self-determined and based on the individual's own values. Efforts to force choices based on the values of others are often strongly resisted by the individual because of the psychological discomfort they elicit. These authors conclude that the need to express uniqueness and autonomy is a major motivational force of the human being. On the other hand, Rotter (1954) indicates that some people want to make their own choices and some do not. Rotter's social learning theory is based on the idea that the potential for behavior in certain situations is related to the expectation of reinforcement and the value that reinforcement holds for the individual. The two reinforcement patterns of general expectation are (1) rewards that are contingent on internal resources such as effort and (2) rewards that are externally related to such factors as chance and fate. This general expectation is referred to as the locus of control. The locus of control concept has been used in the study of the effects of choice and increased personal responsibility of the aged (Langer and Rodin, 1976) and in the study of the relationship of locus of control to other variables and morale of the elderly (Chang, 1979). Locus of control is viewed as affecting the motivation of older adults toward health care behaviors (Carlson, 1976). Motivation may be influenced by persons perceived to hold positions of power.

Incentive is a motivational term used to describe something that stimulates action. An incentive is often learned from experiences; it serves to direct behavior toward specific goals (Elias, Elias, and Elias, 1977). For a child the incentive may be a gold star for perfect spelling. For an adult the incentive may be a bonus for productivity on the job or lower insurance rates for safe driving. For the older adult self-care can be an incentive for adhering to a medical regimen. Different types of incentives are used to stimulate action among individuals in various developmental stages.

Still another motivational term is *goal*. A goal is defined as the outcome of a sequence of behaviors; it is something toward which behavior is directed. A goal is a tangible outcome expected to result from satisfaction of a need (Elias, Elias, and Elias, 1977). An example of a goal is the higher level of wellness achieved by exercising and giving up smoking.

In summary, a number of motivational terms have been defined. Although these terms are used to refine the definition of motivation, they are used differently by various individuals. "Drive" and "need," for example, may be used interchangeably or defined as separate entities. In any case, these terms indicate internal motivational factors of the individual, whereas "goals" and "incentives" refer to external motivational factors. "Need" is commonly used for physiological and psychological factors affecting the individual's level of wellness (Woolf, 1981). "Drive" is often defined as a need of instinctual nature having some urgency, such as a sexual need. Needs or drives vary in type. They may or may not be essential to physical survival, but they are important for the high-level wellness characterized by the well-integrated human being.

Selected Theories of Motivation

Since motivation is a phenomenon that is not clearly understood, it is not surprising that varying theories on motivation have been proposed. Nor is it surprising that these theories are evolutionary in nature, since theory development is a process of new information continually refining ideas. Although a definitive theory of older persons' motivation is lacking, the need for knowledge and understanding of the motivation of older adults is urgent. Theory should lead to the discovery of relationships between events or variables previously unobserved. Development of theory is a means of logically organizing and integrating empirical findings about a set of related events. Another function of theory is to specify parameters or limits of the observed phenomena. Without such limits crucial elements of the phenomena might be lost in the myriad of details surrounding the phenomena.

Theory of motivation is based on ideas about what impels the organism to act. Ideas about human motivation include the affective component, which refers to the goal or incentive that pulls the individual to action and the physiological component, which refers to the drive or need that pushes the individual into action. This is to say that the individual may strive toward a desired goal or be stimulated to act by an incentive such as a bonus. In addition, the individual may be impelled to act because of a drive or need arising from within the self, such as the need to satisfy hunger. Varying ideas about motivation indicate differing and changing viewpoints, which occur with growing acquisition of information about human behavior.

A Historical Overview

In the following paragraphs a summary of the historical development of theories of motivation is presented. This summary includes a brief review of selected theories of motivation and closely related theories of personality development. The focus is on selected theories of the mid-twentieth century because of their recency and influence on the motivation of older adults.

Two models from the history of psychology have continued to influence contemporary psychologists (Allport, 1955): the lockean and the leibnitzian.

The lockean view assumes that the human mind at birth is a *tabula rasa;* that is, it is considered to be blank until it receives impressions through the senses. The individual experiences through the senses whatever is to become a part of the intellect; the intellect is passive in nature. Since the mind is blank, its response is triggered only by an external stimulus. Stimulus-response (S-R) psychology is representative of this view. Early development, according to this model, is assumed to be more fundamental than later development; what happens in childhood is of greater importance for personality development than what happens in later life.

The leibnitzian view maintains that the person is the source of acts. Activity comes from purpose; it is not simply an agitation in response to internal or external stimuli. Understanding the person requires reference to what the person may be in the future, since the total state of the person is directed toward becoming. Becoming is the striving aimed at self-preservation and self-affirmation. The process of becoming is open ended because of the belief that seldom, if ever, is the full potential of the human being achieved. This view is represented to some extent by Goldstein's (1940) emphasis on self-actualization and the postulate that the primary motive in life is development of the potential of the human being.

Goldstein postulated that the individual is motivated by a master tendency toward self-actualization. This theory of motivation exceeds the limits imposed by the drive theory. Individuals act in ways that indicate the likelihood that motivation arises from forces other than those emanating from instinctual drives aimed at physical survival. An example is the behavior of the unidentified man who briefly survived the 1982 plane crash in the Potomac River in Washington, D.C. Although would-be rescuers tossed a line to him several times, he quickly passed it to others afloat in the icy waters. This man sacrificed his life to rescue others; his motivation cannot have been survival.

Selected Theories of Motivation and Personality Development

Early theories of motivation tended to be based on organic drives as the stimulus for behavior, such as hunger, thirst, and sex. These theories, however, failed to explain the motivation underlying behaviors that are not directed toward satisfying a physiological need or ensuring physical survival. Nor was the hedonic theory based on the pleasure-seeking, pain-avoidance principle sufficient to explain the complexity of human behavior. The evolution of theories of human motivation reflects the complexity of motivation underlying human behavior.

Young (1949, 1955) presented a hedonic theory of motivation in which affective processes are the primary motivation. He suggested that an individual tries to maximize positive affective arousal, such as delight and enjoyment, and to minimize negative arousal, or distress. McClelland (1955), on the other hand, spoke of a hedonic theory that points out the significance of novelty. In this case, affective arousal is said to occur when a stimulus results in a change in the adaptation level of the individual. Small changes result in a pleasant affect and a tendency to proceed, but large ones result in unpleasantness and a tendency to avoid. Thus, whether the results of motivation tend toward pleasure or displeasure, the individual is moved to act by an affective need. This action is energized apparently by a need for variety or novelty.

C.R. Rogers (1951) organized a theory around the idea that a healthy person is motivated by a single need. The person, according to this theory, is motivated by a fundamental need for actualizing, maintaining, and enhancing the self. In the beginning, the tendency toward actualizing is directed more toward the basic physiological needs: air, water, and food. With maturation and growth, however, the process of actualization increases, rather than decreases, the tension level of the person.

May (1953) says that the person's primary need is to fulfill potentialities. Achieving this task requires deliberate planning and choosing. Each person must make choices, since consciousness of the self is unique. May's view of motivation tends more toward the cognitive aspect of motivation than the views of the theorists previously cited.

Maslow (1954, 1955) refers to the need to take growth motivation, such as development of self-esteem and self-actualization, into account in addition to physical needs. Maslow's theory, which is elaborated on later, is organized around the holistic concept of human beings.

Woodworth (1958) contrasts theories of need-primacy and behavior-primacy in motivation. Basically, his idea is that human behavior seems directed to a great extent toward affecting the environment without concern for any aroused organic need. Keeping drives in perspective through consideration of the whole person is emphasized. Woodworth illustrates the need for a broad perspective by describing the person as one who engages in activities constantly during periods of wakefulness. He builds on the theories of others rather than discounting previous work or ignoring other forces that may be important in human motivation. Woodworth provides additional support for theories that take nonphysical needs into account.

White (1959) argues that motivation is stimulated by the need for competence. Competence, according to White, refers to the person's capacity to adapt to the environment. Interacting effectively with the environment requires learning. Since learning contributes toward development of competence over time, competence may be considered to have motivations. Thus motivation is based on more than organic drives.

Competence is acquired through organic drives and self-initiated exploratory behaviors. Exploratory behaviors involve direction, selectivity, and continuing interaction with the environment. These activities are conceived by White to be motivated in their own right. White proposes the term *effectance* for this type of motivation. Effectance motivation leads to transactions that produce change in the stimulus field and thus create a sense of satisfaction. The person learns how the environment can be changed and the consequences of such a change. For example, the individual may seek additional stimulation through manipulating the environment by moving to another location. Or the individual may seek to decrease environmental stimulation by retiring to a quiet place and playing solitaire. The direction taken and the selection made depends on the individual's perceived need. Whether it is for more or less stimulation, the individual continues exploring ways for effectively interacting with the environment.

An example of someone who has acquired *competence* is Mr. G., a 68-year-old widower and retired tool maker. Faced with being a right-sided hemiplegic (because of a cardiovascular accident) and already an insulin-dependent diabetic, Mr. G. set a *goal* of returning home to resume his independent life-style. He *selected* objectives necessary for self-care, such as learning to measure and administer his own insulin. Although he was right handed, he had to learn to use his left hand because of the paralysis. He achieved *effectance* by acquiring the requisite skills in 3 days, an achievement some persons never accomplish.

Obviously there are differing views of human motivation. Those that have contributed most toward knowledge of human motivation deserve fuller examination.

Allport (1955) commented that few theories have been developed from the study of human beings striving to make life worth living (as opposed to those striving to preserve life). He proposed a theory describing the process of becoming. The individual in the process of becoming experiences organic sensations, thoughts that can be remembered, social interactions, and so on—all of which contribute to the individual's self-identity. Allport points out that the process of becoming has many forms, some of which do not require a self-image. These forms include certain aspects of cultural learning and the means of adjusting to the environment. He discusses the nature of motivation in terms of peripheral and propriate motives.

At the elementary level, impulses and drives, immediate gratification, and reduction of tension determines behavior. When personality development progresses to the stage of self-image, motives reflective of propriate striving are postulated by Allport. Propriate, or ego-involved, behavior differs from the more elementary type of non-ego–involved behavior. Allport describes peripherally initiated behavior as that aimed at reducing tension or restoring equilibrium (lockean tradition). The passive individual depends on the reception of impressions and responds to external stimuli. In the opposite view the individual is seen as resisting equilibrium and maintaining tension (leibnitzian tradition). In this case the individual plays an active role. Neither of these views of motivation, however, is sufficient to explain human motivation, according to Allport.

Propriate striving is differentiated from the other types of motivation by the goal of the individual: to unify the personality. Striving is characterized by a future orientation. Terms closely related to striving include "tendency," "interest," "disposition," and "planning." Allport stresses the importance of psychological functions being admitted as data in the scientific study of personality. Examples of these functions are warmth, unity, and a sense of personal worth. He holds that the self or soul of the transpsychological character is unacceptable, since it is unavailable for psychological analysis.

Allport uses the term *proprium* to indicate all regions of life regarded as unique to the self. The term is used to describe those functions that reflect the unity and distinction of the personality. It represents what seems subjective, intimate, and important. Proprium evolves over time; therefore it can be considered developmental. Because of this developmental nature of the proprium, it is important that conflict between stages be dealt with as effectively as possible—otherwise the unity of the personality is compromised.

In spite of the conflict that may arise, the individual motivated by propriate striving persists toward a goal and maintains tension. Integrity is maintained by continuing to work toward long-range goals that are central to personal existence. An example is the older gentleman, Mr. Truman, who chose to remain in his home when Mount St. Helens in the state of Washington began erupting. Although Mr. Truman apparently lost his life in the wake of the volcanic eruption, until then he steadfastly strove toward the goal of remaining in his home. He evidently placed a higher value on being at home than on preserving his life. In spite of the conflict he may have experienced in making the decision, Mr. Truman was highly motivated to maintain his integrity as a person.

The major difference between the traditional views of motivation and the propriate striving form proposed by Allport lies in views of tension states of individuals. Allport describes these differences on the basis of motives, or forces, that energize behavior. Differences arise in the deficits and growth aspirations of individuals. The normal person, for example, responds to the discomfort of prolonged pressure on a body part by shifting position. This action reduces the tension and the individual returns to a relatively inactive state. The aspiration for growth, in the propriate striving proposed by Allport, keeps the individual in a state of tension to facilitate progress toward long-term goals, for example, maintaining independence. These goals may or may not be attainable. Thus the major difference between the more traditional view of motivation and the propriate striving view is tension reduction versus tension production.

The process of becoming, according to Allport, is not only governed by the effect of stimuli on drives but by the disposition to become human. One of the most crucial capacities is individualization, or the development of an individual life-style that includes self-awareness and self-criticism. This capacity is essential, since becoming is a lifelong process and the individual requires assistance with the process. Striving toward ego development is typical of the thinking human being. Motivation, from Allport's point of view, is strongly influenced by the individual's disposition to strive toward becoming human.

Another way of viewing motivation is through Lewin's field theory (Hall and Lindzey, 1957). This theory is based on a set of concepts representing the psychological life space, which is composed of the person and the psychological environment. Behavior, according to this theory, is a function of the field that exists when the behavior takes place. Underlying forces are determinants of behavior, with emphasis on psychological facts. (Nonpsychological facts can, however, alter psychological facts.) In any case, the individual is motivated by various facts coexisting in the field at the time of the behavior.

Representation of the conceptual framework is achieved through the use of various diagrams. For example, the person is portrayed by the letter "P" placed within a circle (Fig. 6-1). Everything within the circle represents the person; everything outside the circle is nonperson. The psychological environment of the person is illustrated by placing the circle representing the person within an ellipse. The space around the circle circumscribed by ellipse represents the nonperson or environment (Fig. 6-2). The person and the environment compose the life space represented by this equation: P + E = Life space, L.

Fig. 6-1. **The person.**

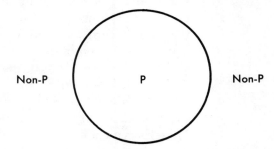

Fig. 6-2. **The life space.**

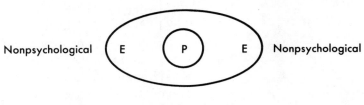

(P + E = Life space, L)

Fig. 6-3. **The foreign hull.**

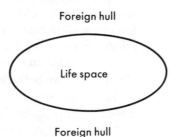

Foreign hull

Life space

Foreign hull

From Hall, C.S., and Lindzey, G.: Theories of personality, New York, © Copyright 1957, John Wiley & Sons, Inc., p. 211.

Life space is the total psychological reality influencing the behavior of an individual. Beyond the boundary of life space is the nonpsychological or physical environment referred to as the foreign hull (Fig. 6-3). The life space is made up of a network of interconnected systems; permeability is one of the properties of the boundary. The differentiated person, composed of an inner-personal region encompassed by a perceptual-motor region, is in turn surrounded by a differentiated environment. Facts in the psychological environment can produce changes in the physical world and vice versa. Permeability of the boundary between the life space and the outer world eases communication between the two realms.

Regions are connected, according to Lewin's theory, by facts in the communication from one region to another (Hall and Lindzey, 1957). These facts include observable things, such as a table or baseball game, and something unobservable that can be inferred from the observable, such as the desire to maintain an independent life-style. These facts are described as empirical (or phenomenal) and hypothetical (or dynamic). In other words, a fact may be sensed or inferred. Interaction of these facts is referred to as an event.

An example of an event is the behavior of an elderly resident in a high-rise apartment dwelling for the elderly. This lady lived on the fourth floor of the high-rise, which limited her activities. She became particularly dissatisfied with her living arrangement because of the inability to sit on the porch in the summer, an activity she had enjoyed in her previous location. Although her income was meager, this lady set about finding housing that would afford greater freedom of mobility and opportunity for sitting on the porch during warm weather. The event occurred when she experienced a need for a change in her living arrangement. The need in the inner-personal region released energy and increased tension. The valence in the psychological region was of positive nature; therefore the force, or vector, pointed toward the potential for more suitable housing. This situation necessitated a great deal of problem-solving, since the functional ability and financial circumstances of this older lady were limited. Examples of events such as this one are multiplied many times over in the daily lives of older individuals. Through the process of communication, according to Lewin's theory, the individual can change the environment and be changed by the environment.

To elaborate further, principal facts of the inner-personal region and valences occupy a separate region in the psychological space. Lewin defines need as a motivational concept equal to such other motivational terms as motive, urge, drive, or wish (Hall and Lindzey, 1957). A need results in an increase in tension and a release of energy. Valence, associated with a need, is defined as the conceptual property of a region located in the psychological environment (Hall and Lindzey). The valence gives value to the psychological environment, positive or negative. For example, the hungry person needing food has a need, which becomes associated with a valence in the psychological environment. If the psychological region contains food, it has a positive valence for the hungry person. The valence serves as a guide to the person seeking to find a way through the psychological environment. The relationship between needs and valences becomes more complex, if other factors such as the type of food or the particular type of food preparation have to be taken into account. Need and valence are important in motivation of the individual, according to Lewin's theory.

A force, or vector, is also coordinated with a need. Conceptual properties of force include direction, strength, and the point at which force impinges on the outer boundary of the person. The strength of the force depends on the strength of the valence, the distance between the person and the valence, and the strength of other valences in the psychological environment. When a force of sufficient strength acts on the person, locomotion occurs. Locomotion is the property of the psychological environment, since it occurs there. Locomotion does not necessarily involve physical movement; it can include social locomotions, such as joining an organization, or intellectual locomotions, such as solving problems. Locomotion, like communication, is considered an event, since it results from an interaction of facts.

Lewin further explains concrete behavior in a psychological situation by using the dynamic concepts of energy, need, valence and force, or vector. He assumes the person to be a complex energy system. Energy, in this case, is that required for psychological or psychic work. This energy is released when the person attempts to regain a state of equilibrium after a period of disequilibrium. Disequilibrium, with an increase in tension in one part of the system relative to the rest of the system, may occur because of external stimulation or internal change. When a need such as for food is satisfied, tension is reduced and energy is no longer released for activity directed toward acquiring food. When the person becomes satiated, food tends to lose its positive valence. Interaction among these dynamic concepts focuses primarily on the need to explain the individual's behavior, according to Lewin.

Tension is another component of Lewin's theory that influences motivation. Tension is a state of an inner-personal region in relation to other inner-personal regions, or systems. Tension in a given system tends to equalize with that in other systems within the inner-personal region. Equalization of tension accomplished by psychological means is referred to as a process. This process may include such activities as thinking, remembering, feeling, perceiving, and acting. For example, the task of solving a problem creates tension in an inner-personal region, in which the person then becomes involved in a thinking process. When a satisfactory solution is achieved, tension in the inner-personal systems becomes equalized. According to Lewin's theory (Hall and Lindzey, 1957), tension always moves in the direction of equilibrium in the whole system rather than in the various subsystems. A certain degree of tension is essential to life. Changes in the amount of tension in the subsystems contribute toward motivation of the person who, in turn, strives toward equilibrium.

Locomotion occurs in the psychological environment, involving little if any activity in the surrounding physical environment. It may occur because of something coming into the individual's awareness that has a stronger valence than the matter previously under consideration. For example, the attention of an older person in a clinic may be diverted from self-care instructions by the arrival of the person providing transportation for the trip back home. Motivation of a tension-reduction nature is a complex process affected by many variables. Locomotion, as defined in Lewin's theory, is the most often used method for returning to a state of equilibrium.

Lewin's field theory gained recognition because it presented a more humanistic view of man; it tended to be favored over the behaviorist approach, which viewed man more as a robot. Lewin perceived the individual as an energy field motivated by psychological forces and as one who makes decisions and demonstrates creative ability in dealing with life events.

Frankl (1963) points out the inescapable individual responsibility to the self in his account of life in a concentration camp. Stripped to "naked existence" by the loss of all his family except for a sister, and faced with the likelihood of death, Frankl explored the meaning of his life and the will to continue living. This exploration brought him to realize that every person must find the purpose of his own life, including suffering and dying. He came to appreciate the freedom to maintain an attitude even when facing nonbeing or death. Discovering and exercising this freedom gave Frankl the desire to identify a purpose in life and to continue personal development in spite of great deprivation. He chose life rather than suicide (which could have been achieved by running into the electric fence). Frankl believes striving to find meaning in life is the primary motivational force of the person.

According to Frankl, "Values do not drive a man, they do not push him, rather they pull him." Values involve freedom to make choices, to determine what one will do. Frankl indicates, however, that the person's will to find meaning can be frustrated. This frustration can be experienced on three levels: existence itself, the meaning of existence, and seeking to discover a will to meaning. This interpretation of values and their motivational impact on the individual provide the basis for differentiating Frankl's view from that of others.

Frankl discusses the meaning of life, which differs from person to person and from time to time. He indicates that what matters is not the meaning of life in general, but the specific meaning of a person's life at a given moment. Frankl seems to be expressing a premise basic to Lewin's field theory: that the person's behavioral response depends on what the person is experiencing at the moment. The uniqueness of the individual is implicit in this theory. A variation of responses might be anticipated in human behavior, and the meaning of life subject to constant change.

Frankl, on the other hand, differs from Maslow in stating that the real aim of human existence cannot be found in self-actualization. Human existence, according to Frankl, is essentially self-transcendence. Self-transcendence is achieved through the fulfillment of the meaning of life. Self-actualization is an impossible goal from Frankl's point of view; rather, self-actualization is a by-product of self-transcendence. Real meaning in life, according to Frankl "is to be found in the world, rather than within man or his own psyche as though it were a closed system." This view supports the concept of the person as a social being. Meaning in life is to be found through transcendence of the self and an appreciation of others who share the human condition.

Frankl thinks that a human's main concern is not merely seeking pleasure or avoiding pain but finding meaning in life. Frankl recognizes potentialities within human beings; what is actualized depends on decisions rather than on conditions. Humans are ultimately self-determining; they have the capacity to rise above surrounding conditions.

Elaborating on Frankl's theory, C.R. Rogers (1964) refers to the valuing of mature persons as movement in the direction of personal growth and maturity. This movement is toward being the real self, owning feelings of the self, and believing that the self and its reactions have worth. In acquiring appreciation of the self, the individual begins to accept and appreciate others as they are. Positive value is placed on deep relationships, which seem to be a need of every human being, according to Rogers. This movement toward psychological maturity is received as enhancing the self and others. Rogers, like Lewin, focuses on the psychological aspects of motivation; valuing is viewed as a motivational force.

Since values are viewed as acts, beliefs, ideas, and traits to which the person attaches worth, the potential influences of values on individual behavior are apparent. Rogers hypothesizes that persons moving toward increasing openness of the self tend to promote development not only of self but of others. Rogers suggests that the possibility of universal human value direction arises from within human beings who find a base for valuing within themselves. In other words, the individual's value system has the potential for influencing individual behavior and interpersonal relationships. Values contribute toward a philosophy of life; they influence the person's will to find meaning in life.

Jourard (1964) points out that the spiritual dimension of the person should be examined with respect to the older adult's motivation toward high-level wellness. The spirit is defined as an intangible dimension that arises, for the most part, from within the individual (Dunn, 1959). Jourard (1964) discusses possibilities for resolving the mind (or spirit) and body dualism. He suggests that man be looked at as an organized whole composed of interlocking systems that can be observed and described through appropriate techniques. With this conceptualization, the spirit can be regarded as a means of organization and the mind as a perceptual cognitive system. Jourard considers the worthwhile goal as an important factor for mobilizing the spirit and channeling energy into effective behavior. He speaks of a general hope syndrome characterized by a rising titre of spirit which, in turn, contributes toward a higher level of wellness. Jourard describes a spirit-titre as being like a scale ranging from zero to 100. The degree to which a person functions as an integrated person and behaves effectively can be scored according to the units on the scale. Jourard suggests that it is unlikely that individuals would score 100 except for brief intervals. The normal person leading a life characterized by accepted and socially patterned behavior would probably be scored between 30 and 60. If the person's spirit-titre drops below the designated wellness level, to about 20 to 30 units, the person would be described as depressed. This reading would be of importance, since it is believed that the depressed person is more vulnerable to illness than the content or happy person. With hope and a reason for living, the individual is moved to act in such a way that a higher level of wellness is realized. Motivation arising out of the spiritual dimension of the person can be influenced by internal and external factors. According to Jourard, acceptance of one's personality and honoring it is likely to be inspiriting. With the positive, inspiriting influence the person tends to view the self more positively and to accentuate the positive aspects of life experience. The person's self-concept influences the level of motivation and the outcomes of goal-directed behavior.

Another theorist, Maslow (1970), cites a hierarchy of basic human needs and the "wanting" individual as the basis of a theory of human motivation. He indicates that human life eludes understanding unless its highest aspirations are taken into account. Widespread and perhaps universal tendencies of human beings are growth, self-actualization, striving toward well-being, search for identity, desire for autonomy, and yearning for excellence. Although this list is not exhaustive, it represents an aspect of an individual's motivation toward achievement, according to Maslow.

Maslow asserts that the individual has a right to become fully human and to actualize potential. He, like Allport, refers to the process of becoming human, in developmental terms. The infant is viewed as growing into humanness within the family and its culture. Humanness cannot be fully achieved by the infant; self-actualization requires a greater measure of life experiences and maturity.

Maslow proposes a hierarchical order of basic human needs. These needs, physiological requirements, safety and security, love and belongingness, self-esteem and self-actualization, are ordered on the basis of their prepotency as motivators. Once the basic physiological needs such as oxygen and water are at least partially satisfied, the next level of needs, safety and security, begins to emerge; the process continues until the highest level of needs, for self-actualization, begins to emerge. The individual, according to this theory, is always wanting and striving to satisfy basic human needs. Satisfying these needs facilitates becoming a fully human person. In adulthood the individual has the capacity for at least partially satisfying the higher level of needs essential to humanness and personhood.

In addition to the needs just cited Maslow acknowledges the highest of human values, beauty, truth, justice, harmony, and so on, as motivators. These motivators are based on needs beyond those for physical development and survival. Such motivators display the complexity of needs that include the underlying cognitive and affective aspects of human behavior. In essence, needs of the total being—physical, psychological, sociological, and spiritual—must be at least partially satisfied if human development and self-actualization are to be achieved.

Although most behavior is considered to be motivated, Maslow points out that not all behavior is motivated by need gratification. Rather, with respect to maturation, expression, and self-actualization, behavior may better be thought of as expression than as coping. Expressive behavior is believed to reflect 'the personality and is not goal directed. It may be observed in the characteristic gait or in the countenance of the person. A great degree of differentiation may be observed in the expressive behavior of older individuals.

Satisfaction of the lower levels of human needs frees the individual's more creative level of being. Although older adults experience self-actualization on this level, expressions of creativity may vary from one individual to another. The developmental nature of the theories of Maslow and Allport is evident. Maslow speaks of the need for a certain level of maturity before self-actualization can be achieved. Allport, on the other hand, describes the tension-reducing behavior of the infant and child, which gives way to the propriate-striving or ego-developing behavior of the mature adult. Behavior seems to be motivated by the desire to persist in the process of becoming human. The unique nature of each individual is revealed by the creative approach taken in the process of becoming human.

M.E. Rogers (1970) presents yet another view of human motivation. A human, according to her theory, is a single-system human being whose characteristics encompass the biological and psychological dimensions, consciousness, and creativity that are integral to wholeness. A human is a unified whole, a complex electrodynamic field interacting with a unique environmental field.

Capacity for experiencing the self and the world identifies the humanness of a person from Rogers' point of view. A human is in a state of becoming that is characterized by a constant interchange of matter between human and environment. A human is affected by and affects the environment. Implicit in this concept is the notion of a human as an active participant in life rather than a passive recipient of life experiences. A human tries to organize and make sense of experience through feelings and rational thought. Motivation, or the will to do, in this case arises from within the individual, energizing the ongoing developmental process.

M.E. Rogers (1980) uses three basic principles in her conceptualization: resonancy, helicy, and complementarity. The principle of resonancy describes the change that occurs through the rhythmic flow of waveforms in a space-time dimension. These waveforms result in the ordering and reordering of the unique human and environmental fields. Waveforms occur as a result of previous learning and experience. The life process is described as proceeding rhythmically along a spiraling axis and having cyclical continuity. Rogers (1970, 1980) views humans and the environment as having a complementary relationship in which biological rhythms are interwoven with rhythms of the universe.

The principle of helicy relates to the nature and direction of change. Change is characterized by the increasing complexity and variety of the human field pattern and organization and the increasing frequency of the waveforms. The increasing complexity and variety, according to Rogers, is not synonymous with health. Health and illness are viewed as being on the same continuum rather than as separate entities having a separate continuum. All conditions are considered probabilistic expressions of the interaction occurring between person and environment.

In Rogers' theory (1970) a person is an open system. The life process is characterized by unidirectionality, which evolves along a space-time continuum with a certain amount of predictability. Repatterning occurs as a result of the person-environment interaction and the increasing complexity of organization. The person always strives toward wholeness.

A brief summary of selected theories of motivation has been presented. A major difference among motivational theories arises from the view of the individual. The individual is viewed as a passive organism motivated by sensory input or as an active organism who is self-directed and goal oriented. The view of the person is important to health care providers from whom the older adult seeks assistance.

Developmental Aspects of Motivation

Motivation, like other aspects of human development, changes with the passage of time. According to Kuhlen (1968), psychological needs affect the person's attention and response to environmental factors. They also affect the responding individual's intensity of involvement with those factors. Wigdor (1980) points out the need for understanding the motivation of the older adult in mainstream activities of daily life. Although the motivation of persons changes over time, older persons may be highly motivated generally and may become highly motivated to pursue new personal goals. For example, learning how to maintain high-level wellness may be motivated by the desire of older persons to continue an independent life-style.

Developmentally, motivation has been conceptualized as occurring in two or three phases over the life span. These phases are identified as (1) the growth phase, (2) the realization phase, and (3) the constriction phase (Buhler and Messarik, 1968); or, according to Kuhlen (1968), (1) the growth expanding phase and (2) the growth contracting phase. Jung (1933), in turn, has described the importance of developing the inner self in the second half of life. He believes that the goal-directed life is more satisfying than the aimless life. Inherent in his work is the notion of the continuing development of the person and the importance of this development for wellness. These concepts of motivation support the idea that motivation changes over time.

Consideration thus should be given to developmental motivation in the older adult. If these individuals are viewed by others or view themselves as being in the contracting phase of the late middle years, the potential for further growth may be limited by this perception alone. Because of life events such as retirement, declining health status, or widowhood, health care providers and older people themselves may disengage rather than maximize potential for continuing development (Buhler and Messarik, 1968). Counteracting these limits requires careful assessment of the motivation of older people and of the options for maximizing potential for both a higher level of wellness and a continuing development of personhood.

Assessing the motivation of older persons may be accomplished in several ways. Subjective data may be obtained by asking older people about their goals and aspirations, how they expect to achieve them, their expectancy of success in achieving them, their perceptions of their skills for achieving them, their sense of efficiency in organizing energies and resources needed for achieving them, and their perceived locus of control. Objective data on motivation may be obtained by observing the behavior of older adults, obtaining a history of their interests and attainments, and gathering additional information from family, friends, and other significant people. These data should provide clues to the psychological motivations of the elderly.

Concern about motivation is evident shortly after the birth of an infant. The physician, midwife, or nurse and parents anxiously await the cry that signifies the infant's initial response to the external environment. The infant's behavior is closely monitored to determine whether he or she can breathe independently. At this point the infant is very dependent on others for physical needs and state of well-being. There is further watching for evidence of the infant's reaching out to its unfamiliar environment.

The normal, developing infant soon begins to look around, reach for objects, and jump at noises, even when its physical needs are met and comfort is provided. Parents attempt to elicit a verbal response from the infant by talking as if he or she understands what is being said. Mobiles are often suspended above the crib to encourage attention to the physical environment (an example of the "pull" phenomenon of motivation). Gradually, the infant begins to differentiate between the self and the environment and initiates a search for identity as an individual. This search, intensified during adolescence, continues throughout the life course. The normal individual persists in a thrust toward self-development throughout life (Kuhlen, 1968), although goals and the level of energy invested in pursuing goals may change during later adulthood. Decline in older persons' involvement is not necessarily caused by a lack of capacity or ability; it may be caused by lack of opportunity to participate in meaningful roles or failure to see the purpose of various activities.

Rosow (1976) discusses role change as it occurs throughout the life span and the changing social role of older people. He cites the empty social role of the aged and the discontinuity that occurs because people are not socialized into the later stage of maturity. According to Rosow, society does not provide a role for the aged because it does not assign them major responsibilities. Older people thus tend to lose value solely because of age. They must attempt to adapt to a change in life-style with little to guide them—in contrast to the socialization process that preceded their entry into previous developmental stages.

The Decremental Model of Aging

Differing concepts of aging lead to varying approaches to the aged. The decremental model of aging has widely influenced the attitude toward the aged and approaches to their care. In this model the individual has achieved a maximum level of functioning during early adulthood and thereafter experiences an irreversible downward decline (Birren and Schaie, 1977). Unfortunately, the decremental aspects of aging have been emphasized with little attention given to the capacity and reserve strengths that can be used in adapting to changes of aging.

The trouble with the decremental model of aging is that health care needs and problems of older adults may be attributed to aging and therefore considered untreatable (Sadavoy, 1982). Butler (1969) coined the term *ageism,* which refers to prejudices and stereotypes based simply on chronological age. Butler and Lewis (1982) acknowledge that sometimes there are limits as to what may be possible in treatment of older persons. However, they also remind us that "the right to treatment is more than a moral obligation—it is a legal right and requirement." They refer more specifically to mental health care, but the holistic approach makes it impossible to ignore the other dimensions of the person's health care needs. The decremental model of aging requires the exercise of judgment, if mistreatment of older people is to be prevented.

Older people themselves subscribe to the decremental model of aging and fail to explore available options for health care. Health care providers subscribing to the decremental model may be remiss in promoting health care services that they consider of questionable value for older adults. Too often troublesome conditions are believed to be part of the aging process and something with which older people simply must learn to live. Thus the decremental model of aging tends to be discriminatory and may inhibit use of approaches directed toward the promotion of high-level wellness among older people.

The Developmental Model of Aging

More recently, the developmental model of aging has been gaining acceptance (Jourard, 1964; Kuhlen, 1968; Neugarten, 1968; Timiras, 1972, Laslett, 1976). In this model aging is seen as a natural process occurring throughout the life span of the individual. This model is more positive than the decremental model. Development is viewed as occurring in stages, including the later stage of maturity. Individuals in various stages of development learn to perform tasks that in turn prepare them for the next developmental stage. Successful achievement of these tasks facilitates adaptation to change and life events (Havighurst, 1953; Duvall, 1977). Butler and Lewis (1982) describe the major task of old age as clarifying, deepening, and finding use for what has been experienced over the years. The developmental model is nondiscriminatory; the older individual is believed to have the same potential for continuing development as the younger individual. This model provides a guide for examining the unique needs and problems of older adults and their motivation for dealing with life experiences.

The concepts of aging described in the models just cited can be examined within the systems theory frame of reference referred to previously. The individual can be viewed as an open system composed of subsystems (or parts), such as cells, organs, and organ systems, which function in an interdependent relationship as part of the whole system (Hazzard, 1971). The whole system develops toward either increasing order and organization or differentiation and disintegration. Throughout the life span, the person or system continues exchanging matter, energy, and information with an everchanging environment. Energy within the system, entropy, is incapable of work and contributes toward disorder, whereas negentropy or negative entropy is the energy available to do work. Negentropy is described as contributing toward the organization of the system. When the anabolic process exceeds the catabolic process, growth of the individual occurs. Aging occurs when the entropy, or disintegration process, exceeds the negentropy, or building-up process, according to the systems theory.

The concept of the aging person will not be further discussed here, since it was examined in Chapter 3. However, the value and rights of the older human being are not to be minimized. The older person is entitled to live out the allotted years in the peace and dignity befitting a human being.

Motivation and High-level Wellness

High-level wellness of the older person depends to a great extent on the motivation of the individual and the intensity of that motivation. Just as in the earlier years, the physiological source of energy responding to internal and external stimuli is intracellular metabolic activity (Birren and others, 1981). Expenditure of this energy is, however, influenced by multiple variables. Much of the older person's purposive behavior results from the "push" of unmet physiological needs such as drives for food and water. The older person may also be "pulled" into action by such factors as the need for achievement, novelty, or variety. The individual who continues to strive toward a goal in spite of pain and frustration is highly motivated. Although little is known about the subtleties of motivation among older persons, attention is increasingly being focused on the motivation of older adults toward a higher level of wellness and responsibility for self-care.

Motivation of older adults takes on added significance in view of the rapidly increasing number of older persons, the current emphasis on personal choice and individual responsibility for self-care, and the use of health care resources.

In 1980 the average life expectancy in the United States was 73 years. And the elderly population is expected to double to 50 million within the next 50 years, when approximately one in five persons will be above 65 years of age. Moreover, the "old-old," those above 75 years of age, will increase at an even more rapid rate (Besdine, 1982). In 1981, an estimated 25.6 million people in the United States were age 65 or above—slightly more than 11% of the population (Butler and Lewis, 1982). About 33% of this population were 75 plus, and about 9% were above 85 years of age. Those 75 plus are in the fastest growing segment of the population. This graying of America and the fact that elderly persons more often require assistance with health care needs are significant in pointing out the need for learning more about the motivation of older adults with respect to health care and the effective use of health care resources. Health care resources include the elderly themselves; hence there should be focus on health education and on personal responsibility for health care.

Knowles (1981) has pointed out that the next advances in the health of Americans will be contingent on what the individual is willing to do for self and society. He conceptualizes health holistically—that is, with respect to its relationship with such areas as educational attainment, housing, and values of the health care system. He cites examples that have improved health, such as a program aimed at improving the self-care of individuals with diabetes mellitus and a health education and preventive medicine program that resulted in a better informed public, improved dietary habits, and decreased smoking among a high-risk population.

The locus of control concept has been used to gain understanding of psychological aspects affecting motivation of the elderly (Carlson, 1976; Reid, Haas, Hawkings, 1977). Locus of control is defined as internal or external (Rotter, 1966), depending on whether the individual believes events and rewards are outcomes of his or her own efforts (internal) or outcomes determined by chance, fate, or influential people (external). Carlson explored the association between selected variables and preventive health behavior by using Papanicolaou smear examinations of postmenopausal women as the preventive measure. She found that the percentage of subjects classified as having regular Papanicolaou smears infrequently increased significantly for older subjects (60 to 89 years). The percentage of subjects who perceived themselves as having an internal or medium locus of control also increased with age. These findings suggest that internal locus of control could lead to maladaptive behavior when assistance is required from health care providers. Carlson also found that the subjects' perception of their vulnerability influenced their behavior. Motivation toward mastery over the environment and one's personal affairs tends to remain strong in most older persons.

Recently an 80-year-old widow with diabetes expressed her perception and concerns about the future. This lady, aware of her changing health status and desiring to maintain control over her destiny, commented, "I can will myself to die, you know." This lady went on, "I will not be moved from this place [a high rise for the elderly]." In essence this lady is highly motivated to maintain control over her living arrangements. Knowledge of this motivation may be useful in helping her to adhere to the preventive aspects of care essential to her well-being and independent living status.

Motivation cannot be measured directly but may be inferred from behaviors of individuals. Motivation is often referred to in a global sense, for instance, as the will to do or not to do or the will to live or die. However, the concept needs to be examined in terms of more specific behaviors, since the individual may be highly motivated toward certain goals and apathetic about others. The intensity of motivation toward certain goals may change over time. For example, the young person may be relatively unconcerned about health care, whereas the older person may be highly motivated toward learning about health care by the desire to maintain an independent life-style.

One of the more commonly used methods of determining motivation is to check clients' compliance with prescribed therapeutic regimens, particularly medication regimens (Marston, 1970; Sackett and Snow, 1979). Little attention has been given to the influence of the health care provider on client compliance. Compliance has recently been examined within the health belief model (Becker, Drachman, and Kirscht, 1979), which is based on motivation theory. In this model, emotional arousal is considered an important variable in the health-seeking behavior of the individual. This behavior, in turn, is believed to depend on two additional variables: (1) the person's perceived vulnerability and (2) the value the person places on the prescribed action. Older persons having recurrent bouts of angina, for example, realize their vulnerability and the need for assistance. The relief from pain afforded by application of nitroglycerin pads provides immediate positive reinforcement for the behavior and elicits continuing adherence to the medical regimen. Motivation, from a holistic perspective, is affected by the perceptions of older adults and by those seeking to assist with health care needs.

In some cases family disagreement leads to conflict about the older person's health behavior. For example, the 85-year-old lady driving home from the beauty shop was shocked by the "for sale" sign in her yard. Her only daughter and another relative had decided that Mrs. W. was no longer able to live alone. Mrs. W.'s ability to participate in deciding matters affecting her state of well-being was totally disregarded, and external control was assumed by these well-intentioned relatives. The action reflects how easily an older family member can be relegated to the depersonalized status of social nonbeing.

An important consideration with respect to motivation of the older person is the possibility of learned helplessness (Seligman, 1973). This helplessness arises out of the individual's realization of living in a helpless situation, such as enforced institutionalization. Motivation of the individual who heretofore had been functioning independently in a semi-independent role is repressed with the advent of institutionalization. In such a situation the older person often becomes needlessly dependent in many areas of daily living. Assessment of functional ability in personal care and of motivation for performing activities of daily living may not be carried out in a discriminating manner. Needless dependence is to be prevented primarily because of its effect on the personhood of the individual and secondarily because of the cost of helplessness and the drain on health care resources.

There are many examples of older persons having an internal locus of control and a high-intensity motivation for mastery over their living arrangements. Mr. B., an 82-year-old bachelor who lives alone, apparently decided to have a hernia repair recently because he values his independent life-style. He was able to pay health care costs above Medicare coverage through supplemental insurance. The benefits of his determination to continue living in his own home with respect to his personhood and sense of independence are immeasurable. The elderly lady who chose to leave a comfortable fourth-floor apartment in a high-rise for the elderly evidently was highly motivated by the desire to live where she could sit on the front porch in the summer, as had been her previous custom. In spite of physical and financial limitations, she managed to achieve her goal with minimal assistance. Both of these individuals can be described as having an internal locus of control; both maximize their strengths and minimize their limitations to achieve personal goals. When such individuals seek assistance, their strengths and motivation should be carefully assessed. Otherwise the outcome could result in needless learned helplessness, dependence, and depersonalization.

Assessing the motivation of older adults is essential to the process of formulating and implementing individualized plans of health care. If the role of the health care professional is regarded as assisting older persons in self-care and health promotion, then anticipatory guidance and health education become important functions. Older persons fearful of becoming mentally incompetent can learn to make decisions regarding their care when the use of extraordinary measures is under consideration or if they wish to donate their bodies or body parts for research or transplants. These wishes should be formalized through such means as the living will or other legal documents. Although such documents are not always legally binding, the wishes of the individual are more likely to be respected in this form than when unexpressed. Prenuptial agreements can be made by the elderly couple who plans to marry if they want to protect their individual futures and the inheritances of their respective families. Inherent in the concept of the meaningful life is the concept of the whole person interacting with a constantly changing environment and being motivated to maintain mastery over the environment. Freedom of choice is one of the most prized freedoms, and older persons are usually highly motivated to exercise that freedom. Acknowledging the personhood of older individuals requires respect for the rights of these persons and an appreciation of the underlying motivation directed toward achieving those rights.

Henderson's definition of nursing can be used as a guide to nurses and other health care providers:

The unique function of the nurse is to assist the individual, sick or well, in the performance of those activities contributing to health or its recovery (or to peaceful death) that he would perform unaided if he had the necessary strength, will or knowledge. And to do this in such a way as to help him gain independence as rapidly as possible.*

Nurses and other caregivers can identify needs of older persons based on this definition and assess the individual's motivation within this frame-

*From Henderson, V.: The nature of nursing: a definition and its implications for practice, research, and education, New York, Copyright © Virginia Henderson, 1966, The Macmillan Company.

work. It is important to keep in mind that the seeming lack of motivation of the older person may be related to depression rather than to an underlying biopathology. With minimal assistance the older person may regain hope and optimism and become highly motivated to perform activities that contribute toward a higher level of wellness.

Motivation of older persons has only recently become a priority of researchers. This priority has been stimulated in the United States to a great extent by the rapidly increasing population of the elderly and declining health care resources. Much of the previous research has been done on animals, which although important is limited in terms of human motivation. Moreover, research on human motivation has generally focused on such areas as learning, cognition, and social interaction. Studies of differences between older and younger persons in cognitive functioning and performance have not necessarily identified differences in motivational states. Differences in performance of older persons may relate to their life experiences rather than reflect their motivational state, according to Elias and Elias (1977). Little attention has been given to physiological mechanisms affecting age-related changes in motivation (Elias and Elias, 1977).

One of the areas of motivation frequently under study is compliance, particularly compliance with medication regimens (O'Connell, 1982). According to O'Connell, many persons do not follow their prescribed medical regimen strictly and yet report they have complied. O'Connell is attempting to determine why individuals do not accurately report their taking of prescribed medications. She is intent on learning what individuals are thinking and feeling about their illnesses, medications, and relationships to their physicians. Ultimately O'Connell hopes to learn how health care providers can improve their relationships with clients and thus promote increasing responsibility for self-care among clients.

Motivation sometimes refers to the process whereby behavior is initiated to satisfy a need or to overcome a lack in the individual (Kaluger and Kaluger, 1979). In this context, behavior is viewed as stimulated by a need, which leads to goal-directed action. When the desired goal is attained, the need is satisfied and the individual's equilibrium is reestablished. An example of this motivational process is the sensation of thirst, which gives rise to the need for fluid intake. Drinking a glass of water satisfies the need, relieves the sensation of thirst and maintains the hydration of tissue essential to the individual's state of well-being.

Laboratory studies of human motivation toward task performance have pointed out many variables affecting motivation. These variables include task difficulty and task pacing (Elias, Elias, and Elias, 1977). Impairment of the performance of older persons can be caused by excessive motivation, which may be as decremental as too little motivation (Burnside, 1976; Elias, Elias, and Elias, 1977). What the "therapeutic" level of motivation should be for older persons is yet to be answered. However defined, motivation is an abstract concept important to those working with older adults.

In summary, the concept of motivation as it relates to older adults is becoming increasingly complex. Although the physiological source of energy for motivation remains, with later development psychological factors increasingly influence the intensity of motivation and the consequent behavior. Whether the older person is pushed into action by bodily needs or pulled into action by aspirations of a cognitive nature, the potential for increasing an involvement in new and varied activities is great; this potential often remains relatively undeveloped. Motivation of older adults is often repressed because of the negative attitude toward the aged held by others. This attitude tends to arise out of the value placed on material productivity, but ironically older persons tend to be barred from opportunities to be materially productive. This situation contributes to low self-esteem and often toward a state of learned helplessness, which becomes a vicious downward cycle with respect to motivation and high-level wellness.

The concept of productivity needs to be reexamined. Productivity in such areas as moral and emotional support and counseling, which may come from older persons who have acquired a great deal of experience over the years, has yet to be fully appreciated. This lack of appreciation can contribute toward feelings of worthlessness and lack of purpose and low-intensity motivation. In turn, this situation affects the will of older persons to engage in health promotion and undermines their present level of wellness. Thus motivation of the elderly depends not only on their locus of control but on the concern and compassion of influential others.

Given the importance of motivation in the lives of older persons with respect to personhood and the potential for achieving a higher level of wellness, assessment of it is imperative. Of equal urgency is the need for assessing environmental factors affecting the motivation of older persons. This environmental assessment should include assessment of health care providers who may, albeit unwittingly, be contributing to a less than adequate environment for the realization in the elderly of higher-level wellness.

The literature has little on the assessment of motivation of older persons, but opportunity abounds for observing behaviors from which motivation may be inferred and for gathering useful data from other sources. The paucity of material on motivation of older persons does not negate the need to assess their motivation and its intensity. This assessment is essential to health care providers seeking to assist older persons in their strivings toward personhood and away from the constriction and constraint leading to depersonalization.

References

Allport, G.W.: Becoming, New Haven, Conn., 1955, Yale University Press.

Becker, H.M., Drachman, R.H., and Kirscht, J.P.: Motivations as predictors of health behavior, Health Serv. Reports 87(9):852-863, 1972.

Beland, I.L., and Passos, J.Y.: Clinical nursing: pathophysiological and psychosocial approaches, ed. 3, New York, 1975, Macmillan, Inc.

Besdine, R.W.: The data base of geriatric medicine. In Rowe, J.W., and Besdine, R.W., editors: Health and disease in old age, Boston, 1982, Little, Brown & Co.

Birren, J.E., and Renner, V.J.: Research on the psychology of aging: principles and experimentation. In Birren, J.E., and Schaie, W.K., editors: Handbook of the psychology of aging, New York, 1977, Van Nostrand Reinhold Co.

Birren, J.E., and Schaie, W.K., editors: Handbook of the psychology of aging, New York, 1977, Van Nostrand Reinhold Co.

Birren, J.E., and others: Developmental psychology: a lifespan approach, Boston, 1981, Houghton Mifflin Co.

Burnside, I.M., editor: Nursing and the aged, New York, 1976, McGraw-Hill Book Co.

Buscaglia, L.F.: Personhood, Thorofare, N.J., 1978, Charles B. Slack, Inc.

Buhler, C., and Messarik, F., editors: The course of human life, New York, 1968, Springer Publishing Co., Inc.

Butler, R.N.: The effects of medical and health progress on the social and economic aspects of the life cycle, Industrial Gerontol. 1:1-9, 1969.

Butler, R.N., and Lewis, M.I.: Aging and mental health: positive psychosocial and biomedical approaches, ed. 3, St. Louis, 1982, The C.V. Mosby Co.

Carlson, L.B.: Association between perceived control, perceived vulnerability, and perceived behavior: postmenopausal women and Papanicolaou tests, master's thesis, 1976, University of Kansas.

Chang, B.L.: Locus of control, trust, situational control, and morale of the elderly, Int. J. Nurs. Stud. 16(2):169-181, 1979.

Dunn, H.L.: What high-level wellness means, Health Values: Achieving High-level Wellness 1(1):9, 1977.

Duvall, E.R.: Marriage and family development, ed. 5, Philadelphia, 1977, J.B. Lippincott Co.

Elias, M.F., and Elias, P.K.: Motivation and activity. In Birren, J.E., and Schaie, W.K., editors: Handbook of the psychology of aging, New York, 1977, Van Nostrand Reinhold Co.

Elias, M.F., Elias, P.K., and Elias, J.W.: Basic processes in adult developmental psychology, St. Louis, 1977, The C.V. Mosby Co. .

Frankl, V.E.: Man's search for meaning, Boston, 1963, Beacon Press.

Goldstein, K.: Human nature in the light of psychopathology, Cambridge, Mass., 1940, Harvard University Press.

Gove, P.D., editor: Webster's third new international dictionary of the English language (Unabridged), Springfield, Mass., 1971, G. & C. Merriam Co.

Hall, C.S., and Lindzey, G.: Theories of personality, New York, 1957, John Wiley & Sons, Inc.

Havighurst, R.: Developmental tasks and education, New York, 1953, David McKay Co., Inc.

Hazzard, M.E.: An overview of systems theory, Nurs. Clin. North Am. 6(3):385-393, 1971.

Hilgard, E.R.: Introduction to psychology, ed. 2, New York, 1957, Harcourt Brace & Co.

Jourard, S.N.: The transparent self, New York, 1964, D. Van Nostrand Co.

Jung, C.G.: Modern man in search of a soul, New York, 1933, Harcourt Brace & World.

Kaluger, G., and Kaluger, M.F.: Human development: the span of life, ed. 2, St. Louis, 1979, The C.V. Mosby Co.

Knowles, J.H.: Responsibility of the individual. In Cowart, M., and Allen, R.F., editors: Changing concepts of health care: public policy and ethical issues for nurses, Thorofare, N.J., 1981, Charles B. Slack, Inc.

Kuhlen, R.G.: Developmental changes in motivation during the adult years. In Neugarten, B.L., editor: Middle age and aging: a reader in social psychology, Chicago, 1968, The University of Chicago Press.

Langer, E.J., and Rodin, J.: The effects of choice and enhanced personal responsibility for the aged: a field experiment in an institutional setting, J. Pers. Soc. Psychol. 34:191-198, 1976.

Laslett, P.: Societal development and aging. In Binstock, L.H., and Shanas, E., editors: Handbook of aging and the social sciences, New York, 1976, Van Nostrand Reinhold Co.

Marston, M.V.: Compliance with medical regimens: a review of the literature, Nurs. Res. 19:312-323, 1970.

Maslow, A.H.: Motivation and personality, New York, 1954, Harper & Row, Publishers, Inc.

Maslow, A.H.: Deficiency motivation and growth motivation. In Jones, M.R., editor: Nebraska symposium on motivation, Lincoln, 1955, University of Nebraska Press.

Maslow, A.H.: A theory of motivation. In Baller, W.R., editor: Readings in the psychology of human growth and development, New York, 1963, Holt, Rinehart & Winston.

Maslow, A.H.: Motivation and personality, ed. 2, New York, 1970, Harper & Row, Publishers, Inc.

May, R.: Man's search for himself, New York, 1953, W.W. Norton & Co.

McClelland, D.C., editor: Notes for a revised theory of motivation: studies in motivation, New York, 1955, Appleton-Century-Crofts, Inc.

Newcomb, T.M.: Human motivation. In Baller, W.R., editor: Readings in the psychology of human growth and development, New York, 1963, Holt, Rinehart & Winston.

Neugarten, B.L., editor: Middle age and aging: a reader in social psychology, Chicago, 1968, The University of Chicago Press.

O'Connell, K.: Dr. O'Connell studies patients' drug compliance, The Bulletin 33(4):8, 21, 1982 (University of Kansas Press).

Reid, D.W., Haas, G., and Hawkings, D.: Locus of desired control and positive self-concept of the elderly, J. Gerontol. 32(4):441-450, 1977.

Rogers, C.R.: Client-central therapy, Boston, 1951, Houghton Mifflin Co.

Rogers, C.R.: Toward a modern approach to values: the valuing process in the mature person, J. Abnorm. Soc. Psychol. 68:160, 1964.

Rogers, M.E.: The theoretical base of nursing, Philadelphia, 1970, F.A. Davis Co.

Rogers, M.E.: Nursing: a science of unitary man. In Riehl, J., and Roy, C., editors: Conceptual models for nursing practices, ed. 2, New York, 1980, Appleton-Century-Crofts.

Rosow, I.: Status and role change through the life span. In Binstock, R.H., and Shanas, E., editors: Handbook of aging and the social sciences, New York, 1976, Van Nostrand Reinhold Co.

Rotter, J.B.: Social learning and clinical psychology, Englewood Cliffs, N.J., 1954, Prentice-Hall, Inc.

Rotter, J.B.: General expectancies for internal versus external control of reinforcement, Psychological Monograph 80, whole 609, 1966.

Sackett, D.L., and Snow, J.C.: The magnitude of compliance and noncompliance. In Haynes, R.B., Taylor, D.W., and Sackett, D.L., editors: Compliance in health care, Baltimore, 1979, The Johns Hopkins University Press.

Sadavoy, Joel: Treatment of the elderly in general psychiatric practice (editorial), Can. J. Psychiatry 27(1):1, 1982.

Schuster, C.S., and Ashburn, D.S.: The process of human development: a holistic approach, Boston, 1980, Little, Brown & Co.

Seligman, M.: Fall into helplessness, Psychol. Today 7(6):43, 1973.

Timiras, P.S.: Developmental physiology and aging, New York, 1972, Macmillan, Inc.

White, R.B.: Motivation reconsidered: the concept of competence, Psychol. Rev. 66(5):297, 1959.

Wigdor, B.R.: Drives and motivation with aging. In Birren, J.E., and Sloane, R.B., editors: Handbook of mental health and aging, Englewood Cliffs, N.J., 1980, Prentice-Hall, Inc.

Woodworth, R.S.: Dynamics of behavior, New York, 1958, Henry Holt.

Woolf, H.B., Editor-in-Chief: Webster's new collegiate dictionary, Springfield, Mass., 1981,
    G. & C. Merriam Co.
Young, P.T.: Food-seeking drive, affective process, and learning, Psychol. Rev. **56:**98, 1949.
Young, P.T.: The role of hedonic processes in motivation. In Jones, M.R., editor: Motivation,
    Lincoln, 1955, University of Nebraska Press.

Chapter 7 Theories of Self-care and Personhood

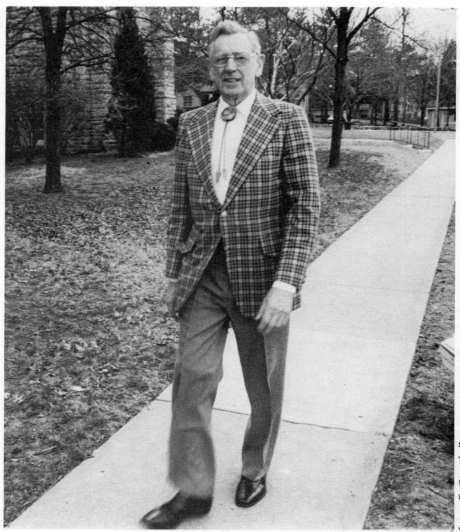

Leroy E. Campbell

Self-care for the older person is a phenomenon of recent origin in the United States. It is emerging as an innovative and challenging dynamic within the health care system generally and within gerontological nursing specifically. Health professionals and consumers alike spawned it after having reviewed needs and resources for health care. In the past the medical profession was the entity totally responsible for the health of individuals. This custom is now giving way to a general consensus that the major responsibility for health maintenance resides within the individual. The individual is capable of and, indeed, is becoming enthusiastic about the gift of health; he or she is taking measures to preserve the health status that allows for well-being, activities of daily living, goal achievement, and, in the last analysis, a full life.

This reversal of trends resulting in the self-care movement has elicited theories from many health professionals. Along with other health professions, nursing demonstrates its unique position in the health care system by putting the theoretical framework of self-care into practice with clients seeking nursing care. Examination of the self-care theory and the theories of care by Orem (1971, 1980) and Kinlein (1977) has led to their application in gerontological nursing and other health care of older persons.

Theory Building and Health Care

The complexity and magnificence of the human body have inspired numerous theories regarding its health and maintenance. These theories reflect scientists' comprehension of what is believed to be the cause and effect relationship in the dynamics of the human body. These theories allow a measure of insight into the highly complex components responsible for health. Each small element of knowledge leads to a greater appreciation and understanding of the intricacy of the human organism. What then is a theory and how does theory building aid in comprehending health?

Theory and Theory Building

A theory is a projection that attempts to characterize some event, situation, or phenomenon for the purpose of understanding it. Stevens (1979) notes that a theory is really a philosophical statement about the salient components of a phenomenon, which separates the critical factors from the nonessential factors. Thus the theory brings into focus the components comprising the phenomenon and allows for analysis of those components.

Stevens (1979) classifies theories as follows:

1. Descriptive theory, in which the identification of the major events in a phenomenon is the main focus
2. Explanatory theory, which attempts to explain factors, such as cause and effect relationships or interaction among the theoretical components

Descriptive theory is the first step of theory development. It is essential for it to be taken, to appreciate at the outset what is within the phenomenon. The second step of theory building is explanation of those relationships, moving more toward causes and effects within the relationship. For example, when element Y interacts with element C in manner R, then event Q occurs; when element Y interacts with element C in manner J, then event P occurs. When these events occur consistently, then a formulization of certain rules begins to emerge in this particular situation. Thus theories deal with the probability of events occurring in a specific situation rather than with specific rules. This approach suggests once again that theories are an approximation of truth; they are attempts at obtaining greater insight into events that demand investigation and analysis.

Within the explanatory theory categorization, several approaches to theory may be taken. One is a predictive approach, which suggests what may occur once the theory is applied. Another is a situation-producing, or proscriptive, approach, in which elements within a given event are controlled according to the theory rule (Stevens). Both of these approaches to theory are used for predictions in health care. Examples of predictive and proscriptive theories relating to health care regimens currently being investigated include the following:

1. Nutritional effects on central nervous system functioning
2. Cholesterol effects on efficiency of cardiovascular functioning
3. Estrogen replacement therapy as a possible carcinogenic agent

Health Care

Theory building provides insight and understanding of—and procedure for—health care. Wellness, the epitome of good health, as described by Dunn (1973), is considered to be high-level; that is, it integrates the mind, body, and spirit to such an extent that a person is able to function in all aspects of living with a certain degree of vitality and enthusiasm. When this philosophy of health care emphasizes caring, the health professional views the client not just as another number or recipient of care but as a unique individual with particular needs, life history, health practices, self-beliefs, and attitudes toward life. Mayeroff (1971) indicates that caring is the orientation toward helping another individual grow, so that actualization of the person can occur. Caring is the process by which mutual trust and a deepening of the relationship occurs. This approach helps the individual to feel needed, appreciated, and fulfilled, with all potential recognized and actualized. Health care is enhanced by application of more efficient regimens.

Nursing: a Caring Profession

Nursing's main emphasis is on caring. In a caring environment nature can do its healing (Nightingale, 1859). In the nursing process each individual is appreciated as unique and precious regardless of age, creed, color, or occupation. In implementing the nursing process format, the health professional recognizes that caring includes knowledge, patience, honesty, trust, humility, hope, courage, and give and take (Mayeroff, 1971). Caring, incorporated into the health care plan, helps the client improve in health and ultimately regain high-level wellness. Knowing the individual makes the health professional realize that his or her unique personhood is to be preserved at all costs. Through caring, the health professional does not make decisions for the individual but allows that individual access to all the information needed to make intelligent decisions regarding treatment. By encouraging patience, humility, honesty, trust, hope, and courage the health professional aids the client in working with nature instead of against it. As Nightingale noted, working with nature allows natural healing in an individual.

Theories and theory building belong in the health care delivery system. Because everyone is unique, many theories are needed to understand the dynamics inherent in each person as he or she moves through the health care system.

Nursing theories promulgating the concept of self-care have emerged in recent years and have had a marked impact on nursing practice and health care. An overview of self-care, both as concept and as social movement, is necessary to appreciate its applicability to nursing care.

Self-care: an Overview

Levin, Katz, and Holst (1976) describe self-care as an old movement in society. Self-care is defined as "a process whereby a lay person can function effectively on his own behalf in health promotion and [illness] prevention and in disease detection and treatment at the level of the primary health resource in the health care system" (Levin, 1978, p. 17).

According to Norris (1979), self-care is defined as "those processes that permit people and families to take initiative, to take responsibility, and to function effectively in developing their own potential for health." The self-care movement began in the 1960s as a way of protesting against health professionals who were too controlling of the health care system. The emphasis in self-care is caring for another within the community, family, and neighborhood, as well as for self.

This self-care movement attempts to incorporate both the personal health behavior skills and the social and political skills of lay persons to aid in the acquisition of proper health care. The lay person's control of decision making helps to ensure that the right kind of health care is received. A barrier to self-care, according to Levin, is that the self-care movement is a lay movement in direct conflict with professional dominance of the health care system. Another barrier is that health care professionals fail to appreciate the need for health education so that the lay person can make more intelligent decisions about health care. Problems also arise when individuals fail to accept responsibility for self-care. Larson (1983) reports that 50% of all mortality in the United States results from unhealthy behavior or life-style. Within the other 50%, 20% is attributable to environmental factors, 20% to human biological factors, and only 10% to inadequate health care. With the large percentage of deaths attributable to insufficient self-care practices by individuals, Somers (1980) suggests that policy regulating self-care and health promotion can come only when the general public endorses and embraces such practices. She notes that the trend toward personal responsibility for health is growing in the nation, but that millions of citizens continue practices having deleterious effects on their health.

Self-care has high return for the lay person: health and a full life. When the self-care of the individual is emphasized, the health care system can be more responsive to the individual client than the current system of institutionalized health care delivery mechanisms is.

The basic activities within self-care, according to Norris,* include the following:

1. *Monitoring, assessing, diagnosing.* This activity includes breast self-examination or monitoring cancer warning signs for early detection of disease.

2. *Supporting life processes.* Examples in this activity include routines such as brushing teeth, washing hands, using Kleenex, and eating regular meals.

3. *Therapeutic and corrective self-care.* This activity includes treatment in the home without professional intervention of many minor illnesses. Such treatment may involve forcing fluids and extra rest for colds and influenza, regulating fluid intake, and controlling invasive procedures at the time of a terminal illness.

4. *Prevention of disease and maladjustment states.* Examples include: instruction regarding maintenance of one's physical, mental, and spiritual health; activities such as walking, jogging, or exercise to maintain one's cardiovascular fitness; and instruction about the aging process.

5. *Specifying health needs and care requirements.* People are interested in evaluating their own health needs and seeking the kind of care that will be helpful in overcoming difficulties. When the health care system is open to practitioners who may give a broader overview of health, such as acupuncturists, hypnotists, podiatrists, and nurse practitioners/clinicians/clinical specialists, then better health care can be delivered to all people.

6. *Auditing and controlling the treatment program.* A variety of population

*From Norris, C.M.: Self-care, Am. J. Nurs. **79:**486-489, 1979.

segments are asking for more control of the treatment program. For example, older persons are demanding better care in the community, in nursing homes, and in hospitals; if possible, they want to remain in their own homes instead of being institutionalized.

7. *Grass roots or self-initiated health care.* A variety of models have developed in the self-care movement by citizens who are interested in promoting their own health without the intervention of a health professional. Groups such as Weight-Watchers, programs for smoking cessation, and support groups to help a variety of people (widowed, divorced, bereaved) are prominent examples of the grass roots movement.

Levin, Katz, and Holst (1976) perceive self-care participants as active rather than passive in maintaining their own health status through personal behavior and health practices. Assuming responsibility in taking over-the-counter drugs, maintaining a nutritional balance, and regulating blood pressure, weight, rest, leisure activities, mental health practices, spiritual well-being, and social activities is to control one's health in all dimensions. As primary health care gains prominence, so too does the self-care movement gain in importance, prominence, and respectability. As fewer resources are available in society to underwrite soaring health care costs, the self-care movement becomes even more important in the health care field.

Two major theories emerging within the last decade and having an impact on the health care system are Orem's self-care theory and Kinlein's theory of care. Each of these theories is analyzed in terms of their major components and applied to the nursing process.

Orem's Self-care Theory

Orem, a nurse, educator, researcher, and theoretician, promotes a theory that is having marked effects on self-care practitioners. As a theoretician, Orem identifies key philosophical constructs that emphasize the importance of preserving the individuality of each person who comes to the health care system for assistance. Through formulizations comprising the essence of nursing, Orem suggests that the variety of nursing theories constitute nursing knowledge. All theories regarding health, therefore, are important components in understanding self-care as a nursing modality. With this modality the health professional preserves the right and responsibility of the individual to continue at a level of wellness compatible with the chosen health status. Orem defines self-care as "the practice of activities that individuals personally initiate and perform on their own behalf in maintaining life, health, and well-being."*

*From Orem, D.E.: Nursing: concepts of practice, New York, 1971, McGraw-Hill Book Co. By permission.

In past decades a controlling factor in nursing was the medical care model; that is, the nurse's responsibility for health care was primarily suggested by medical orders. Little attention was given to self-care. Orem, however, in describing the essence of nursing, promotes the theory of self-care; that is, each individual has the responsibility and the right to a chosen health care status. For Orem, self means the total being (Orem, 1980). Self-care, then, means taking care of one's self—mind, body, and spirit—through a variety of daily practices conducive to health preservation.

Self-care Agent

Orem (1980) identifies the provider of self-care as the self-care agent; the self-care agent performs activities that promote his or her own health and well-being. If an individual is unable to carry out health care practices, for example, an infant dependent on a parent for care or an older person whose health deteriorates to a point at which dependence on another for care is necessary, that individual is known as a dependent care agent. Health practices put into operation either by the self-care agent or dependent care agent are self-care. Optimum self-care is continuous and voluntary. It is based on deliberate and thoughtful judgment. It meets the requirements for basic, universal human needs. Self-care behavior evolves through a unique combination of the individual's interpersonal relationships, culture, and cognitive and social abilities. Based on these various components, self-care is unique to the individual; since no one experiences life in the same way as another, self-care practices are particular to each individual. Because self-care is so individualized, it contributes to the self-esteem and self-image of the individual.

Universal Self-care Requirements

The universal human needs that must be maintained to have health, according to Orem (1971), include the following:

1. Air, food, fluids
2. Elimination
3. Solitude and social interaction
4. Activity and rest
5. Protection from hazards
6. Normalcy

These universal self-care requirements (Fig. 7-1) are the essence of nursing practice. The nurse must aid the individual in understanding the importance of these universal self-care requirements for promotion of health.

Therapeutic Self-care Demand

Therapeutic self-care demands are a specified set of actions to be performed by the self-care agent to maintain health and well-being. These demands are determined by universal self-care requirements, life cycle events or health deviations that emerge in one's life, and by available health technology (Joseph, 1980).

Fig. 7-1. **Universal self-care requirements.**

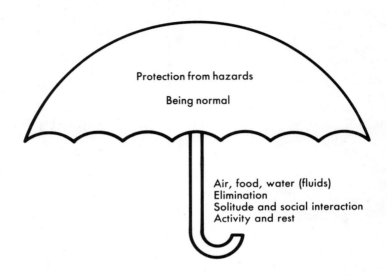

Protection from hazards

Being normal

Air, food, water (fluids)
Elimination
Solitude and social interaction
Activity and rest

From Joseph, L.S.: Self-care and the nursing process, Nurs. Clin. North Am. **15**(1):131-143, 1980.

Whether the self-care agent can meet needs depends on his or her self-care agency. The nurse must perform an assessment of the individual's assets and limitations in knowledge, motivation, and skill that may facilitate or hamper the self-care agency.

Agency

Self-care agency is the ability of an individual to perform self-care. This agency includes the knowledge, ability, and power to carry out activities necessary for maintenance of health, affective feelings, and psychomotor development—all coordinating into a whole that allows the individual to perform beneficial and healthful activities (Jacob, 1980). The quality of self-care agency depends on knowledge, skills, beliefs, attitudes, values, and motivation.

Orem thinks that the self-care agent exercises self-care agency only to the extent that he or she holds a positive self-concept. A negative self-concept may interfere with health-promoting activities. If the individual's self-concept is positive, a health care problem may be alleviated or resolved.

The self-care agency is an open system; that is, the individual interacts with the internal environment as well as with the external environment. This interdependence influences the impact of knowledge, motivation, and psychomotor skills on the self-concept. Fig. 7-2 describes the self-care agency as an open system.

Fig. 7-2. **Self-care agency as an open system.**

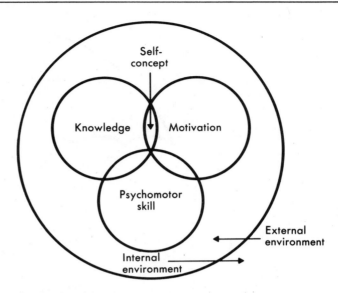

From Joseph, L.S.: Self-care and the nursing process, Nurs. Clin. North Am. **15**(1):131-143, 1980.

Determinants of Self-care Agency

Orem considers a variety of factors to be important determinants of one's ability to engage in self-care. They include the following:
1. Age
2. Developmental state
3. Life cycle event
4. Sex
5. Sociocultural orientation
6. Health state
7. Health care situation
8. Organic/behavior diagnosis
9. Family system
10. Other factors (Joseph, 1980)

These are important elements for the nurse to evaluate as they relate to the health care status of the individual. Each of these factors affects how well the individual can assess his or her own particular health care needs and initiate activity that promotes well-being.

Self-care Deficit

When an individual cannot meet certain health demands, self-care deficits may emerge. Because of a lack of knowledge, skill, or motivation, there may be insufficient health care agency to meet the demand of that individual. This inability to meet self-care demand may come from any of the determinants of self-care agency. The nurse focuses, therefore, on any real

Fig. 7-3. **Therapeutic self-care demand and self-care deficit.**

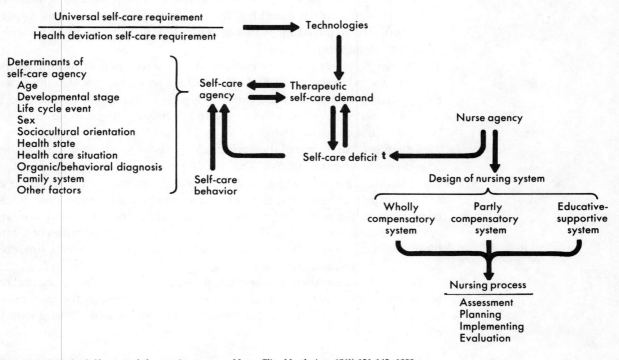

Universal self-care requirement

Health deviation self-care requirement

Determinants of
self-care agency
  Age
  Developmental stage
  Life cycle event
  Sex
  Sociocultural orientation
  Health state
  Health care situation
  Organic/behavioral diagnosis
  Family system
  Other factors

Technologies

Self-care agency

Therapeutic self-care demand

Self-care deficit **t**

Self-care behavior

Nurse agency

Design of nursing system

Wholly compensatory system

Partly compensatory system

Educative-supportive system

Nursing process

Assessment
Planning
Implementing
Evaluation

From Joseph, L.S.: Self-care and the nursing process, Nurs. Clin. North Am. **15**(1):131-143, 1980.

or potential deficit. Nursing's objective is to assist clients with actions that they are unable to do for themselves. Fig. 7-3 suggests the relationship between therapeutic self-care demands and self-care deficits.

For Orem, the nursing system is generated by the nurse and the client in meeting the client's self-care demands, overcoming deficits, and putting into operation certain nursing actions promoting the well-being of the individual (Orem, 1971). Orem names three types of nursing systems meeting the therapeutic self-care demands of the client. These nursing systems are different combinations of assistance. They include the following:

1. Wholly compensatory system, in which the client, because of lack of resources, is unable to meet the therapeutic self-care demands, and these become the responsibility of the nurse.
2. Partly compensatory system, in which the nurse and the client together perform health care measures.

3. Educative supportive system, in which the client has the resources to meet demands but needs the assistance of the nurse in decision making, behavior control, or acquisition of knowledge or skill. In this approach the client has the ability to perform or learns to perform the required measures of self-care but is unable to do so without assistance at times.

The nursing system is a very controlled and structured approach with a constant focus on the client and needs. Only when the client cannot perform independently does the nurse intervene directly. Thus self-care is always uppermost in the mind of the nurse helping to promote the well-being of the individual client.

The interrelationship of the various elements of nursing with the theory of self-care is seen in Fig. 7-4. The nursing process of assessing, diagnosing, planning, implementing, and evaluating is based on a foundation of the self-care requirements, determinants of self-care agency, and deviations from self-care requirements that necessitate an individual nursing system design. This nursing system results in the implementation of a care plan designed conjointly with the client for that client's health (maintenance and promotion) and well-being.

Orem's self-care theory is another innovative and dynamic orientation to the nursing system and process. When the client remains the focal point of nursing, then the boring and repetitive routineness of nursing care is eliminated.

Kinlein's Theory of Care

Another individual who has been instrumental in changing nursing from the medical model to a true nursing orientation is Kinlein. Kinlein's theory of care is substantially based on Orem's self-care theory and is an-

Fig. 7-4. **Self-care concept of nursing.**

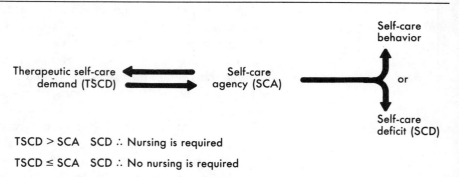

TSCD > SCA   SCD ∴ Nursing is required

TSCD ≤ SCA   SCD ∴ No nursing is required

From Joseph, L.S.: Self-care and the nursing process, Nurs. Clin. North Am. **15**(1):131-143, 1980.

alyzed in terms of independent nursing practice with clients.

Kinlein, a member of the Nursing Development Conference Group (NDCG) at Catholic University of America in Washington, D.C., was a participant in the initial development of the self-care theory promulgated by Orem and the NDCG in the 1960s. The theory stressed that self-care emphasizes an individual's responsibility and right over his or her own actions. Caring for an individual became more and more prominent in Kinlein's thinking.

In 1971, Kinlein became the first independent nurse practitioner by opening her own practice in her own office in Maryland. What has emerged is an entirely different orientation and definition of nursing. For her, nursing is "assisting the person in his self-care practices in regard to his state of health" (Kinlein, 1977). This nursing definition is the basis of her practice, and the total focus for Kinlein's practice is on the client. Consequently, the initial contact with the client, providing in-depth knowledge about the client, is a crucial portion of her nursing practice. The information offered by the client in a free-flowing manner is extremely valuable to Kinlein in understanding the individual's concept of health, self-care practices, demands, deficits, and needed nursing interventions. Kinlein's concept of nursing focuses on health not merely on the absence of illness; therefore any information the client offers in the initial contact is vital data. Fig. 7-5 demonstrates the concept formulated by Kinlein.

Kinlein notes that the formal object of nursing is the total person—that is, the incorporation of body, mind, and spirit (or soul) as the main focus for nursing care. As she has progressed in her practice, she has clarified her theory of care, as noted in Fig. 7-6. This approach to nursing gives the client full control of health; the nurse moves only as directed by the client. The planning of care, projection of goals, and evaluation of outcomes rest solely with the client; the nurse is an assistant. Dependence on the nurse becomes apparent in situations in which the individual, because of lack of

Fig. 7-5. **Initial client contact with nurse.**

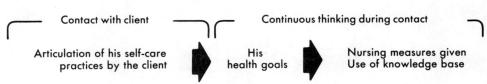

From Kinlein, M.L.: Independent nursing practice with clients, New York, 1977, J.B. Lippincott Co.

Fig. 7-6. **Kinlein care concept.**

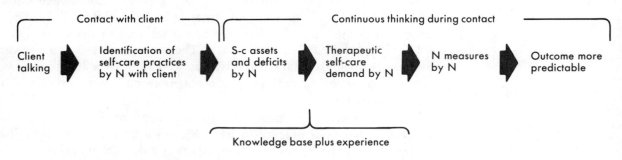

From Kinlein, M.L.: Independent nursing practice with clients, New York, 1977, J.B. Lippincott Co.

resources—mental, physical, or spiritual—is incapable of making the correct decision regarding his or her own health status.

The major concept underlying Kinlein's theory is care. Care means concern: any aspect of the client's life is of concern to the nurse who practices Kinlein's theory of care. In essence caring really means love. Love of the client is essential for a nurse totally committed to the client's needs. This loving approach precludes boredom and nursing by rote. To really care is to love each client as a member of humanity with special physical, mental, and spiritual needs. Each dimension of the client's total composition merits attention from the nurse. If the client is experiencing a spiritual problem, that self-care deficit becomes the focal point of nursing intervention in conjunction with the client. If needs are prominent in the other dimensions, priorities are set to help meet those needs. The client, however, always remains the one who directs the nursing care.

Kinlein identifies the use of the caring concept in six phases of the nursing practice. These phases demonstrate the use of nursing knowledge and at what point judgments are made about the needs of the client. The six phases, according to Kinlein (p. 59), are as follows:

Phases	In the nurse's mind
1. Greeting the client	No judgment made; knowledge base active
2. Narration by client	No judgment made; knowledge base active
3. Clarification by nurse	No judgment made; knowledge base active
4. Identification of self-care assets and deficits	Judgments made; knowledge base active

Phases	In the nurse's mind
5. Therapeutic self-care demand	Judgments made; knowledge base active
6. Prescription of nursing measures	Judgments made; knowledge base active

In each of these phases the nurse is an extremely careful listener. To hear more than the word demonstrates a caring attitude. Intense listening is extremely reassuring to the client. It also aids in identifying therapeutic self-care demands as well as deficits.

Kinlein's theory of care, with its foundation in Orem's self-care theory, could revolutionize nursing practice. Numbers of nurses who subscribe to this nursing theory are beginning to move into independent practice, changing the decades-old nursing practice formed on the medical care model and based on control by the medical profession. With this new vista opening, professional nurses are beginning to stand as advocates for their clients. A truly caring professional promotes well-being and health rather than supporting the client only in times of illness.

In the United States the health care scene is moving more and more toward self-care; individuals are taking the responsibility for their own health by bettering their knowledge of body, mind, and spirit. The nursing profession is grateful to Orem and Kinlein for having courageously promulgated this excellent theory as a basis for nursing practice.

The Professional Nurse: a Role Model for Health

The nurse who hopes to put into practice the concept of self-care as promoted by Orem and Kinlein must be a model of health. In such role modeling a nonverbal message suggests to the client that health truly is a gift to be appreciated and preserved at all costs. The nurse examines practices that may or may not promote high-level wellness and well-being and initiates change if necessary. The nurse realizes that health practices promoted in early childhood are the foundation for health in old age. The nurse as the primary health care provider is important in the life of the client, especially those who are older. The nurse, therefore, must introduce into his or her daily living health care measures that foster energy and professional enthusiasm. These health measures include dieting for ideal weight, obtaining sufficient rest, allowing for recreation and social activities, and allowing for solitude, to regain equilibrium and perspective. The nurse must appreciate the totality of personality to truly be a role model for the client, especially the older client. Aging is a process that has many dimensions. A nurse who is a good health model is better able to help older people appreciate the effort it may take to implement health measures. Activities of daily living are thus accomplished without effort and the older individual sees the nurse as truly interested in health. This approach helps the older person initiate good health practices.

Application of Self-care Theory to Gerontological Nursing: Promotion of Personhood

The independence of the older individual is a major goal of gerontological nursing. Self-care should be the theoretical framework for gerontological nursing, for it is in self-care that the ultimate independence, decision making, is incorporated into one's life. The older person is capable of initiating self-care and self-help and should be strongly encouraged to do so by the gerontological nurse.

In the assessment of each older person the approach to obtaining a detailed history is important. Included in this historical overview is information about (1) self-care practices, (2) definition of health, (3) health beliefs, (4) cultural components that may influence health practices, (5) life-style, (6) sleeping patterns, (7) food preferences, (8) social contacts, (9) amount of daily exercise, and (10) periods of solitude. Information on all of these factors is important for the gerontological nurse to obtain from the older client.

As Kinlein notes, initial observation and continuing reflections throughout the interview help the professional nurse make a valid assessment. The gerontological nurse should continuously think about the older person in terms of what is said, what is not said, appearance, gestures, facial expressions, loudness or softness of voice, and so forth. There are cognitive questions the gerontological nurse should reflect on during the initial client contact, such as the following. Is the older person stooped in posture, giving some evidence of possible kyphosis or osteoporosis? Is this posture indicative of low self-esteem or a poor self-image? Are statements such as, "I don't want to be a burden to you. I really don't need much" made by the older person indicative of feelings of worthlessness? These are crucial points at the outset of client contact and should be recorded for further reference and clarification, to help build the nursing care plan in conjunction with the older person.

The gerontological nurse, in using the self-care theoretical framework for interacting with the older person, focuses on the client's resources. What is available within the inner environment that would motivate the person to continue a daily regimen of activity that promotes health? Are there sufficient vision, hearing, and psychomotor skills to enable the older individual to function at an adequate level without interference or assistance from others? Is an exercise program possible so that there is a modicum of physical fitness (Price and Luther, 1980)? How restful is the sleeping pattern? When does the individual sleep best? How nutritious is the dietary intake over a 24-hour period? Who are the significant others in the life of this individual? Are there moments of solitude or weeks of isolation from social interaction? How does the older person meet the needs for spiritual growth? Resources from both inner and outer environments need thorough assessment before the gerontological nurse has enough knowledge of the older client to project a plan of self-care.

A key component for maintaining health is control over decisions that affect one's life. Gerontological nursing standards of practice identify the importance of having the older person promote, in conjunction with the gerontological nurse, certain goals and priorities. Self-care theory requires that the older individual always retain control of the environment, decision making, and health practices. The older person realizes that caring does mean loving by the gerontological nurse in the self-care modality. The concern and respect for personhood is an attitude that cannot be denied to the older person. Self-care as a theory in nursing promotes the individual's personhood in body, mind, and spirit. To neglect any area or dimension of personhood is a violation of the trust placed in the gerontological nurse by the older person. To assist the elderly person in maintaining integrity and self-respect as aging takes place is a responsibility of the gerontological nurse.

When self-care is initiated, the older person has a futuristic orientation to health goals (Kosidlak, 1980). To give the elderly client hope and optimism is extremely important in promoting self-care. Self-belief is crucial for believing in others and helps to dispel older persons' feelings of being a burden to society, to their families, and to the nurse.

Summary

Self-care aids all population segments. Of particular interest is the development of self-care practices among older individuals. The self-care movement helps to dispel the attitude that once people retire, their access to health care is curtailed because they lack financial resources. Each older person is unique and has the right and responsibility to promote well-being fully. The gerontological nurse has the responsibility to ensure that the older person's right to self-care is never violated within any setting where the nurse has control over the quality of care. Self-care theory holds a challenge for the older person but a greater challenge for gerontological nursing. To help older people fulfill their potential will profit society at large. A healthier older population generally and each older person specifically are on the brink of self-actualization. What greater goal could gerontological nursing ask?

References

Dunn, H.L.: High-level wellness, Arlington, Va., 1973, R.W. Beatty.

Jacob, L.S.: Self-care and the nursing process, Nurs. Clin. North Am. **15**(1):131, 1980.

Joseph, L.S.: Self-care and the nursing process, Nurs. Clin. North Am. **15**(1):131-143, 1980.

Kinlein, M.L.: Independent nursing practice with clients, New York, 1977, J.B. Lippincott Co.

Kosidlak, J.G.: Self-help for senior citizens, J. Gerontol. Nurs. **6**(11):663-668, 1980.

Larson, P.: Health strategy: Americans told prevention best disease fighter, The Kansas City Star, Jan. 21, 1983, Kansas City, Mo.

Levin, L.S.: The lay person as the primary care practitioner, Nurs. Digest **6**(1):17, 1978.

Levin, L.S., Katz, A.H., and Holst, E.: Self-care: lay initiatives in health, New York, 1976, Prodist.

Mayeroff, M.: On caring, New York, 1971, Harper & Row, Publishers, Inc.

Nightingale, F.: Notes on nursing: what it is and what it is not, London, 1859, Harrison.

Norris, C.M.: Self-care, Am. J. Nurs. **79**:486-489, 1979.

Nursing Development Conference Group: Concept formulization in nursing: process and product, ed. 2, Boston, 1979, Little, Brown & Co.

Orem, D.E.: Nursing: concepts of practice, New York, 1971, McGraw-Hill Book Co.

Orem, D.E.: Nursing: concepts of practice, ed. 2, New York, 1980, McGraw-Hill Book Co.

Price, J.S., and Luther, S.L.: Physical fitness: its role in health for the elderly, J. Gerontol. Nurs. **6**(9):517-523, 1980.

Somers, A.R.: Regulating personal behavior: health promotion's goal, Hosp. Prog. **61**(8):58-66, 1980.

Stevens, B.: Nursing theory: analysis, application, evaluation, Boston, 1979, Little, Brown & Co.

Chapter 8   A Celebration of Life

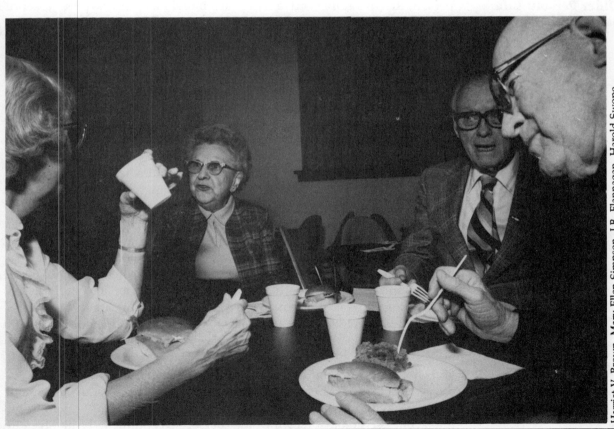

Harriet V. Brown, Mary Ellen Simpson, J.B. Flannagan, Harold Swope

A major goal of the health professions is the preservation of life. Inherent in this concept is the sacredness of life in all stages of development. The older person has all the potential, basic needs, hopes, and expectations that any other individual has. The health professions have a special interest in the older person's unique needs. Resources readily available to a younger person—physical strength, financial resources, spouse and family support—may not be available to the older person. Because of limited resources, the challenge of aiding the elderly person to promote health maintenance may become staggering at times; it stimulates health professionals to seek creative and innovative approaches to holistic care of the older person. When this challenge is met, the result is a fulfilled, self-actualized, healthy, and happy older person.

Promotion of Personhood of the Older Person: Life Satisfaction

When the health care professions, in implementing standards of care, continue to strive for the goal of a healthy, happy, self-actualized older person, then what they strive for in each individual is the inherent essence of human nature, that is, the promotion of personhood. In doing so the health professional provides for the continual development of the individual's potential. When that individual sees himself or herself as developing more talents and capabilities, then he or she becomes joyful and positive. Life, then, does not become a burden but an opportunity to live each day fully to the best of one's capability and to find satisfaction in the life lived.

In the therapeutic review of one's life, peak experiences can be pinpointed and their joy analyzed. This joy can be a way of life for the older person who has no regrets, because the joys and sorrows that make up life's peaks and valleys have been survived and are claimed as a part of the life history. When that life history is seen as continuing to move the individual toward a meaningful goal, then all of life can be placed into proper perspective. The health professional uses that life perspective in helping the older individual make meaningful goals for life. (For example, the goal of using time profitably may be established.) Everyone needs goals to make life meaningful. When the older person who has a major emphasis on work retires, then he or she may feel roleless—as if there are no other roles that need to be fulfilled once the work role has been terminated. The health professional helps the older person realize capabilities that are of value to others, opportunities for using those talents that should be investigated, and choices that should be made for directing energies toward a goal. So, the joy that is to be experienced in the so-called last trimester of life is really a test for living. Living does not just happen automatically. Living is an intelligent decision made by the older person to continue to be involved in life events and to meet challenges directly with full realization that disappointments and rejection may be experienced but that many happy moments also occur. This test for living is really what health promotion has as its main objective.

Health: Goal for Living

Health is not an end in itself but an opportunity to live life as the individual chooses. With health energies can be directed toward that goal; when illness occurs, goal achievement is interrupted. Therefore health enables the older person to be joyful about living: to demonstrate enthusiasm, to project goals on a year-to-year basis, and to evaluate the achievement of past years. The health professional is in a key position to help older persons realize that many of their lifetime goals have been met. For example, if the individual had reached a goal of gaining meaningful employment, to realize it will be remarkably pleasant to the older person. To get a good job and, despite lack of formal education, to be a success in the business world and to enjoy retirement based on the profits made in business is a cheering accomplishment. Another example is realizing that one of the personal goals in life—to enjoy a deep, intimate marriage, to have children, to see those children succeed in their own lives, and to enjoy grandchildren—has been met. When the health professional aids the older individual to perceive life in a meaningful framework, then joy, although not measurable in scientific terms, can be felt. Joy of living is a qualitative entity. It cannot be measured, but it is evident when one interacts with another person. That sense of peace of mind, the taking of life as it comes, the enjoying of each moment for the beauty it holds—all describe a particular quality in the life of the older person. These qualities should be inherent in each older individual whose life truly has been lived instead of merely tolerated, and able to be perceived by the health professional.

Coping and Adapting Processes

Celebration of the wholeness of life—physical, psychological, social, and spiritual—demands the elderly to continue on a life-style similar to that initiated in the earlier phases of life. There are some very important coping and adapting processes that allow this to continue into later years: relationships with friends, family, health professionals, and significant others; a variety of communication techniques; a zest for living. Each of these coping and adapting processes is explored to demonstrate that adaptability, flexibility, creativity, and dynamism are all attributes of the older person as life progresses toward the end-points of self-actualization and death.

Relationships

For the older person as for all individuals a major factor in life is relationships. Relationships are founded on lovability. Lovability is openness, freedom, appreciation for another individual, and enjoyment of spiritual rather than physical beauty. Lovability, according to Buscaglia (1982), is the human quality of need inherent in each human person. Relationship is the reaching out to others in a loving manner to meet the essence of another human being.

Therapeutic relationships. In the client–nurse/health professional relationship a therapeutic milieu allows the older person an atmosphere for sharing. The therapeutic relationship, then, should be initiated in a warm, friendly manner so that the older person becomes aware immediately of a caring attitude in the health professional. Many times, the elderly person responds much more readily if touched on the hand or shoulder by the health professional. This helps the older person feel lovable and attractive to the nurse or health professional. With this approach the health professional conveys a feeling of comfort in the relationship with the older person and with the aging process in general. This is an important element in establishing a good relationship with the older client.

Listening is a key component of the relationship. The health professional should learn to listen not only to what is said but to what is not said. Many times in the pauses and silences that occur in an encounter much communication takes place. The relationship is enhanced by an understanding of those pauses and silences by the health professional (Wahl, 1980).

For a therapeutic relationship to be established, rapport with the older person is essential. Rapport is enhanced if the health professional is closely positioned by the older person's side. By so doing, the older person, who may be experiencing visual or hearing difficulties, is given an opportunity to hear and see the health professional better. This rapport, then, is to be fostered for the sake of aiding a very important relationship in the life of the older person. To discuss one's health in the four dimensions—spiritual, social, physical, and psychological—to a caring health professional is a key component in the celebration of the wholeness of life. Health is needed by the older person to carry out daily living activities as well as to achieve goals.

Family relationships. Another important relationship for the older person is familial. In the family the supportive network is enhanced by a positive relationship with each member: children, grandchildren, and great-grandchildren, as well as cousins, uncles, and aunts. Coming together at periodic intervals for family reunions and other celebrations (anniversaries, birthdays, and significant days in the lives of the family) is important for the older person in keeping an important role within the family. To be a participant in these activities helps the older person appreciate his or her own significance to these family members.

Friends. Another relationship important to the older person is friendship. Friends are those who come into the life of the older person at various points, provide a loving, caring attitude in times of joy, sorrow, disappointment, and pain, and help to create those beautiful moments that are shared only by people who know each other very well.

Wade (1982) indicates that friendship between older persons is extremely important, not necessarily for romance but simply for companionship. Because retirement and deaths of friends and relatives may leave older adults lonely, companionship is important. Freedom in their relationship, with no demands or pressures for seeking a commitment beyond friendship, allows for enjoyment of life. Life is enhanced by being shared in such a way that romance may enter but is not expected. A good relationship gives a sense of belonging, of being wanted and found attractive by another person. Social interaction and the sharing of common interests enhances the quality of life. Sometimes this kind of relationship is not appreciated by the friends or children of the elderly person entering into such a relationship, but that is not a deterrent in many cases (Wade, 1982). Senior citizen centers, church activities, and other social programs for the elderly are excellent means for meeting people and making friends. The friendships made in the later years widen one's circle of acquaintances and make possible relationships that can be extremely valuable in living life fully. A case in point is an elderly woman of 83 years of age, a widow for approximately 5 years, living alone in a small town, having moved there from a farm 20 years ago. An elderly male acquaintance, 84 years of age, lives several houses away. His wife died 2 years ago. To fill the lonely evenings, the elderly woman called to suggest that they spend an hour or so together playing cards, which was a longstanding social activity when each of the spouses was alive. The man readily agreed and came to enjoy the card playing. This was very fulfilling for him and for the elderly woman. They enjoyed each other's company; they enjoyed the card playing in itself and as a vehicle for communication. As time went on, the man offered to do some small repair work around the home and to provide transportation for shopping and church activity—he offered to be a good friend in the truest sense of the word. Each of these two elderly people are in excellent health, enjoying life and activity; it is apparent to the children in each of their families that this relationship has done wonders for their outlook and their enjoyment of life. This kind of relationship is extremely important for an older couple for raising the level of depression and loneliness to a level of joy and fulfillment.

Marriage commitments. Finally, a look at that intimate friendship—marriage—for the older person is important. It is noted that marriages lasting 50, 60, or 70 years are as strong today as marriages were in the past. For the older couple in a "golden sunset marriage," several key factors aiding the continuance of a happy marriage include:

1. Strong commitment to the spouse as a person
2. Good communication
3. Shared decision making or power
4. Mutual respect and support*

Each of these factors are very important for a relationship with intimacy and commitment. Commitment is extremely important because through it the older person celebrates the wholeness of life. Commitment needs a goal that is all-consuming in the life of the individual. In marriage there is a strong commitment to its continuance, and there is a positive determination on the part of both spouses to weather the storms that may come with the aging process as well as with the intimate relationship. With renewed effort the relationship deepens as each day passes, so that there is a beauty exhibited by each partner in the very lives they live. Because their communication is free, they enjoy each other's opinions and look forward to interactions that move them beyond the status quo to new ideas. Through shared decision making or power, they demonstrate the importance of making decisions together for a couple relationship. And finally, mutual respect and support demonstrates the unique qualities in the husband and wife that have been complementary through their lifetime. This gives rise to a stability in the marriage that fosters happiness.

Relationships, then, of the older person with health professional, family, friends, and spouse aid in the celebration of life for the older person. This coping and adapting process continues the process of self-actualization—that is, fulfilling all four dimensions of personhood.

Communication Techniques

One of the key components for celebration of life is communication. Humans can communicate through words. This communication offers the opportunity for sharing ideas, feelings, perceptions, creative notions, and theories. Only humans have this privilege of sharing their inner world. Communication for the older person is extremely important in continuing relationships with others and in helping to shape the life-style to that degree that he or she can be an individual and yet share self with other people. Through communication a sense of reality is shared by two or more persons.

A very important means of communicating is through touch. Touch shows that a caring attitude is present. The sense of touch, be it a hug, kiss, or a light touch on the hand, shoulder, or forehead, conveys to older persons that they are real, and that their presence is appreciated, wanted, and needed. The use of communication through touching can enhance the

*From Sweeney, J.: Taking the long view of marriage, June 21, 1982, Los Angeles Times.

celebration of the wholeness of life for an older individual. Touch can become an extremely essential and powerful communicator with and for the elderly.

Health professionals who use touch as a means of communicating with the elderly have found it to be extremely valuable in establishing an optimum therapeutic relationship. Through touch they demonstrate that there is an opportunity for feedback. Touch may help a lonely person to come out of isolation and begin interaction with other persons.

Zest for Living

Zest for living is a feeling that life is worthwhile. The older person who continues to live life with zest has a sense of joy, vitality, and enthusiasm for each day. An example is demonstrated in the following description of a woman who, at the age of 91, continued to live fully:

Woman, 91, celebrates each year with zest

When Mayme Blink was a child, she was told that children are to be seen and not heard.

Now that she is about to turn 92, she is making up for lost time.

"At 92, I'm doing what I wanted to do at 22," she said.

Mrs. Blink has attracted national attention with her birthday celebrations. She tries to do something special each year and has ridden a motorcycle, gone on a hayride, been in a helicopter and gone up in a hot-air balloon.

"I don't really know what it's like to be old," said Mrs. Blink, whose birthday is Oct. 15.

Her balloon trip in August coincided with the picnic at Colonial Manor Retirement Home, where she has lived for five years.

"The balloon was really hard to get up to," Mrs. Blink said. "I had to hang on to the necks of all the men on the thing. I thought I'd choke them. . . . None of the other old ladies would go on it. I've never seen such a bunch of sissies."

The tradition of celebrating her age with something new each year began four years ago when she jokingly told some retirement home officials that she had never ridden a motorcycle and would like to. The ride was arranged through friends and, before she knew it, Mrs. Blink found herself astride a motorcycle, clutching the waist of its owner.

She said she took that first ride to show people that they can do new things, even if they are old or handicapped. Mrs. Blink herself is legally blind.

"You see, I really am old, but I don't want to be. I do all these things so I don't have to be," she said.

Mrs. Blink has a beauty and health regimen that she follows to keep from growing old before her time. She eats carrots every day at noon, massages her hands before bedtime and exercises.

"And right before I go to bed, I have a little brandy over ice because I don't like sleeping pills," she said.*

Health Care: Striking a Balance

The health professional helps an older person celebrate the wholeness of life by ensuring that each dimension of the person receives equal atten-

---

*From Associated Press News features: At 91, woman celebrates each year with zest, Kansas City, Mo., Sept 9, 1982, The Kansas City Times.

tion. The four dimensions, physical, psychological, social, and spiritual, are brought into focus and incorporated into a plan of care and intervention, helping the individual to find a sense of reality and a meaning to living, and to make the necessary modifications in life-style that promote a zest for living. When health care takes into account the total person, that individual is assured of receiving the kind of care required to help the aging person maintain control over his or her chosen life-style. Therefore health care actions are extremely important in upholding the individuality of the older person, whose particular life history, culture, and ethnic origins exist to make this older person unique. The health professional who can appreciate each individual's beauty helps to prove that there is only one such individual in the world. If an individual continues to live beyond the body in a spiritual dimension, he or she can continue to celebrate life in the fullest sense. It is the privilege of the health professional to help the older person achieve that wholeness of life that all wish to have.

Several older persons we know are beautiful examples of the celebration of the wholeness of life and zest for living. They consented to interviews that display their life histories, philosophies of life, insights into the aging process, continuing contributions to humanity, and expectations for continuing the celebration of life. It is with pleasure that we present the entire interviews for your enjoyment and edification.

**Case Histories
Demonstrating Zest
for Living**
**Life Review
of Sam Reaves**

Nurse: It is my pleasure to introduce to you Mr. Sam Reaves, a highly influential and prominent individual in the greater Kansas City area who has helped shape community policies and programs for the elderly citizens residing in the metropolitan area. Because Mr. Reaves, an 88-year-old gentleman, is a role model for successful and graceful aging, it is my good fortune to have this opportunity to interview a celebrity who has graciously consented to share his beliefs about the aging process.

Mr. Reaves, as a nurse, I am interested in your health status. How would you describe your health?

Mr. R.: Very good. My gallbladder was removed a year ago; and since that time I have had some reaction but nothing of any consequence. I have problems with my hearing and sight, but I guess for my age that is to be expected. Maybe not to be expected—but I know that many people much younger than I have the same problem and even more serious than I.

Nurse: That is very true. Would you please share with us where you were born?

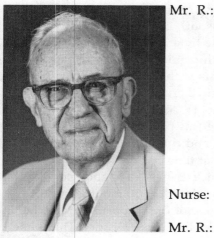

Mr. Sam Reaves, Executive Director, Mid-America Resources and Training Center on Aging, Shepherd Center, Kansas City, Missouri

Mr. R.:   I was born in southeast Missouri in a place that, as far as I know, no longer is in existence. The town was, at that time, the little town of Vincent in Dunklin County. A second cousin of mine and I, a year ago this last summer as a matter of fact, tried to find that community and it is no longer there. I am assuming that it has either been blown off the map or people have moved away. My parents were sharecroppers, which means that they didn't own any land at that time and did not own any land until my father passed away in 1904. Mother, then, used the little money that my father left to buy a farm. We became farmers and landowners then.

Nurse: Could you tell me how many were in your family? How many children?

Mr. R.:   There were eight of us all together. Five girls and three boys. Three of us lived to maturity; my brother who was 6 years older than me and my sister who was 2 years younger than me. Only the three of us lived to maturity.

Nurse: That meant you had a lot of work to do in your lifetime.

Mr. R.:   That is for sure! But very pleasant.

Nurse: Education is an important component of one's life. Could you talk about your educational background?

Mr. R.:   My elementary education was in the rural school. As I indicated a moment ago, my mother bought the farm. Later, in 1907, just 3 years later, she sold the farm and we moved to Cape Girardeau, Missouri, which is a college town. It was a teachers' college in those days, and the three of us, mother and we three children, kept a boarding house for college students. It was this income that allowed the three of us to get a college education. So all three of us were graduates of the Southeast Missouri State Teachers' College at that time. It is now Southeast Missouri State University at Cape Girardeau, Missouri. All three of us did get a college education.

Nurse: That is excellent! What did you major in in college?

Mr. R.:   I majored in secondary education primarily. I presume that would be what I would consider my major. I became principal at the ripe old age of 18 of a school in Pemiscot County, which is adjacent to and part of the boot heel of Missouri, in 1913. A year later I became principal of a three-room school; the school actually that I had attended in Pascola, Missouri, before we sold the farm and moved to the

Cape. At the end of that year I became principal of a high school in Caruthersville, Missouri, in Pemiscot County, and spent 2 years there. All of the time I was a principal, I was teaching subjects dealing with mathematics and science. Those were my major interests at that time.

Nurse: Very good! You were a principal and a teacher—

Mr. R.: And a superintendent of schools. As a matter of fact, while I was in Caruthersville where I was principal of the high school, going back and forth and continuing to work on my degree at the university at that time, World War I broke out. In 1917 I became a part of Uncle Sam's Navy and spent 20 months in Uncle Sam's Navy. After my 20 months in the Navy, I became principal of one of the schools, a rural school in St. Louis County, the Rock Hill School District. That same fall, the community, now Brentwood, Missouri, decided they wanted to incorporate, to pull itself away and incorporate a separate school district. So we organized a school district, and Brentwood School District in the town of Brentwood at the same time, and I became the superintendent of that school district.

Nurse: Very good! You emerged as a leader very early in your lifetime.

Mr. R.: In 1919, that came about. Well, I was an old man to the kids. I still hear from those kids, come to think of it. I got a letter from one of the boys who is now out in Burbank, California, last Saturday. A young man, 76 years of age.

Nurse: You must have had a tremendous influence in his life as well as your other students.

Mr. R.: Hopefully so.

Nurse: Did you go on for further education beyond college?

Mr. R.: Oh, I took some special classes at Washington University in St. Louis after I came back out of the service and settled there in Brentwood, or in Rock Hill. I lived in Rock Hill but was teaching in Brentwood. I took some special classes at Washington University that I was not able to get at the Teachers' College, particularly in the field of genetics and heredity. As a matter of fact, one of the subjects that I had in college was World History, Ancient History, but I didn't get very much out of it. I blamed the teacher rather than myself. There was a chap at the Washington University teaching a course in World History; I took that also just to brush up on it.

Nurse: Good! That gave you some appreciation of the geographical regions you visited as a Navy man.

Mr. R.:   Right.

Nurse: You have told me about your work career as a faculty member, a superintendent, a principal. You have also been involved in some other careers since I have known you. Could you tell us of other career involvement?

Mr. R.:   Actually, in 1919, when we started this new school system, the Brentwood School System, the boys and parents in that community wanted to have a boy scout troop, so that they would not have to go to Clayton or University City or Kirkwood or some of the other neighboring communities. We organized a scout troop and I became its scoutmaster. Then within 5 years, the scout executive from the St. Louis Council, a fellow by the name of Earl Beckman, invited me to join his staff. In January, 1926, I became a field executive of the Boy Scouts of America and served there, in Omaha, Nebraska, as a scout executive, and then back here in Kansas City, Missouri. This period spanned from 1926 until the time I retired in 1959. I spent almost 33 years as a scout executive. Upon my retirement, while I was working in Kansas City on the staff here, we worked very closely with the Community Chest and later the United Fund. Because of those relationships, I made contacts with the top people of the community and various agencies and organizations. One of the agencies which really appealed to me was the Kansas City Chapter of the American Heart Association. A young fellow by the name of Ed Stollenwork, who was at that time chairman of their Board of Directors of the Kansas City chapter of the American Heart Association, with whom I had worked actively in the United Fund and Community Chest, invited me to appear before their executive committee. I accepted that invitation and the first of September, after I retired at the end of August, I became the executive director of the Kansas City Chapter of the American Heart Association and served there for 5 years. Then Dr. Cole became the pastor of my church, The Century United Methodist Church, and invited me to become the business administrator of my church. I served there from 1965 until 1973. In 1973, I said to Dr. Cole and my wife, "I think I am going to hang up my shingle and I am going to quit work." Well, at the end of about 6 months, my wife said, "Sweetheart, you have got to get a job. There isn't room for both of us in this kitchen." So, I ended up by going back and becoming the Director of the Mid-America Resources and Training Center on Aging. It was called the Resources and Training Center on Aging at that time; but, later it became a not-for-profit corporation on its own in the state of Missouri, known as the Mid-America Resource and Training Center on Aging. I have been the director of that organization since the fall of 1973 when they launched the program.

Nurse: It has been almost 10 years now since you have retired and you have taken on this position.

Mr. R.: Right.

Nurse: Very good! Could you tell us about the training center?

Mr. R.: Basically, we provide opportunities for people all over the country, in fact, around the world, to come to Kansas City and hear about the Shepherd Center, learn about the Shepherd Center. We provide this opportunity for people coming to Kansas City to actually rub shoulders with, come in contact with, the people, 400 to 500 elderly people, who are part of the Shepherd Center, the volunteers who give leadership and participate in it, so that they can go back to their community and use this same concept in administering to the elderly of their community. The Shepherd Center is an ecumenical project involving 25 churches and synagogues in the southwest Kansas City area as participants in this Shepherd Center program. Wherever there is a Shepherd Center, wherever they use the Shepherd Center concept, it is ecumenical. So, we in the Shepherd Center say that where there are people that care, there can be a Shepherd Center, and we have proven it. There are at the present time some 60 Shepherd Centers in the United States of America and one up in Brockville, Ontario, Canada, all resulting from people coming to Kansas City and participating in the seminars. We have had people from Hong Kong, Johannesburg, South Africa, several cities in Australia, London, England, Hawaii (Honolulu), and a place I have never heard of before in England. We have had people from around the world that have heard about the Shepherd Center. As a matter of fact, I am going to tell you a very interesting story. I will cut it short. A young man from Starke, Florida, wrote me about 5 years ago and said, "I want to be a volunteer for the Shepherd Center." I wrote this young man and found out later that he was incarcerated in the penitentiary in Starke, Florida. The Shepherd Center has been heard of in all sorts of places, even behind the prison walls. He is now in Leavenworth, and I am corresponding with him there.

Nurse: To know that you have been able to help the elderly have a better quality of life is so extremely important.

Mr. R.: That is what it is all about.

Nurse: It was your input, along with Dr. Cole's, that shaped Shepherd Center to what it is today!

Mr. R.: I would say, yes! The idea came out of the Shepherd Center Board. They decided that their staff, a limited staff of three people at that time, did not have the time to answer all of the requests coming in, first from Kansas City and then from around the area, and then from the states. Therefore, the Board of Directors of Shepherd Center decided there ought to be a component of the Shepherd Center; so, we became a component the first year of the Shepherd Center. The title of our agency is Mid-America Training and Resource Center. Then, at the end of our first year, we became a separate not-for-profit corporation. But really, we had people like Dr. Mays, Dr. Cole, Dr. Kermit Phelps, Dr. Neil Bull of the University of Missouri in Kansas City, Dr. George Spear of the University of Missouri in Kansas City, and Dr. Warren Peterson. So all of those people were on our Advisory Board the first year. We were a component of the Shepherd Center, but we had these people, involved in one way or another in the field of aging, working with us as our advisory board.

Nurse: And they helped give the input; but you were the responsible person for putting the ideas together and implementing them.

Mr. R.: Most definitely! My role is that of the director to see that things happen. We have, as you know, a library, book library, with something like 800 volumes, all of which are in the field of gerontology, and a library of films, cassettes, tapes, and slides. We are, I think, on the mailing list of all the organizations and agencies over the country that, even in Canada, send out any kind of publication dealing with gerontology. We think that we have one of the best libraries in this whole field. As a matter of fact, some of our friends over at Lawrence-K.U. have come over and viewed our library, have gone back to Lawrence and used some of the ideas and material in developing their library.

Nurse: Excellent! What do you perceive as the future of the Shepherd Center?

Mr. R.:   I think it is going to continue to thrive. I don't think there is any question about it. At the present time, they have 25 programs available to the elderly, some of which are directed to the homes themselves—that is, actually, to make it possible for the elderly to continue to live out their lives in their own home. You know, of course, better than I, the percentage of people that never enter into any kind of long-term care. Those 95% that don't enter any kind of long-term care need to be gotten out of the home so that they don't dry up and blow away. Eighteen of the programs are for that purpose.

Nurse: Very good! Could you present a brief overview of those programs?

Mr. R.:   The programs started in January, 1972, before there was a Shepherd Center, with a group of men of our church delivering Meals-On-Wheels. Some half a dozen men delivered Meals-On-Wheels to men and women of our church who couldn't get to the church or attend fellowship dinners and that sort of thing. As they delivered the meals, they discovered some things that ought to be done in the homes: light fixtures, plumbing fixtures, doors, windows that needed to be repaired. They suggested that the church ought to start a Handyman Program or a Home Repair Program, which they did. Some of the women in whose homes the meals were being delivered said, "Well now, listen, my husband was a chauffeur. I never did learn to drive; and, at my age, it would be foolish to try to learn to drive. If somebody could take me shopping, or go shopping for me, I could prepare meals. It wouldn't be necessary for you to bring these meals in." They started the Shopper's Service and one thing lead to another.

            In 1972, Dr. Cole and this group of clergy from the 25 churches in the southwest part of the city said, "Let's get together and work this thing out together." They started a task force of some seven or eight people, which later became the Board of Directors of the Shepherd Center. That's the way the whole thing started. At the same time that this was going on, some of the men and women of our church and the community, who had become involved with the Meals-On-Wheels and Handyman Programs, said, "Now, you have told us that less than 5% ever go into any kind of long-term health care setting, so let's do something about the other 95%." They conceived the idea, after a series of meetings, of an Adventure in Learning Program, a college education type of program that would pull the people out of their homes and bring them again to the Central United Methodist Church. Here they would use volunteers, elderly people themselves, and some university professors and Elliott Berkley from the International Relations Council; and they started, in the fall of 1972, an Adventures in Learning Program. These clergy—rabbis, priests, and ministers—began to talk about some of the problems they were encountering with some of their elderly parishioners they couldn't deal with. So, they conceived the idea of what is now the Life Enrichment Program. Dr. Cole hired a lady, a former YWCA Executive Director, who had originally been the Director of Religious Education of our church and had just retired and moved back to Kansas City. Dr. Cole and she got together with Dr. Kermit Phelps and out of that discussion came the Life Enrichment Program initiated in 1974 as a personal-goal program. Dr. Phelps, a psychologist, indicated, "None of us use more than 15% of our potential and what we ought to do is give these people an opportunity to increase that at least 5%." That formed the basis of the program. The clergy of the area gave Helen Humphreys a list of about 25 people who had had some rather traumatic experiences and therefore needed this kind of program. Helen contacted each one of them and said, "We are going to launch a new program, a pilot program, and we would like you to help us." She didn't say, "We want you to be guinea pigs"; she said, "We want you to help us." And almost without an exception they agreed. And that program continues every Tuesday morning. There is another program on Thursday morning, which is made up of new people. People who have been identified with the program since the fall of 1974 still come back on Tuesday mornings and are part of the program. It is a beautiful thing!

Nurse: I agree that it is really an outstanding program to assist the elderly to maintain themselves in the home, as well as giving themselves to other people, which is such a basis for happiness.

Mr. R.: A couple of rather recent programs have been enlarged. The Health Enrichment Program has been enlarged and expanded recently to the point that one of your graduates is a part of it, whom you know, of course. Kathy Bock is the Director of this Health Enrichment Program. David Shepherd is the coordinator of the Health Enrichment Program, but it is now expanded into a full-fledged geriatric/gerontological nursing program through 5 full days of the week and sometimes even on Saturday. It is outstanding! For my money, it is the finest thing that has been added to the Shepherd Center since it began. Recently, the Hospice Program has been established, part of which involves the training of 20 people in the fields of theology, psychology, sociology, to work with the family of those who have a terminal illness. There are some beautiful stories that have come out of that. It is just, well, it makes you bubble over with enthusiasm to hear about the real outcome, the real value of the Hospice Program. This particular program is designed for health professionals to go into homes and help these people bear their burden—so valuable.

Nurse: I would agree that it is a very outstanding program; and it is really a role model for other programs in the greater Kansas City area.

Mr. R.:   One of the things that has impressed me, also, is the interest of the elderly in knowing more what they themselves can do to keep themselves physically fit. Now, being one of those people, I am aware of many of the things that I need to do in order to keep myself physically fit. I don't do all those things that I should; I guess none of us do. But as a part of the Health Enrichment Program, the elderly, the people who have these health problems, become aware of what these things are and what can be done. Several different programs have resulted, having come out of this awareness on the part of the elderly themselves.

Nurse: I think so much focuses in on the mental attitude of the individual; that they are not to be resigned to a rocking chair kind of philosophy, but that there is much they can do even after retirement.

Mr. R.:   Right! Actually, the Shepherd Center idea is not to duplicate something that has already happened. If a church, an organization, or center in the area is doing something, we find out about what that is and tell the adult members, the retired members, the older people of the community, what these programs are and where they can be found. It's not

only a center of actually doing things but also referring
people to where they can get the help they need; for
example, preparing their income tax return every year. The
Shepherd Center has available places in the community
where these elderly people can get the kind of information
they need.

Nurse: Your description of the Shepherd Center demonstrates your
enthusiasm for the program.

Mr. R.:   As far as I am concerned, my whole life has been filled! Oh, I
have had my ups and downs. I have had my concerns, but I
have also been blessed. The Lord has been good to me all of
my 88 years. He has thrown me into contact with such lovely
people as Sister Bahr, Lucille Gress, and these other nice
people that I know over here at the University of Kansas.

Nurse: Thank you! You exude such enthusiasm for someone who has
been retired for 23 years.

Mr. R.:   The personnel policy of the Boy Scouts of America did
require, and still does, that you retire at 65 to give someone
younger a chance, and this is good. I have never ever taken
any exception to that part of it. But 23 years ago I retired as
the scout executive.

Nurse: That is outstanding! Well, Mr. Reaves, you have been
describing the program at Shepherd Center and what it does
for the other person, as far as their aging process is
concerned. Let me shift the discussion to yourself. What are
some of the beliefs that you have about the aging process that
have enabled you to continue working so hard?

Mr. R.:   It would be pretty hard to really select the things that have
been important to me. I think a major fact is that the
Shepherd Center believes in the whole person, administer to
the whole person. I have been a member of my church, of *a*
church, ever since I was a youngster. As kids we had our
own vesper services in our own home. Mother was our Bible
teacher, our song leader. I presume that a key factor is that
the Shepherd Center believes in administering to the whole
person as an extension of my upbringing. I think probably
that would be number one belief if I were to select any one
thing. Secondly, the fact that they (the Shepherd Center) give
such direct interest to utilizing the skills, the expertise of the
elderly themselves. In other words, they don't say to the
elderly, "Now, here are a bunch of young kids around that
are going to do these things for you." They say to the elderly

people, "What are the things that you need, what are the things that you need to have done, what are the things that you see that need to be done by people like yourselves?" Once they begin to get these things out on the table, they have a pretty good idea of what the elderly of that particular segment of the city are interested in having done. Then they say, "Would you be willing to give leadership, and, if you are not capable, do you know somebody that can?" In other words, they utilize the knowledge, the expertise, the know-how of the people themselves. They administer to the whole person; at least, if that person is willing to be administered to. And being ecumenical would be another factor because I believe so strongly in that. My dear little ol' mother, bless her heart, many times said, "Now, don't forget there are other people, you know. there are Catholics, Protestants, and Jews, and we all are going to the same place. We are using a different road, but we are going to get there. If we ever get there at all, all are going to get there."

Nurse: She was the first person that really emphasized the faith dimension in your life and how important that is?

Mr. R.: No question about it! I mentioned, I think, the fact that my father died when I was a youngster, 7 years of age. When you are 7 years of age, you don't remember a whole lot about your parents unless they are around later. I remember he was a very handsome individual with a beautiful moustache, but that's about all I remember. He had to be a swell guy for my mother to have married him.

Nurse: I am sure that is very true. Your life, then, was shaped a great deal by your mother?

Mr. R.: No question about it!

Nurse: Her emphasis on faith, that other people are to be appreciated, and that there is an opportunity for everyone in this world helped shape your thinking.

Mr. R.: I do emulate her in my own life in dealing with my children and with my grandchildren and my six great-grandchildren. I don't think there is any question about the relationship enjoyed between my son and daughter and I. I lost the mother of my two children when my boy was 11 and the girl was only 3. So I became the father and mother of my two children until I remarried 14 years later. They were grown when I remarried. I think having seen my mother go through that same role of becoming both the father and mother, I became a mother and a father. You can't really do justice to both. I attempted to be a true father to my boy. And there was hardly a day passed when he didn't call me to be sure that I was O.K. when my second wife passed away, that I was getting over my grieving period. His idea was not only to check up on me, but to assure me that he and my daughter-in-law were very close to me and loved me. Then, after he passed away, my daughter-in-law continues to keep in touch; we are very close, just as close as if she were my own flesh and blood. Then, on top of that, my grandson and granddaughter, who live here in Kansas City, have been very lovely to me. They are trying to take the place of my second wife and are doing a beautiful job of it.

Nurse: That's tremendous! What gives you the motivation to have such zest for living?

Mr. R.: There again, I guess it comes by nature. I love living. As I indicated a moment ago, the Lord has been good to me. I don't deserve, I don't think any of us deserve, all the blessings He showers on us. Maybe we do, but the Lord has been good to me, and I am trying to measure up to what I think my responsibilities have been. I know I have not always done so. I am aware of that, I am human. I am not immortal, so I know that I have fallen short. I read my Bible morning and evening and read a lot of other religious material. I belong to the Fellowship Foundation of Christian Living. I'm a card-carrying member, a life member of the United Methodist Men, a national organization. That group decided to make me a life member some 7 or 8 years ago. This honor occurred because of some work I did in the Kansas City South District of the United Methodist Church. I had chaired a committee that provided a Lenten breakfast by the men of the district for some 10 or 12 years, so this group of men said, "Well, that guy deserves something." So, I got this little ol' pin.

Nurse: Very good! That's a very attractive pin also.

Mr. R.: Probably another point to be made: I learned from working with the youth! You stay young by being open-minded, and I know I am stubborn in many respects. My son-in-law says, "Dad, if you ever quit working, you ought to become a taxi driver in New York City." In other words, I don't want to

	give the right-of-way to anybody. I think probably the fact that I have spent so many years working with youth has given me a youthful point of view. I hope I always have it.
Nurse:	And I think you will.
Mr. R.:	I hope I always have it. My doctor tells me that he is going to keep me alive until 100, and I am going to hold him to it if I can! He is a very fine young Filipino, and he said to me quite recently, "Your cholesterol count is much better than mine." I said, "Doctor, you ought to get a good doctor."
Nurse:	That is a good piece of advice! Well, what advice would you have for those of us who are trying to grow old gracefully? You have mentioned open-mindedness, orientation to full living through the total being of mind, body, and spirit. Anything else?
Mr. R.:	I think primarily to remain active, and I mean with meaningful things. I don't mean just sitting down knitting and crocheting. I mean to remain active, be active in things that are worthwhile, helping people. Most of all, be active in participating in worthwhile things, active in your own church primarily. If I weren't up in my own church early on Sunday morning, I would feel like I had missed out on something. There are so many worthwhile activities you can participate in that it would be hard to be inactive. But, at any rate, to remain active, be active! Live as long as you live!
Nurse:	I think that's an important comment. Do you have any other comments you would like to make that we have not touched upon, as it relates to successfully aging and enjoying life for as long as the Lord will give it to us?
Mr. R.:	I think we have touched on the important things. I think we need to continue to study the Lord's word, whatever our religious faith may be. But I also think we need to know something about the other religions so that we are not too opinionated. I don't know what the proper word would be, but I remember how my mother used to talk about it. She said it was almost suicidal to our church to take the position that we were the only church around. Now maybe that's going a bit too far, but that was my dear little ol' mother's point of view. That these other people have their right to believe the way they wish and practice their religion.
Nurse:	You have given me extremely excellent and informative material. I have enjoyed this very pleasurable experience of visiting with you about your own life, Mr. Reaves, in terms of

what you have done since retirement. Most people, when they get to be 65 will say, "Well, I deserve to rest." You have been active since your retirement 23 years ago, including being the executive director of a highly successful organization. As you commented, it has reached not only to the national borders but international borders as well. It must give you a tremendous mind-expanding experience every day to realize that you have touched many lives.

Mr. R.: I am honored to have a chance to be with you, and to be a part of your book. As far as I am concerned, this, to me, is a delightful experience. Any way that I can help you is important to me. I want to help. As long as I am physically and mentally capable of doing so.

Nurse: You have been extremely helpful.

Mr. R.: I just appreciate the opportunity to be here.

Nurse: Mr. Reaves, you are a man who has been extremely valuable to all of us through your life-style and orientation to life itself. Thank you for sharing information about your life.

Life Review of Marion Lincoln

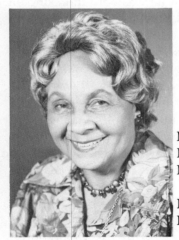

Mrs. Marion Lincoln, President, Board of Directors, Mid-City Towers, Kansas City, Missouri

Nurse: It is my pleasure to introduce to you Mrs. Marion Lincoln, a highly prominent and influential individual in the greater Kansas City area who has helped shape community policies and programs for elderly citizens residing in the metropolitan area. Because Mrs. Lincoln, a 73-year-old black woman, is a role model of successful and graceful aging, it is my good fortune to have an opportunity to interview a celebrity who has graciously consented to share her beliefs about the aging process.

Mrs. Lincoln, please tell me where you were born.

Mrs. L.: I was born in Kansas City, Missouri, on February 16, 1909.

Nurse: How many were in your family?

Mrs. L.: I had one brother and two sisters. One sister is living in Flint, Michigan. She is an elementary school teacher.

Nurse: Are your father and mother still living?

Mrs. L.: No, they are both deceased. My father died when I was quite a young girl. I was about 13 years old; and my mother died in '56.

Nurse: What kind of work did they do while you were growing up?

Mrs. L.: My mother was always, more or less, a cook working for different families; my father worked at the Union Station at night as a janitor.

Nurse: You know that one of the things that shapes our lives is education. Could you tell us what kind of educational background you have? Did you go to elementary school? High school?

Mrs. L.: Yes, I went to elementary school and high school until the senior year, when I got married in 1925 to William R. Lincoln.

Nurse: You have 3 years of high school! Did you have any extra kind of education, like workshops or seminars?

Mrs. L.: No, not at that time. In those days you didn't hear of workshops and other programs like they have now. I just went right on through life, and what I have picked up, as far as education is concerned, is by reading and working with other people and studying different things. I really wanted to be a nurse. That is what I wanted to be. When I was a little girl that was my calling, I thought, and I always played with things pertaining to nursing. Then I met my husband, and he said, "We are going to have a big family." We had only one child. I never did get to go back and finish my high school. In those years you had to have a high school education before you could take up nurse training.

Nurse: So your husband was very much a major part in shaping your life. Where did you meet him?

Mrs. L.: I met him here in Kansas City, but he was born in Lexington, Missouri. My father was born in Lexington, and his whole family was from down there. My aunt, my father's sister, knew him when he was just a little boy. He came to our house after my father passed and I was 13 years old. He didn't know me and I didn't know him because I was just a kid and still in school. I didn't see him any more until I was 16, but the first time I saw him, I said, "Oh, I'm going to marry him some day." When I was 16, he was 21. He had changed, and I had too. He had really forgotten me. I went to Lexington and met him there. That was in May; we married on December 14th of 1925.

I was going to go on to school but in those days, the woman was supposed to stay at home. Things were different. You didn't hear of a lot of women working like we do now. In later years I felt that there was something that I should do. I felt there was something else in my life that I should do because I had always wanted to help people. I think that is what nursing is, helping other people. I started out working in the community. At first I organized a neighborhood club, 26 years ago. I felt there was a need for the neighbors to be a little closer together. I am still their president after 26 years. I like to do outreach work in the community. When model cities started in Kansas City in 1967, it tempted me to work in the community with people. There were a lot of people that were not organized; and I vowed that I would work to get the people organized in the community before model cities started. That way they would be eligible to get a lot of things they didn't know they were to receive.

After we began to get the people organized pretty good, then we felt a need for a formal organization. That's when The Mid-City Community Congress of Representatives came on board. We started working with St. Joseph Hospital, trying to revitalize the community that we live in. Then in 1968 we purchased the old St. Regis Hotel at 1400 Linwood and turned it into a senior citizens residential building for the elderly. We have done quite a lot of work in the community. Of course, I work in other phases of the community doing many different things—anywhere where I am needed.

Nurse: I know that you are very much involved.

Mrs. L.:   Anywhere that I feel I am needed. There is a need to help people, because you would be surprised the people that are not aware of the different things that are available to them. You think that they know, but they don't. For the last 4 years, I have worked within the paint-up program in the city. All the work I do is volunteer. I don't get a dime for anything that I do. I do get the satisfaction of knowing that I am helping somebody. God always blesses me in other ways. This past year, I think I got about 10 or 12 houses painted for elderly people that were not able to paint their homes. The city will give them the paint. If they are not able to paint it themselves, and if they qualify, you can get someone to paint it for them for free. I felt that was a pretty good record. So I have worked with that program pretty hard this past year.

I work also in the key coalition area. I am on the advisory committee there. There are just so many things that I do, I couldn't begin to name them all. I work also with the Harold Thomas Center, a reconciliation center named after our minister drowned in the 1979 flood and located at 3210 Michigan. Many agencies work out of that building. I have charge of the kitchen. I do the cooking for a lot of the Presbyterians when they have retreats and other functions. I do keep quite busy.

Then, I am on the Board of Directors for Mid-City Towers I and II, high-rises for inner-city elderly. We worked to get those buildings. We were turned down a number of times, but we didn't give up. We continued to put in our applications. Finally, we got it. We have beautiful buildings there. But I don't take up as much time at Mid-City Towers II as I do Mid-City Towers I. I feel a little closer to Mid-City Towers I.

Nurse: Because you fought so hard for it.

Mrs. L.: Yes! We had quite a hard time getting Mid-City Towers I, and in a different way from the time we had getting Mid-City Towers II. So, as I say, there are a lot of things that I do. I am always doing something.

Nurse: What would you say has motivated you to get that involved?

Mrs. L.: Well, I think really the need of the people! That has really motivated me to get involved because there are a lot of people that really don't know how to go about getting things. Not that I know a whole lot more, but I have had a little more experience in some of it. I think there is a need there for someone to help people that really don't know.

Nurse: How did you get that experience?

Mrs. L.: Well, I guess, just working. I can't say how I got it because I had no professional training. The only thing that seems clear is that it was my calling—because I do enjoy working with people and helping other people. I think that God has all of our lives planned for us. I just go on. I am kind of a go-getter! I don't give up very easily! You have to have something to do and that's what helps you. That's what helped me because I have to keep doing something. I can't sit and hold my hands. And that's what I try to tell the people at Mid-City Towers: they must not give up, because age doesn't mean anything. It's the way you feel inside, I think. There are a lot of people in their 80s that are doing beautiful work.

Nurse: That's right, that are very active and very healthy and have a good outlook on life.

Mrs. L.: That's right! And I think you have to have that outlook. You can't just give up and sit down. So that's what I try to do each day of my life. When I wake up I thank God and ask him to let me do some good today that I would feel that my living this day will not be in vain. So, that's just my life. It's just something I like to do and I don't mind doing. I am not afraid of work. Work doesn't bother me.

Nurse: You must have had some very beautiful parents that gave you this orientation of helping others and this faith in God.

Mrs. L.:   Well, I did! I can't say too much about my father because he died when I was quite young. But my mother was the type of person that liked to help other people. And I had some very beautiful grandparents.

Nurse: That you knew?

Mrs. L.:   Yes! My grandmother taught me a lot of things about life. Maybe that's where I got it. Just like the cooking, people say, "Oh, how do you do this? How can you do that for all those people?" I have cooked for 100 people at one time myself. I had help to serve it, but I did the cooking. For example, we had a fish and chicken dinner as a fund-raiser last week. It isn't a hard job for me because it is something that I like to do. If you enjoy whatever you are doing, it doesn't bother you. If you have to do something that you don't want to do, that's when it bothers you.

Nurse: For what purpose did you prepare that dinner?

Mrs. L.:   For their Christmas! We always give the elderly a little Christmas at Mid-City Towers. Everything has gone up so sky-high and money is quite tight with the government. It takes all of the monies that we get in to help keep up our buildings. I decided, instead of asking the management for money to give our people a little Christmas, that I would just plan this dinner. And we were very successful! There were a lot of people that I wasn't able to serve because I ran out of food, and it was getting late; I couldn't get the food that I wanted. I was quite tired. I get tired; but it doesn't bother me. If I can get home and get my rest, I am all right.

Nurse: I know that you are the president of the Mid-City Towers organization. Could you describe your duties?

Mrs. L.:   Well, as president of the organization, I have to talk to the tenants about different things and to the nurses. We have a nursing service, you know.

Nurse: Mid-City Towers I holds about how many tenants?

Mrs. L.:   We have 85 units there, really 88 persons because we have three couples who are married.

Nurse: And what are their age ranges?

Mrs. L.:   One or two people are around 62. I think the oldest person we have is 93 some years old. But we don't take them under 62 unless there is a reason. If they are handicapped in some way, we can't refuse them. That is really an independent living place and they are supposed to be able to look after themselves. When they get to the point where they can't, we

advise the family. That's when I have to come in sometimes
and call in the family with the resident manager and talk to
them. If they don't take them, then we advise that they be
put into a home or some place where they will get care. The
nurse comes once a week, as well as student nurses. But we
have nobody in the building that can look after the elderly at
all times. I prefer that the family takes them, but some
families do not want to be bothered. You know how that is.
It's just something that you have to deal with.

There are quite a lot of things to do, working with the
senior citizens. People think it's easy, but it isn't. It is quite a
burden on you sometimes. Because they can get kind of set in
their ways, which makes it kind of bad for us; but we have to
deal with them as best we can.

Nurse: Now, how do people learn about Mid-City Towers I and II?
Do you go out yourself and speak to groups?

Mrs. L.:   No! They advertise in the local papers, and a lot of people
hear about the building, and they always have a waiting list
of people who call in.

Nurse: Very good! So that brings a large number of names?

Mrs. L.:   That's right! And in those buildings we are supposed to have
so many white and so many black, any nationality.

Nurse: So there is no discrimination?

Mrs. L.:   There is no discrimination. We do have a white lady that has
been with us ever since we purchased the building. I get
along very nicely with the tenants. I don't make myself
common with them; but any time that they need anything,
need my help in any way, I am right there to help them. I
don't try, because I am president, to boss them. We have a
white managing agent who has been managing our building
for the past 2 years. I am very pleased with the progress that
has been made since they have taken over. To tell the truth,
my thinking is that that was the best thing that could have
happened. You know, sometimes a change is good! You need
a change. I think this is the best thing that could have
happened to us, because they have been able to accomplish
far more than we did during our trying to manage it. We
were very inexperienced. We didn't know, but we did pretty
good.

Nurse: The very fact that you got the building started is, I think, a
tremendous contribution.

Mrs. L.:   Yes!

Nurse: Now, I know that you have done a tremendous piece of work there as far as helping the black elderly to have a very nice home in their retirement years, their years of aging.

Mrs. L.:   Yes! We tried. I think most of the people that are there are quite happy. Of course, now times have changed quite a bit. There is a lot of vandalism, and that keeps us kind of upset. To hire a guard there costs so much money. So I hope and pray we will be able sometime in the near future to have someone there on duty as a guard 24 hours a day. That is what I would like to see before I jump down.

Nurse: Very good. Well, knowing you, Mrs. Lincoln, you definitely will get that goal achieved.

Mrs. L.:   Well, I hope we can.

Nurse: That's right. But you have a lot of hope—that I know.

Mrs. L.:   Well, I do. I think that's the only way you can go through life. You have to have hope that something good will happen. I try not to be a pessimist.

Nurse: And you are not! Let me ask you just several more questions. What practices do you use to maintain a hopeful and optimistic outlook on life? Now, you mentioned that you have a sense of hope for better things to come, but that must stem from something. What is that stemming from? What motivates you there?

Mrs. L.:   I really can't say what it is, but it is something there. It's got to be.

Nurse: That's right. Would you say it's your faith in God that good things are going to happen?

Mrs. L.:   It must be. I'm not a religious fanatic, but I do believe in prayer and faith. I think that if you have faith, you can overcome a lot of things. So, it must be my faith in God.

Nurse: That gives you that sense of zest for living. As you said, every day you wake up and thank God for another day to do some good.

Mrs. L.:   That's right! I try each day as I live to do something. It may not amount to much, but I try to do something that is worthwhile. And I feel in the evening that this day I haven't lived in vain.

Nurse: It gives you a sense of satisfaction that the strength that you have has been used for someone else.

Mrs. L.:   Yes! Something, someone else! Not that I have any more than anybody else, but I don't mind sharing what I have. If I had gone on to school and finished my education, I probably could have been far along; but I didn't. God has helped me to do the things that I do because I couldn't do them if He didn't.

Nurse: That's for sure! From what I know of you, Mrs. Lincoln, and what you have shared through this interview now, I would say that you have a tremendous faith dimension. Despite all odds, you just move right along even though you didn't have a lot of formal education. You educated yourself in what needs to be done and—

Mrs. L.: And I do quite a lot of reading. I think that has helped me a lot. I read an awful lot; all kinds of books and things. That has taught me a lot of things.

Nurse: Certainly! That you are a self-educated person.

Mrs. L.: You know, I must be, because I didn't finish my high school.

Nurse: That's right! You have the self-assurance of going out and asking questions where you need to to find out what needs to be done.

Mrs. L.: And I have to say that anything that I started out to do, I seem to be pretty successful in it. It has to be my calling!

Nurse: I think you are very right. I think that title is extremely valuable. It is a calling! It's much more like a vocation for you to do some things for others than just a job.

Mrs. L.: I feel that when I do things for other people that helps me in many ways.

Nurse: Yes, that's true! Well, one final question. What advice would you have for those of us who are aging to get to the point where you are now?

Mrs. L.: Just keep on working and having faith in God! You will make it.

Nurse: And you will make it. So, the idea of activity . . .?

Mrs. L.: Activity. Keep active, don't give up! You have to be involved. The way life is today, you have to be involved.

Nurse: That is very true! As you said, there are many people who have not been as blessed and don't understand what they can do to help themselves. They need others to help them.

Mrs. L.: That's right! Some of the people up there in our building have a good education, far more than I, but they just seem to give up. But you can't give up. You have to just keep fighting; eventually, you will come out on top.

Nurse: Very true! If I might just summarize, you are saying, then, those of us who are aging are to keep an open mind, keep involved, have a sense of motivation that something good will come out of our activities, put it into a prayer format, and to have faith in God. Would you say that those are the things that have helped you?

Mrs. L.:   That's right. Those are the things that have helped me.

Nurse: They have helped you to come to this point in life at 73 years of age where you have a lot of energy and are willing to do a lot for other people.

Mrs. L.:   And then another thing, I think, that has really helped me: I had a beautiful marriage, all the 57 years. I think we have had an understanding; and I have no complaints with my marriage at all. He has been a beautiful husband to me, and I hope, at least, I have tried to be a good wife to him. So I think that has helped me. Of course, we all have problems in life. I mean there is no perfection in life, and you don't go through life without having some problems. But I haven't had the marriage problems that some people have had. I think that's because of a lot of people are not happy. I am not an unhappy person. I don't let myself get unhappy. If I feel depressed, I start doing something or reading.

Nurse: And that helps balance things out so you can get a different perspective on life once again.

Mrs. L.:   That's right.

Nurse: Very good. Now, Mrs. Lincoln, this has been a wonderful opportunity to interact with you. I want to say, "Thank you very much." It has been extremely informative; and it will be very valuable in our classroom instruction for gerontological nursing students.

Mrs. L.:   You just tell them to just keep on, and whatever they do, keep getting their education. Just go as far as they can go because they are going to need it.

Nurse: That is very true! I wish you the very best of success in your endeavors and enjoyment of the aging process. Thank you so much.

Mrs. L.:   Thank you for asking me.

Summary

Life is for celebration! It is a gift to be enjoyed and cherished each day. To live life fully is to celebrate the wholeness of life. Celebrating the wholeness of life brings happiness, zest, vitality, enthusiasm, and gratitude to any life-style.

The interviews with two outstanding senior citizens highlight the potential and talent residing within each older person that needs actualization. To give respect and to allow dignity to each older person is to honor their very essence, their personhood, in its individuality and uniqueness. May each older person encountered in the health care system be given the opportunity to celebrate life in all dimensions. Life is to be lived and embraced fully.

References

At 91, woman celebrates each year with zest, The Kansas City Times, September 9, 1982.

Buscaglia, L.F.: Living, loving and learning, Thorofare, N.J., 1982, Charles B. Slack, Inc.

The test of time: why some marriages pass with flying colors, The Kansas City Star, July 5, 1982.

Wade, D.: Older couple may enjoy a special freedom in their relationship, Kansas City, Mo., June 30, 1982, The Kansas City Star.

Wahl, P.F.: Therapeutic relationships with the elderly, J. Gerontol. Nurs. **6**(5):260-266, 1980.

Chapter 9 Gerontological Nursing: the Emergence of a Specialty

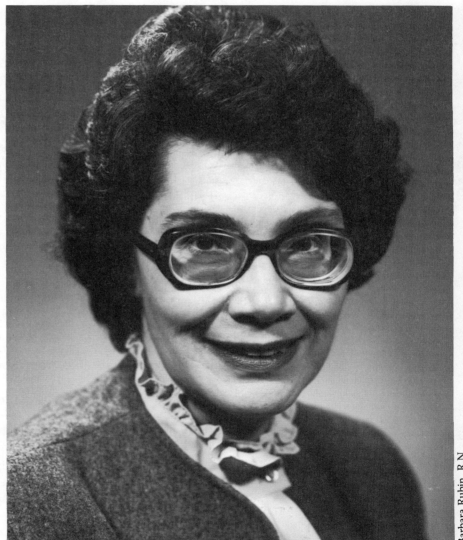

Barbara Rubin, R.N.

Nursing has always cared for older persons and for a variety of reasons is increasingly specializing in this area. In recent years, as societal awareness heightened regarding the population increase of citizens over 65, the nursing profession, recognizing the national trend toward specialization in other career fields as a result of increased knowledge, reviewed its role in providing quality care for older persons. In 1966 the American Nurses' Association (ANA), realizing its responsibility to the aged of the United States, pursued legitimizing the specialty of gerontological nursing. In this specialty professional nurses appreciate the complexities of the aging process and recognize the unique health care needs presented by older individuals in the hospital, home, or community.

Historical Development

Nursing is permeated with the living experiences of many persons who envisioned humanity's need for health care. Such a vision prompted Florence Nightingale to direct energies toward bettering the human condition through care and comfort, which extended far beyond the call to action in the Crimean War. She observed the insufficient knowledge about sanitation, causes of disease, and the constitution of an environment conducive to health promotion during those hectic days and nights spent with war-ravaged soldiers in a makeshift hospital, the first model of modern warfare's Mobile Army Supply Hospital (M.A.S.H.). This concern led Nightingale to seek ways to extend nursing action beyond the military environment to the larger civic community. It was her desire to promote the health and wellness of citizens throughout the world, beginning with her native land of England. Health decisions being made without systematic case findings and the poor quality of data collection, data analysis suggesting trends in disease, and scientific planning of interventions to correct health problems were appalling to her. As a direct response to this deficiency, Nightingale initiated a systematic investigation and presented a statistical report of her findings about conditions within the British Army to the Minister of Health (Kelly, 1981). This report presented facts about existing problems and recommendations pertinent to changes needed by the military establishment and its health care program. With this sophisticated approach, Nightingale, the first nurse researcher, attempted to improve client care and promote nursing as a scientific profession.

After the Crimean War Nightingale started implementing her visionary ideas by educating women in the art and science of nursing. Educating women through a formalized program was countercultural; women of her day were thought to have only one place in society: in the home as wife and mother. Consequently, Nightingale had to set high standards for women aspiring to the profession of nursing.

The nurse, as envisioned by Nightingale in her day, was to be an exemplar of capabilities, qualities, and knowledge. Quain, summarizing Nightingale's thought, gave the following description of the nurse in an 1883 document entitled *A Dictionary of Medicine:*

What a nurse is to be

A really good nurse must need be of the highest class of character. It need hardly be said that she must be—(1) Chaste, in the sense of the Sermon on the Mount; a good nurse should be the Sermon on the Mount in herself. It should naturally seem impossible to the most unchaste to utter even an immodest jest in her presence. Remember this great and dangerous peculiarity of nursing, and especially of hospital nursing, namely, that it is the only case, queens not excepted, where a woman is really in charge of men. And a really good trained ward "sister" can keep order in a men's ward better than a military ward-master or sergeant. (2) Sober, in spirit as well as in drink, and temperate in all things. (3) Honest, not accepting the most trifling fee or bribe from patients or friends. (4) Truthful—and to be able to tell the truth, and nothing but the truth. (5) Trustworthy, to carry out directions intelligently and perfectly, unseen as well as seen, 'to the Lord' as well as unto men—no mere eye-service. (6) Punctual to a second and orderly to a hair—having everything ready and in order before she begins her dressings or her work about the patient; nothing forgotten. (7) Quiet, yet quick, quick without hurry; gentle without slowness; discreet without self-importance; no gossip. (8) Cheerful; hopeful; not allowing herself to be discouraged by unfavourable symptoms; not given to depress the patient by anticipations of an unfavourable result. (9) Cleanly to the point of exquisiteness, both for the patient's sake and her own; neat and ready. (10) Thinking of her patient and not of herself, 'tender over his occasions' or wants, cheerful and kindly, patient, ingenious and neat.*

Nightingale, desirous of promoting these qualities in nursing practitioners, initiated the nursing profession in 1860 (Kelly, 1981) by establishing a school of nursing in St. Thomas Hospital, London, England, a separate but distinct unit from the hospital proper, for educational purposes. Learning, not service, was the primary orientation of Nightingale's nursing school. Her concern was for the care and cure of acutely ill hospitalized patients as well as for the maintenance of their health after discharge.

People of all ages, whether sick or well, were to be cared for by nurses, according to Nightingale. From this beginning a variety of approaches of nursing practice began to emerge, including those for the care of older persons. As noted previously, it was not until the twentieth century that this orientation was known as gerontological nursing, the newest of nursing's clinical specialties.

To appreciate the development of gerontological nursing it is important to understand the models of nursing as perceived by Nightingale and as modified when implemented in the United States in the late 1800s and

*From Kelly, L.Y.: Dimensions of professional nursing, ed. 3, New York, copyright © 1981, Macmillan, Inc.

early 1900s. Many societal factors influenced nursing's development and produced effects that are still evident. Reviewing the models gives a perspective to the development of clinical specialties within the ranks of professional nursing.

Models of Nursing: Nightingale and American

A model is a schematic outline of a series of constructs depicting the universality of an idea or theory. Each component of the model provides input to the comprehensiveness of its design that, when viewed in light of the total scheme, presents insight into the idea or theory. The purpose of the model, then, is to aid understanding of the complexities of ideas. Each segment of the model is presented in a logical, well-organized fashion. Whether viewed singly or intermeshed with all components, each model's segment provides a method of determining the completeness of the purported concept; and, in the contrast of one idea against another in several models, the differences in theory application in various circumstances are seen. In using the model approach to content presentation, commonalities and differences can easily be defined and evaluated in terms of outcomes. Numerous models that promote theory development, organizational design, and nursing practice styles exist in nursing. A review of the Nightingale and American models of nursing aids in understanding societal forces that have influenced nursing generally and gerontological nursing specifically.

Nightingale believed at its initial inception that nursing should be distinct and totally different from its medical counterpart. Her orientation to nursing included such concepts as "health nursing," which included preventive care, and "sick nursing," the care of the ill. She had a client-care orientation and a holistic approach to the role of the nurse; moreover, her nursing process emphasized a scientific approach, not purely the technical aspects of care. When she began modern nursing in 1860 at St. Thomas Hospital in England (Kelly, 1981), Nightingale had a distinct set of eligibility criteria for student admittees. Her educational model for professional nursing included the following tenets:

1. Nursing educators and students carefully selected
2. Nursing taught and controlled by nurses
3. Autonomous and financially independent nursing schools
4. Careful contractual agreements with clinical facilities for purpose of clinical skill training
5. Research-oriented teaching faculty
6. Provision for continuing education and upgrading practice (Lysaught, 1981)

The concept of nursing spread; it was brought to America and implemented in three hospitals in 1873: the Belleview Training School in New York City, the Connecticut Training School in Hartford, and the Boston Training School in the Massachusetts General Hospital (Kelly, 1981). Conditions in the United States were such that a more expedient approach to training nurses was needed; consequently, the concepts of nursing education promulgated by Nightingale were modified considerably. The American adaptations of the Nightingale model of nursing education emerged from prevailing conditions, such as

1. Scarcity of qualified educators; little selectivity of students
2. Nurses nominally in charge of program but obligated to hospitals
3. Nursing schools neither autonomous nor financially independent
4. Student nurse services required by hospitals in exchange for educational experiences and based on institutional needs
5. Little or no research orientation; emphasis on pragmatic skills
6. Little or no provision for education beyond basic preparation*

Nursing education for Nightingale was to be fully under the control of nursing and in the hands of qualified nursing instructors. American adaptation of that model placed more emphasis on a service commitment to the institution that controlled the educational unit through financing. This situation produced a limitation on the education of nursing students because it focused on illness rather than health.

Nursing practice, flowing from the adapted American nursing educational programs, also took on a practice style very foreign to the Nightingale concept. This practice style for the most part has continued in modern times. The nursing practice models have the following commonalities and differences:

Nightingale model	American adaptation
1. Holistic approach to role	1. Task-oriented approach to role
2. Client-centered orientation	2. Institution-centered orientation
3. Two-component system of care a. Health nursing (preventive care) b. Sick nursing (care of the ill)	3. One-component system of care: sick nursing (care of the ill)—based on medical service model
4. Nursing process emphasized as a scientific approach	4. Nursing process emphasized as a reactive process in response to physician orders and institutional regulations

These models (Lysaught, 1981) demonstrate the contrast of a client-oriented, holistic approach to nursing as perceived by Nightingale to a task-oriented, illness focus with nursing's major responsibility being the execution of physician orders and implementation of the institution's regu-

*From Lysaught, J.: Action in affirmation: toward an unambiguous profession, New York, 1981, McGraw-Hill Book Co.

lations. In the American adaptation, control of nursing practice rests outside of nursing; nurses are viewed as employees of the institution.

The comparison of the two models of nursing practice provides a frame of reference for discussing the newly emerging specialty of gerontological nursing. Nurses in the past who worked with the elderly were for the most part products of the American system of nursing education and practice. Elderly clients were viewed as sick and decrepit. This approach to nursing practice is called geriatric nursing (nursing of the ill elderly) in modern nursing.

Historically the elderly became a publicly acknowledged group with special needs with the introduction of Social Security in 1935. Retirement was forced on many older persons who were economically unprepared to live without a work income. A new group was formed—the retired elderly—without jobs or hope for the future. This situation for the most part continues today. Many older citizens, although now allowed to work until the age of 70, are not able to meet the economic demands of daily living. As a result they must often resort to living arrangements not to their liking and seek health care in a variety of settings. When all other options are closed to them, the elderly often view the health care centers, usually called "nursing homes," as the only source of comfort open to them. Once admitted to the health care center, the nursing personnel may not be the competent professionals they had hoped to see; oftentimes the staff consists of unlicensed persons who have not had any special training in the aging process and do not understand the unique health care needs of the older person. As a result, the older person suffers from their insufficiency of knowledge. Even if the professional nurse has completed a baccalaureate educational program in nursing, there is no assurance that the aging process was included in it. This lack of preparation engenders an attitude that anyone can take care of the elderly—that all they need is tender loving care. For this reason and many more, nurses decided there was a need to establish a professional group within the ANA that would focus on the health needs of the elderly.

When the delegates at the 1966 convention of the ANA in San Francisco voted on establishing five divisions of nursing practice in its organizational structure (Davis, 1968), a Division for Geriatric Nursing was included. This was a significant decision because for the first time the nursing profession was recognizing that older persons in the United States were to be given the same consideration for their health care needs as other age groups. Nurses who had been working with the elderly in a variety of settings, such as nursing homes and retirement centers, cheered the decision. It gave them a renewed sense of commitment and a feeling that they no longer were to be considered second-rate nurses because of their care for the elderly in this youth-oriented society. It projected geriatric nursing into the arena of professional nursing, in which improvements in care could be formally regulated and enforced.

The division's elected officers and ANA staff continued the work of promoting the health and welfare of the elderly begun earlier within the ANA by conference groups and interested nurses. With the division as a structural unit established within the national organization (Davis, 1968) the specific and unique health care needs of the elderly population could be focused on with greater intensity, and outcomes of those efforts could be given greater recognition throughout the nursing profession.

A particular need emerged immediately within the Division of Geriatric Nursing to formulate a philosophy that would serve as a guide for the division in pursuing its goals, which included the following:

1. To improve and advance the practice of geriatric nursing
2. To develop nurses in this new specialty professionally

The first philosophic statement read:

> Registered nurses are responsible for meeting the nursing needs of all people regardless of age. The increasing numbers of individuals in the older age group must be a concern of all registered nurses if this segment of our population is to receive appropriate nursing care.
>
> Geriatric nursing is concerned with the assessment of nursing needs of older people; planning and implementing nursing care to meet these needs; and evaluating the effectiveness of such care to achieve and maintain a level of wellness consistent with the limitations imposed by the aging process.
>
> Geriatric nursing practice requires the application of advanced knowledge and research in the fields of nursing and gerontology. Such knowledge provides the basis for continuous improvements of arts and skills of nursing in this area of practice.

This statement (Davis, 1968) heralded a new beginning for the emerging specialty. Since this statement was issued, the membership in the Division of Geriatric Nursing, now titled Division of Gerontological Nursing (so titled to emphasize the wellness and health status of the elderly rather than just illness), is ever increasing. Nurses are responding to the call of society to care for elderly citizens wherever they may be found—in homes, nursing homes, health care centers, adult day care centers, retirement villages, senior citizen centers, or hospitals. Nursing education programs are beginning to develop and teach courses on the aging process with a focus on health maintenance and promotion and, in the practice setting, on completing health assessments of the elderly. More qualified nursing personnel are now being employed by health care centers. Nursing care of the aging has decidedly improved over the last 5 to 10 years.

Another organization was established by the ANA in 1979 called the Council of Nursing Home Nurses. This group was formed to meet the specific needs of nurses employed in nursing homes. Many administrative and resource problems (finances, staffing patterns) face this group of dedicated nurses who desire to provide quality care to institutionalized older persons. The Council of Nursing Home Nurses interacts closely with the Division of Gerontological Nursing in promoting the health and welfare of all older individuals in society.

Standards of Gerontological Nursing Practice

Following the formal acceptance of the philosophic statement by the members of the Division of Gerontological Nursing, the need was raised to develop standards for the newly emerged nursing specialty, to measure quality of care and practice. For nurses to upgrade care for the elderly, in both the institution and the community, it soon became apparent that some uniformity of nursing practice would be beneficial to the elderly. The Division of Gerontological Nursing Practice prepared the *Standards of Gerontological Nursing Practice* in 1976. These standards are measurable guidelines for implementing the nursing process specifically with the elderly person, and they include the participation of the older adult and family. These standards are a legal document. They are rapidly becoming the legal and moral measure for assessing reasonable care for the elderly when lawsuits are filed against health professionals in nursing. The standards are extremely vital to gerontological nursing and are worthy of study by all nurses working with older adults. For example, when an elderly client is admitted to a health care setting, all aspects of health status must be explored; otherwise poor nursing care planning ensues and makes nursing outcomes questionable. Each standard as it appears in the ANA booklet is given with a discussion of its implications for the nursing care of elderly persons.

> **Standard I.** Data are systematically and continuously collected about the health status of the older adult. The data are accessible, communicated and reported.*

This guideline presents key words in the overall initial assessment of the older adult. The word *data* indicates that the information obtained by the professional nurse is treated as scientific information to be studied, evaluated, and interpreted, from which inferences can be formulated regarding the elderly person and his or her demonstrated needs. These data provide insights into the personality type, cultural or ethnic background, health habits, beliefs, and goals of the elderly person, and are reviewed

*Standards I-VI from American Nurses' Association, Division of Gerontological Nursing: Standards of gerontological nursing practice, Kansas City, Mo., 1976, ANA.

often in the interaction of nurse and client for promotion of health. *Systematic* refers to the nurse's possession of the necessary knowledge and skill to thoroughly assess the condition of the elderly person. Using a systems approach in the assessment phase of the nursing process, the nurse is able to detect any deviation (for instance, neurological, cardiovascular, or respiratory) from what is found in healthily functioning older persons in all the bodily systems—physical, social, psychological, and spiritual. *Continuously collected* suggests that since the older person's condition changes daily, current, updated information must be gathered by the professional nurse if accurate care is to be given the person. Outdated or inaccurate information on the older person's health status may constitute negligence. The elderly client controls the information about health status; the self-report of health conditions is paramount in soliciting such information. To perform otherwise would be unprofessional and infringe on the rights of the individual.

If the individual elderly person is unable to communicate information about the health status, responsibility for it moves to the family members. It is essential that knowledgeable persons be contacted to obtain pertinent information before any nursing care other than emergency measures is initiated. Knowledge is power. To know who the elderly person is in all facets of his or her life places the professional nurse in a key position to coordinate all aspects of medical care, supportive care, and nursing care. Errors in clinical judgment are consequently reduced as accurate information about the client's condition is shared by multidisciplinary team members.

Standard I alludes to the accessibility, communicability, and recording of data and is a crucial guideline for the professional nurse. The last portion of Standard I relates to the need for accurate and comprehensive documentation of information, gathered during the initial assessment period and each day thereafter for as long as the client is receiving care in the formal health care system. Legally the professional nurse must preserve all pertinent information in written form so it may be used to provide continuity of care in the nurse's absence. This standard lays the foundation for the remainder of the nursing process, depicted in the following standards.

Standard II. Nursing diagnoses are derived from the identified normal responses of the individual to aging and the data collected about the health status of the older adult.

This normative statement identifies the aging process as a normal part of the life span and recognizes the uniqueness of the process to each individual. *Nursing* alludes to the professional nurse's framework of caring, compassion, and empathy in the assessment of the health care practices of the older person. Another word, *diagnosis*, refers to the utilization of a systematic orientation for the categorization of symptoms relevant to a complete data base and nursing care plan formulation. *Normal responses* indicate that a wide range of responses are acceptable behavior for the older person, which do not deserve the stigma "abnormal" simply because the older person perceives health practices differently than the younger person. *Health status* suggests that each older person has a definition of health. Health includes a wide range of components that must be explored with the older person to obtain insight into a specific health status. With this information nursing specialists may proceed with the nursing care of the elderly person based on a scientific and valid foundation.

Standard III. A plan of nursing care is developed in conjunction with the older adult and/or significant others that includes goals derived from the nursing diagnosis.

This standard suggests the need of the nurse to place all information before the older person and the family or significant others so that they can understand the health status, needs and strengths, approaches to resolving the needs, and the need for compliance with any plans projected. The nurse knows the importance of compliance with the formulated plans, not only by the client but by the family or significant others. Through such health teaching the family become more aware of the health conditions requiring attention, thus increasing their involvement in the total plan of care. This approach places the responsibility for compliance with the plan on the elderly client and the family or significant others and gets input into the plan from the older person, the family, and the nurse. Personal responsibility for health care and independence become more real. With this approach the goals agreed on by client, family, and nurse will be realistic and attainable and have measurable results. Without this type of involvement difficulties arise caused by lack of understanding. With involvement a comprehensive care plan can be formulated, implemented, and monitored.

Standard IV. The plan of nursing care includes priorities and prescribed nursing approaches and measures to achieve the goals derived from the nursing diagnosis.

The key word in this statement is *priorities*. When the older client and the family or significant others become participants in planning health practices, priorities are essential since many aspects of the health status totality become obvious to the client and nurse. When the client perceives what the priorities should be, the nurse can begin to develop an appropriate plan of care. Priorities of care that the nurse perceives may not be the priorities of the client or the family. The preplanning phase and the actual planning is critical to a plan of care being implemented precisely as formulated. Nursing measures to ensure progress toward gaining health are also important for concrete progress in achieving the projected goals; this approach promotes a high motivation in the client to continue toward the goals set. This team approach makes favorable outcomes more likely.

Standard V. The plan of care is implemented, using appropriate nursing actions.

Execution of the health plan requires a depth of knowledge and skill in the gerontological nurse specialist. Creative and innovative approaches not only are necessary to gain the confidence of the elderly person and the family but ensure favorable outcomes. Implementation requires the following:

1. An excellent rapport between the client and the nurse
2. Clinical competence in interviewing techniques
3. Evaluation techniques that provide data for the reassessment of goals and insight into the dynamics of the implementation of the nursing care plan

The evolving dynamics must be continually assessed to improve the health of older persons.

Standard VI. The older adult and/or significant other(s) participate in determining the progress attained in the achievement of established goals.

Evaluation of progress is extremely important when the client is an older person. Subtle changes may occur almost daily, which require the nurse to be attuned to the client's condition constantly. Nursing care plans must be flexible to remain feasible, and it is crucial that the client, who remains the key initiator and recipient of care, be informed constantly about his or her condition, physical, psychological, sociological and spiritual, so that the client's mind-set is always positively directed. The final result of such monitoring and evaluation is the optimum functioning and well-being of the client (Bahr, 1981).

The Standards of Gerontological Nursing Practice are essential legal entities that aid the elderly client and nurse in supplying quality care in a variety of settings. This document has incorporated in it the Code of Ethics for Nurses (ANA, 1976); it states that each older individual has the right to competent care performed by qualified nursing personnel.

The legal aspects of gerontological nursing care are crucial in the accountability of the gerontological clinical nurse specialist to the older client. A discussion on the legal aspects of gerontological nursing must emphasize the development of the legal system within nursing through nurse practice acts and their effects on each nurse in a clinical setting.

Nurse Practice Acts: the Legal Aspects of Gerontological Nursing

Since 1913 nursing leaders have believed that those who choose nursing as a profession should have legal rights. Society demands safe practitioners in any profession. When the first nurse practice act was passed by the legislative body of North Carolina, it was deemed a breakthrough for the profession. The early leaders in nursing perceived the importance of formal requirements for individuals wishing to pursue nursing as a career. For such a general public service major requirements must be imposed to protect the public from unqualified individuals (Kelly, 1981).

Each state has a nurse practice act within the purview of the legislative body. Each act contains the requirements set for professional nurses by that state's board of nursing. The acts define nursing and identify the requirements of educational programs for prospective nurse recruits, requirements for licensure and relicensure, and descriptions of legal aspects for prosecution (such as torts, felonies, negligence, and fee statements). A nurse practice act is the legal statement that governs nursing within a state jurisdiction. Consequently, the ANA comments that:

The primary purpose of a licensing law for the control of the practice of nursing is to protect the health of the people by establishing minimum standards which qualified practitioners must meet. Principles of Legislation Relating to Nursing Practice, ANA, New York, Rev. January 1958 (Creighton, 1975).

The main point of this statement is that the licensing law is for the protection of the public. The public, encountering a professional licensed nurse in whatever setting, should be ensured of a qualified, competent nurse who has the health interests and the personhood of the individual as the top priority. This brings us to a question: what legal requirements affect the gerontological nurse specialist?

Historically in the United States taking care of the elderly has not been viewed in a positive light. It has already been observed that the elderly are usually viewed as nonproductive citizens who require a minimum of facilities, personnel, and resources since they are no longer a vital labor force and contribute little to the economy or the citizenry of the country. In the past, when this attitude was even more entrenched, poor farms and almshouses were established in places remote from the vital centers of activity and population. We recall driving past a poor farm in the early 1940s that was under the auspices of the rural county government and described as the last resort for the elderly who could no longer maintain themselves financially. The large, long building on a huge expanse of land appeared isolated, and little activity was seen in the yard. Scant effort was given to beautifying the grounds with flowers, trees, or other landscaping. The building just sat there, a monument to the old. Little attention was given to the qualifications of personnel hired to attend to the elderly adults' needs; they were mostly lay individuals who needed a job, and the easiest place to acquire employment was in the poor farm. Legal aspects of care were not a major consideration at that time.

That picture has not changed a great deal. Instead of poor farms and almshouses, facilities known as "nursing homes," "long-term care settings" and "health centers" are prevalent. With federal government regulations in effect, some improvement has occurred, primarily in the quality of buildings housing the elderly; but there has been little improvement in the quality of personnel caring for the elderly. There are no legal qualifications for nursing personnel who work with the elderly that specifically require an academic preparation. Nursing homes that qualify for Medicare payments are required only to have a professional registered nurse on call 24 hours. This nurse is not required to minister to the elderly but merely to be available for decision making in crises. No stipulations are made in the Medicare law that the registered nurse in charge of the elderly attain a particular level of education or have any preparation in gerontological nursing. The present legal status of nursing care in long-term care facilities can generally be considered on extremely hazardous grounds. An example of this situation is an investigation currently being undertaken in the southern region of the United States. Nurses in a large long-term care facility with a longstanding reputation for providing only custodial care are being sued for negligence: The major complaint expressed by family members in the lawsuit is the occurrence of decubitus ulcers among many of the elderly clients. This lawsuit, if won in the courts, will have a far-reaching impact on the legal qualifications for nursing home personnel, particularly the nursing staff.

Furthermore a national research study funded by Kellogg and under the joint sponsorship of the American Nurses' Foundation and College of Nursing Home Administrators is seeking strategies to upgrade the knowledge and skill of nurse administrators (directors of nursing) in long-term care facilities. This study, when completed, should provide guidelines and regulations regarding employment of qualified nursing service directors (who give leadership to the nursing personnel for quality care to elderly clients).

What should the legal requirements of gerontological nursing be? To ensure the rights of the elderly to adequate, safe, and competent care as designated in the document prepared by the Federal Council on Aging (1976), it seems appropriate to require, by law, that each health care facility open to the public for care of the elderly have a clinical specialist in gerontological nursing on its staff. In many instances the required staffing pattern for the health care facility may be similar to that of a well-staffed acute care unit of a hospital, since many of the elderly in highly volatile conditions demand specialization of the health care personnel. These clinical specialists should have an accredited master's degree in nursing. Content for a concentration in gerontological nursing should include supervised clinical practicum, which gives the professional nurse the opportunity to utilize models of nursing care based on nursing theory; development of research methods appropriate to the aging population; identification and research of the unique clinical problems confronting the elderly; and understanding of the aging process and the personhood of the elderly individual in all domains: affective, cognitive, and psychomotor. To meet the legal requirements of the specialty the gerontological nursing specialist must be a highly competent and knowledgeable health care provider.

The second legal requirement of gerontological nursing should be that the standard of care utilized in the health care facility meet the ANA's Standards of Gerontological Nursing Practice. Each facility is encouraged to adopt these standards formally as measurements for the evaluation of care. Lawyers are becoming aware of the existence of the standards and are using them in depositions obtained from nurses regarding care in institutions undergoing litigation. Every nurse should not only be aware of the standards but make a commitment to use them as the basis for nursing care plans. The integrity of nursing care for older adults depends on the continual improvement of care and the involvement of client and family in the overall compliance of that care. When each facility makes a commitment to pursue quality health care for the elderly client and uses the legal means to acquire that quality, gerontological nursing will have truly emerged as a clinical specialty making an impact on the health status of elderly adults.

Necessity for Health and Wellness: the Self-care Approach for Older Adults

Until relatively recently the main focus of health care was on sickness. The prevailing attitude was that citizens of the United States have a right to health care but no responsibility for their health status. Consequently a large number of health facilities are in existence to accommodate the many people who, because of limited knowledge of health practices, have lived unhealthy life-styles. What we see now in the elderly population is the consequence of those life-styles: acute and chronic illnesses requiring a large portion of the federal and state dollars to provide hospital care, nursing home care, and community health support systems and services. Home health care agencies for the most part serve the elderly populations of our cities; nursing home beds have far outstripped hospital beds within recent years. It is important to realize that personal responsibility for health care has definite consequences in the future. It has been noted that the practices of youth become apparent as one ages. Accidents, bad nutritional habits, little or no exercise, irregularity of sleep patterns, inability to cope with stress, lung abuse, occupational and environmental hazards—all make a mark on the physical, psychological, and spiritual health of the older person.

The trend, however, is slowly beginning to change as more research into health practices demonstrates the positive outcomes of good life-styles. With promotion of healthful living becoming more prominent in the literature for health professionals, professional groups are beginning to teach the lay public about sound health practices. To live healthfully is no longer seen as a fad; it is becoming a necessity as costs of hospitalization and institutionalization escalate beyond all expectation. Health is an investment, having great economic benefits for both the individual and society.

Health is a highly complex concept connoting a homeostatic balance of the body for promotion of such activities as life-support, work, and play. Health is more than absence of illness; it is a positive force energizing every moment of one's existence, regardless of activity performance. When one is healthy, no challenge to the human body is unmet. Health is necessary to meet life's goals.

In addition to a baseline health state, in recent years different degrees of health have been defined. These different degrees are seen on a continuum of health throughout the life span. Kinlein notes that for the most part individuals are born with health if they have been initiated in excellent health practices by the mother throughout pregnancy. As time passes, brief or prolonged episodes of illness may take place, but the main thrust is always toward a healthy state—a wellness state (Fig. 9-1).

Fig. 9-1. **Health continuum.**

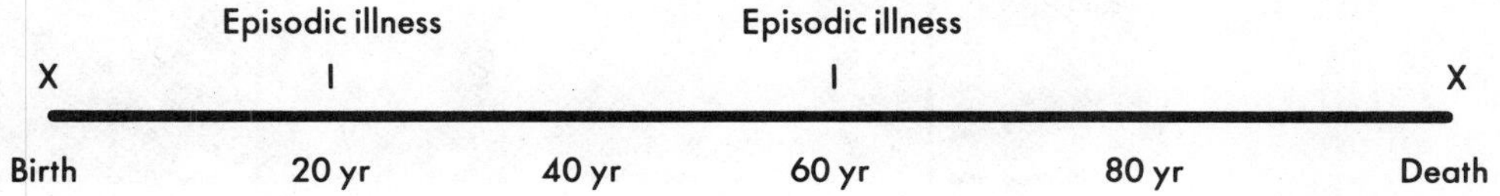

From presentation at First International Assembly of Kinlein Care, Milwaukee, August 1980.

Wellness is described by Dunn (1973) as composed of levels: low, medium, and high. To Dunn, wellness is a rich and comprehensive concept of health based on the integration of mind, body, and spirit. In this holistic orientation each realm of the person contributes to wellness; conversely, each realm, if not progressing toward self-actualization, contributes to a nonwell state. Health enthusiasts embrace this concept of wellness in prescribing therapeutic protocols, such as stress management, body and mind relaxation techniques, nutritional prescriptions, exercise programs, and social interactional schemes. In other words, all components of the human person must be properly cared for if wellness is to be achieved and maintained. Many are now embracing this concept of wellness by assuming responsibility for health care. High-level wellness is necessary for the high-level energy to achieve personhood (Fig. 9-2).

In gerontological nursing wellness of the elderly client is becoming important in formulating nursing care plans. As seen in the discussion of the ANA's Standards of Practice, wellness begins with the elderly client's independent decision-making in his or her own plan of care. This approach fosters energy input into making plans for a healthy life-style,

Fig. 9-2. *Left,* **Kathy Bock, MN, Gerontological Clinical Nurse Specialist;** *right,* **Mary Harrell, participant in the health enrichment program, Shepherd Center, Kansas City, Missouri.**

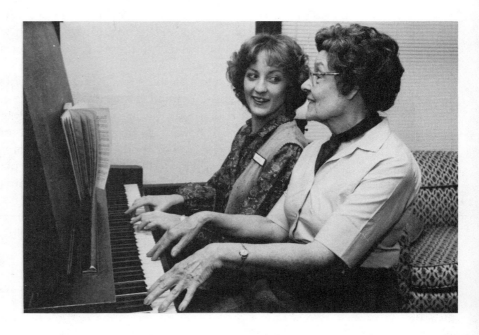

ready and voluntary participation by the elderly in establishing those plans, and evaluating energy put toward the plan. The older client realizes that wellness is initiated with the commitment to it, and continued only by compliance with an established regimen. With personal responsibility the open system of energy within the body continues to be activated, creating more energy as the person perceives its need and utilization. The priorities become initiators and motivators toward continued wellness and optimum functioning.

A major factor that has hampered the acceptance of self-care by the elderly is lack of knowledge. Through health teaching the older client becomes capable of directing his or her own health care. This major service provided by the gerontological clinical nurse specialist facilitates health promotion and maintenance. Wellness practices demand knowledge, skill, and competence in the clinical specialist who must, through his or her own health demonstration, be a health model for the older client. Such a model exemplifies commitment to health. The elderly are impelled to emulate a friend, educator, helper, and confidante.

Wellness, a modern trend-setting concept, is revolutionizing the care of older persons in the community setting. Many programs with wellness as the focus continue to be implemented in senior citizen centers, community service centers, and nursing homes. These activities are increasingly attended and enjoyed by the elderly participants. Fewer palliative measures are needed by the elderly, since their bodies respond positively to the life-style changes; better nutritional and exercise status is evident as bodily functions are actively engaged; and consequently they are more fulfilled and happy. The concept of a healthy older person is imperative to counter the stereotypical picture of the ill and decrepit old adult.

Gerontological nurses can be the pioneers in enhancing the older person's life. This challenge demands an understanding of the roles of the gerontological nursing clinical specialist in the realm of nursing practice.

Gerontological Nursing: Roles in Supporting Older Individuals

At the ANA convention of 1980 the Division of Gerontological Nursing Executive Board presented a draft of the *Statement on the Scope and Practice of Gerontological Nursing* for discussion and comment. This document is an attempt to clarify and amplify various role definitions inherent in the care of the elderly by the gerontological clinical nurse specialist. Many roles are enumerated, including those of educator, researcher, and health promoter. The major roles related to the support of older individuals include advocate, change agent, and leader; these terms need defining.

Advocate

The term advocate is defined as "one who pleads another's cause," or "one who argues or pleads for a cause or proposal" (Webster, 1965). The gerontological nurse specialist–advocate is beginning to enhance life for older persons of the United States. In the 1981 White House Conference on Aging professional nurses were viewed as advocates of the elderly in numerous ways. For example, professional assistance at the conference was provided whenever the need arose by (1) the establishment of sufficient health care centers for the elderly; (2) work with elderly committee members in the development and presentation of resolutions that addressed the health care needs of the elderly; (3) dissemination of health information so older persons were informed of the latest scientific findings in relation to the status of normal aging and of the rights of the elderly to health care; (4) promotion of elderly delegates' self-esteem by supporting their oral presentations in committee work and on the conference floor; and (5) advocacy of the elderly in the highly political environment, ensuring that the major cause for the conference would not be jeopardized and that the elderly would be prevented from becoming a burden on society by an inability to gain their rightful place among the citizenry (Banknecht, 1982).

The gerontological nurse serves as an advocate on the state and local level by becoming involved in the legislative and ethical issues facing older persons. The nurse, by being informed of the vast number of issues confronting the elderly in their daily lives, serves as the spokesperson, friend, colleague, and professional health promoter of the elderly. By involvement in state and local committees on aging the nurse becomes a powerful voice in policy decisions that aid in filling gaps in program provisions. These gaps may be in health or basic needs (such as housing, nutrition, transportation, supportive services in home, or any other life-giving service). Since nurses know the needs of older persons, they should act as their advocates at the national as well as the local levels toward achieving a better quality of life for them.

On the local level gerontological nurses in both institutional and community-based practice settings perform the advocacy role by upgrading the care of all elderly persons—well or in need of high-level intensive care nursing. Custodial care, a remnant of earlier years, can no longer be tolerated in contemporary times. High-level wellness means achieving goals in all dimensions, regardless of age. The elderly must be participants in their health care plans as stipulated by the *Standards of Gerontological Nursing Practice.*

In addition, the nurse assists in teaching other professionals about the unique needs of the elderly so that accurate scientific information is incorporated into whatever administrative policies and procedures are initiated within institutions and community-based health care centers. Nurses continue to play a vital role in improving the health care delivery

Change Agent

system for older adults, and the advocacy role is essential for further progress.

Along with the role of advocate, the gerontological nurse becomes the change agent in situations meriting change in life-style and living situations. Change, according to Bennis, Benne, and Chin (1969), necessitates movement of various parts of a complex organization: persons, places, and resources. To be a change agent, the gerontological nurse specialist must understand the dynamics of the change process. This process is initiated only after the situation or episode needing change has been thoroughly analyzed. In initiating change the gerontological nurse specialist must be assured that all involved personnel understand its purpose, target period, and methods. They should also know what evaluative measures will be used to examine the results.

An example of how the change agent role can be put into effect is given by one gerontological nurse specialist, who had completed her master's degree in nursing with a concentration in gerontological nursing. This nurse, on completion of her master's in nursing degree program, became clinical director of nursing in a county health care institution for the elderly that was based on the philosophy of custodial care. This nurse found that all of the elderly were confined to their beds, force-fed, and deprived of all decision-making powers. In addition, she found that the older persons committed to this institution were perceived by the staff to be nonentities, nonpersons. In assessing the situation, the nurse found that no philosophy of gerontological nursing existed; that the in-service education programs did not emphasize the personhood of the individual older person; and that the administrator believed that the state would not fund anything other than the traditional custodial approach. The nurse discovered, however, that a listening ear could be found for the need to upgrade the care. She figured out how the state would save money in the long run by keeping the elderly more independent, concerned about their own health status, and interested in life. This point of economy was acceptable to the state officials, and the nurse began the change process. Through education, role-modeling, and resource identification the nurse emphasized that institutionalization did not mean the older person had lost the right to independence, decision-making, and participation in life events. After 6 months the staff and administrator were ready to implement the new nursing approach. Resident councils were initiated, with the elderly electing their own spokespersons to lead discussions and make decisions about life in the institution. Nursing staff implemented the nursing care plan, which included calling each older person by their title (such as "Mrs. Jones" instead of "Maggie" or "Grandma"); orienting them to the time of day and date in greeting them; helping them to feed themselves while dressed and sitting in a chair if at all possible; assisting them to participate in making their own health care plan and contracts for their health status; and allowing the elderly to enhance the environment, making the agency their home rather than a cold, austere institution. This latter phase was carried out by allowing the residents to paint murals of their choice on the walls in the halls; to choose paint colors for lounge rooms, dining rooms, and resident rooms; to rearrange furniture in resident rooms and bring in their own furniture pieces; and to introduce ethnic food choices on the menu and to have a kitchenette in resident living areas so residents could cook or bake a favorite food occasionally. In other words it became a home where their independence was supported by the staff. The staff helped bring about the changes suggested by the residents. The nursing staff became accountable to the residents, not vice versa.

The transformation of this institution has been incredible. The elderly are more alive and dynamic. The staff have made a deeper commitment to the elderly and do not view their work as a job but see themselves as partners in the well-being of the elderly adults under their care. Because the psychological, physical, social, and spiritual condition of each older person has improved so dramatically, the cost of care has been reduced substantially. The gerontological clinical nurse specialist demonstrated that the role of change agent is important in the provision of quality care to older citizens.

All nurses who have earned the title of gerontological clinical nurse specialist must assume the role of change agent because of the vast amount of work essential to bring needed changes to places where the elderly live and are cared for. A change agent is necessary in creating a more healthful, useful existence for many older persons who seek the assistance of the professional nurse in a variety of settings.

Leader   Leadership in gerontological nursing is of major importance for the vitalizing of that emerging specialty and the upgrading of care for the elderly in society. Elements of leadership are found in a variety of nursing styles. Each individual nurse has an effect on personnel in the strategies for achievement of goals.

Attitude of staff. In terms of leadership the gerontological clinical nursing specialist enjoys a special challenge because of society's and professional nurses' attitude toward the older population. This attitude may become the primary obstacle standing in the way of the leadership offered by the gerontological nurse. In assessing nursing personnel the clinical specialist must observe the subtleties of negative attitudes toward older persons in many areas: the philosophy of the care practices carried out by the nursing staff, the manner in which the elderly are treated, and the way the elderly are communicated with and about in nursing reports, nursing rounds, and conferences. If a negative attitude prevails, the clinical specialist must seek ways to change it to a positive, humane orientation toward elderly adults; this more professional approach is helpful in ministering to the needs of the elderly. Strategies that may be used to bring about a more positive attitude include the following:

1. In-service education stressing the rights of the older adult (for example, those put forth by the Federal Council on Aging, 1976)
2. Provision of instructional material on primary and secondary changes of aging
3. Instruction on *A Statement on the Scope of Gerontological Nursing Practice*
4. Use of *Standards of Gerontological Nursing Practice*
5. Development of a philosophy of nursing care for older adults
6. Seeking of input from older adults about their preferences for nursing care practices
7. Hiring of role models for strategic placement in designated units
8. Hiring of more staff to meet needs
9. Better salary and working conditions in facilities that care for the elderly

Group dynamics. Elderly clients are adults bringing rich experience from their chosen life-styles; consequently, their wish to be partners in health practices should be honored. The clinical specialist in gerontological nursing plays a major leadership role in initiating groups in which past experiences are shared by each elderly participant for promoting mental, spiritual, and physical well-being. These group discussions may help to achieve objectives projected by the nurse leader for high-level wellness of the elderly.

Decision-making policies. Finally, the nurse as a leader assumes responsibility not only for maintaining the health of older persons through nursing ministrations but for actively pursuing the initiation of policy decisions at organization, community, state, regional, or national levels. It is through policy that permanent improvement of care of older persons can be effected. The gerontological clinical nurse specialist is in a key leadership position to provide current information about the health needs of the elderly to legislators, health planning boards, community health agencies, nursing home administrators, hospitals, regional offices for aging, Grey Panthers, and national congressional groups. A most effective method of leadership is not only to provide written information to these groups but to give oral presentations at hearings on issues affecting the welfare of the elderly (such as transportation, energy costs, and housing). Such participation is essential for enhancing the quality of life of the older citizenry.

Summary

Gerontological nursing is an emerging clinical specialty in the profession of nursing. The number of nurses who pursue a formal gerontological nursing program is growing. As the number of qualified nurse specialists grows, the health care system as it affects the health and welfare of older adults will be more visibly effective. Nurses who assume the role of Advocates, change agents, and leaders will change the attitudes of society to positively value older citizens, which will lead to a higher quality of life for them.

References

American Nurses' Association: Code of Ethics for Nurses and Interpretative Statements, Kansas City, Mo., 1976, ANA.

American Nurses' Association, Division of Gerontological Nursing: Standards of gerontological nursing practice, Kansas City, Mo., 1976, ANA.

American Nurses' Association, Division of Gerontological Nursing: A statement on the scope of gerontological nursing practice, Kansas City, Mo., 1981, ANA.

Bahr, R.T.: An overview of gerontological nursing. In Hogstel, M.D., editor: Nursing care of the older adult, New York, 1981, John Wiley & Sons, Inc.

Banknecht, V.L.: Conferees recommend policy for aged, Am. Nurse 14(1):1-8, 1982.

Bennis, G.W., Benne, K.D., and Chin, R.: The planning of change, ed. 2, New York, 1969, Holt, Rinehart & Winston.

Creighton, H.: Law every nurse should know, Philadelphia, 1975, W.B. Saunders Co.

Davis, B.A.: ANA and the geriatric nurse, Nurs. Clin. North Am. 3(4):741-748, 1968.

Dunn, H.L.: High-level wellness, Arlington, Va., 1973, Beatty.

Federal Council on Aging, Bicentennial Charter for Older Americans: Statement of rights and responsibilities of citizens, Washington, D.C., 1976, U.S. Government Printing Office.

Kelly, L.Y.: Dimensions of professional nursing, ed. 3, New York, 1981, Macmillan Inc.

Kinlein, L.: Kinlein care, paper presented at the First International Assembly of Kinlein Care, Milwaukee, August 1980.

Lysaught, J.: Action in affirmation: toward an unambiguous profession, New York, 1981, McGraw-Hill Book Co.

Webster's Seventh New Collegiate Dictionary, Springfield, Mass., 1965, G. & C. Merriam Co.

Chapter 10 The Nursing Process

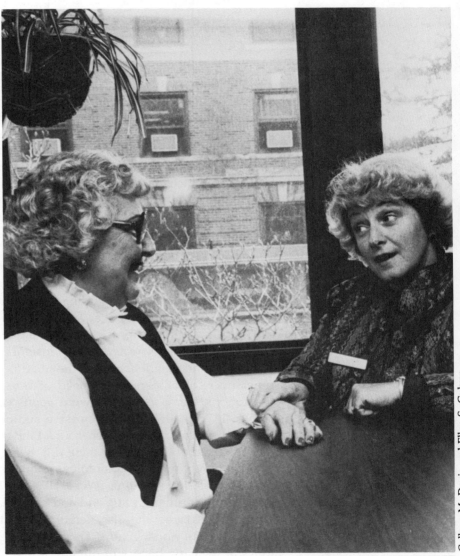

Colleen M. Davis and Ellen S. Culver

The older person is characterized in part by unique health care needs and problems, which are of concern to health care providers. The nursing process is a descriptive framework (Chavasse, 1978) used in the problem-solving approach (McGilloway, 1980) to health care needs and problems. The nursing process can be used with individuals in varying stages of development and experiencing varying levels of wellness. It provides a means of initiating a systematic approach to the health care of older adults in various settings through an individualized plan of care. Documentation of the nursing process's various steps aids in formalizing nursing practice. This chapter focuses on the nursing process as it pertains to older persons.

Historical Perspectives

Advancement of the nursing profession has been achieved through the efforts of many persons. Moreover, the purpose of nursing has been achieved through an interpersonal process that transcends the boundaries of time. Chronological time is of less importance in the overall view of the development of the nursing profession than the noteworthy events that indicate change over the course of time. Philosophies and attitudes expressed by practicing nurses in any given era contribute toward significant events, such as the emergence of gerontological nursing and the development of the nursing process concept, which serve as hallmarks of change. A historical perspective of nursing may be gained by examining the significance of nurses' contributions.

Professional nursing is considered to begin with Nightingale's efforts to improve nursing education and practice; but gerontological nursing, practically speaking, had its beginning within the family unit long before she was born. Historically families assumed responsibility for the care of their members, including the sick and frail elderly. Women have traditionally assumed the caregiver role. In some instances older persons were cared for by friends and neighbors when they had no family to look after them. In other cases older persons in need of care became the responsibility of institutions, some of which were sponsored by religious communities (Wells, 1979). Although an increasing number of older adults have turned to institutions for care (Karcher and Linden, 1974), families continue to provide most of the care for their elderly members.

Initiation of modern gerontological nursing is credited to Agnes Jones, a Nightingale-trained nurse (Wells, 1979). In 1864 Jones began working in a Poor Law institution in England and immediately set about improving the standards of care. She also demonstrated the cost effectiveness of improvements in nursing care. There is no figure corresponding to Agnes Jones in the early history of nursing in the United States (Wells, 1979).

Although the list of nurse leaders in the early history of nursing in the United States has no one who could be considered a gerontological nurse, a number of American nurses are recognized today as gerontological nurses. Virginia Stone, Dorothy Moses, Mary Opal Wolanin, Delores Alford, Barbara Davis, and a number of other nurses have continued to participate in activities that further the development of gerontological nursing. Through research, education, and practice these nurses helped to establish the ANA Division of Geriatrics Nursing Practice (ANA, 1966), which has become a positive force in advancing the nursing profession and improving care of the elderly.

A major influence on nursing practice in the United States was the acute shortage of nursing personnel during and following World War II. Several changes occurring within this period contributed to the formalization of nursing practice. These changes included more systematic use of the nursing process, introduction of team nursing, and use of a more formal communication system.

Although the term *nursing process* is found in the nursing literature of the 1950s, historical evidence points toward Nightingale as the originator of the concept (Dolan, 1978). Nightingale's description of the role of nursing and nursing functions includes assessment and intervention. She emphasized the importance of manipulating the environment as a means of improving the well-being of patients. Nightingale began operationalizing the concept of the nursing process; formalizing the concept has come about largely through the efforts of nurses who came after her.

For Hall (1955) the nursing process was the underlying assumption of a presentation she made on the quality of nursing care. Lewis, while working on a project to define clinical content for higher education in nursing in 1968, became interested in further defining the nursing process (Yura and Walsh, 1978b). Lewis indicated that the focus of nursing is to help individuals cope with reactions to health problems and maintain their integrity during those problems. She defined steps of the nursing process in terms similar to those used by Nightingale.

Although the concept of the nursing process has evolved slowly, it has gained worldwide acceptance as a scientific approach to nursing practice (Chavasse, 1978; Harris, 1979). Practical (Clark, 1978) and legal reasons (Neilson, 1978) are cited for using the nursing process. Acceptance of the nursing process has probably exceeded the dreams of Nightingale for advancing nursing.

Team nursing, a method of providing nursing care to a group of patients, has also served to increase formalization of the nursing process. The nursing team is a group of individuals of varying educational backgrounds and levels of clinical expertise. A professional nurse guides caregivers by assigning them to perform specific tasks according to their ability. This guidance is accomplished through written nursing care plans and daily individual and group conferences. Identification of components of care that can be safely carried out by nonnurses facilitates the nursing process. Although the model of primary nursing is currently being studied and used more frequently, team nursing is still a viable model of nursing practice.

A number of factors influencing gerontological nursing and the concept of nursing process have developed. Change can be almost imperceptible; therefore it can be more readily identified by reviewing events that have occurred over time and examining the impact of those events. Such events as acceptance of the nursing process and the increasing number of older persons are stimulating change in the practice of nursing. The study of historical events can be useful in understanding the role, functions, and development of gerontological nursing.

Philosophy

Consideration of philosophy's influences on human behavior may be helpful in understanding the self and others (Styles, 1982). A philosophy is usually defined as a system of beliefs or values that influences individual or group action. It may or may not be articulated formally, but it is visible through actions of individuals or groups.

Components of a Philosophy of Nursing

A philosophy of nursing contains three basic elements: the nature of the client, the nature of the nurse, and the nature of the interpersonal aspects of the nurse-client relationship (Little and Carnevali, 1969).

Gerontological nursing philosophy focuses on beliefs about the nature of the older person. These beliefs include many ideas that may affect the nurse-client relationship in a positive or negative manner. Examples of these beliefs follow.

The older adult is:
- a unique human being worthy of respect and entitled to dignity
- a being created by an external force, which some refer to as a deity or God
- a being who experiences life, death, and the full gamut of human emotions
- an integrated, organized whole who is interrelated to and interdependent on other human beings
- a being with constantly interacting internal and external environments
- a being who is subject to changes of aging, which alter appearance and functional ability but do not diminish that being's value as a person
- a being who is in a constant state of change

- a being who is interested in learning health-related information that will be helpful in maintaining and promoting high-level wellness*

In the nurse-client relationship there are also beliefs about the nature of the nurse. The nurse is:

- caring
- knowledgeable in the art and science of nursing
- competent in the practice of nursing
- concerned with promoting health
- sensitive to the basic human needs of older adults
- interested in preserving the dignity of older adults
- appreciative of the value of older persons
- concerned with the content of the practice of nursing as well as the structure of the nursing process
- willing to assume responsibility for making judgments, for acting on these judgments, and for the outcomes of the nursing action*

The nature of the interpersonal nurse-client relationship encompasses the beliefs of the nurse and the client about their respective roles with respect to health care needs and services. Some of these beliefs are stated below.

The interpersonal nurse-client relationship involves:

- establishing a relationship conducive to implementing the nursing process
- identifying client health care needs or problems and establishing mutually acceptable goals for satisfying these needs or resolving the problems
- acknowledging client responsibility for self-care in the promotion of health
- teaching or learning principles of self-care
- attending to activities essential to continuity of care
- maintaining an open system of communication*

Although the items listed under each of the three elements of a philosophy of nursing are not all inclusive, they suggest the basis for a philosophy of nursing. A philosophy reflects values held by those formulating the philosophy and is then reflected in the nursing process.

Developing a gerontological nursing philosophy requires soul searching into such areas as the nature of life itself, the concept of aging, the concept of productivity, and the worth of the human being. Aging may be viewed as a natural part of life or as a disease. Either of these views is likely to affect the approach to nursing intervention with an older adult. The right of an older adult to exist, especially if nonproductive in the usual

*Modified from Little, D., and Carnevali, D.: Nursing care planning, Philadelphia, 1969, J.B. Lippincott Co., pp. 22-26.

material sense, may be questioned. Little attention has been given to defining productivity in other than material terms. Can providing moral support, companionship, and a model for living out the later years of life be considered productive with respect to meeting human needs? How might the productivity of older persons, which includes nonmaterial as well as material productivity, be assessed in human terms? Do older persons have a right to exist simply because of their humanness? Consideration of these questions is important, since there is concern by some people for the use of health care resources by the elderly. The nature and value of life should be viewed within the framework of human rights extending across the life span of older individuals. Gerontological nurses are responsible to older persons for nursing action taken with them; quality of care is affected by the philosophy of nurses who provide that care.

The philosophy of the gerontological nurse influences both the selection of a model of nursing practice (Greenberg and Zaranka, 1975) and the definition of nursing that guides the practice. If a scientific base for practice is to be used, the nurse must believe in the importance of knowledge of human development and aging, the behavioral sciences, and the skills requisite for implementing the nursing process with older adults. The nursing model of practice should direct attention to the unique needs of older persons; moreover, it should be useful in defining and interpreting nursing practice.

Definition of Nursing

Over the years many nurses have shared their definitions of nursing based on their particular orientations to and personal experiences in nursing. Some have defined nursing with respect to a particular setting, whereas others have described the functions of the nurse (Yura and Walsh, 1978b). Defining nursing is an ongoing process in which nurses from each era and area of nursing participate. Since nursing is multifaceted and ever-changing, a single definition of nursing is unlikely to be formulated and universally accepted. Each nurse interprets nursing in his or her own practice. This interpretation should be based on a definition of nursing that, even if eclectic, contributes toward improved nursing care.

One of the definitions of nursing frequently referred to is that of Henderson (1966). Henderson defines nursing in terms of the nurse's function:

The unique function of the nurse is to assist the individual, sick or well, in the performance of those activities contributing to health or its recovery (or to a peaceful death) that he would perform unaided if he had the necessary strength, will, or knowledge. And to do this in such a way as to help him gain independence as rapidly as possible.*

*From Henderson, V.: The nature of nursing: a definition and its implications for practice, research, and education, New York, © Copyright Virginia Henderson, 1966, Macmillan Co., p. 15.

Stone's definition is addressed specifically to gerontological nursing (Stone, 1971):

Gerontological nursing is the nursing care of the elderly based on scientific knowledge from the fields of gerontology and nursing. It encompasses preventive care, maintenance, and rehabilitative aspects of health care. It requires an understanding of the process of aging and its relationship to nursing intervention.*

More recently Schlotfeldt (1981) has proposed a definition that she believes would support the concept of nursing as a profession whose members are responsible for the general health of people. Her definition (Schlotfeldt, 1981) is as follows:

Nursing is assessing and enhancing the general health status, health assets, and health potentials of human beings.†

Schlotfeldt thinks this definition has more universal appeal than previously written definitions. In her opinion it is concise and unambiguous; it gives focus to nursing practice, nursing education, and nursing research; and it conveys nurses' knowledge, practice, and scope of accountability.

The ANA Division of Gerontological Nursing Practice describes nursing within the scope of practice as follows:

Gerontological nursing is concerned with assessment of the health needs of older adults, planning and implementing health care to meet these needs, and evaluating the effectiveness of such care. Emphasis is placed on maximizing independence in the activities of everyday living and promoting, maintaining, and restoring health. The learning aspects of health care have significance in achieving and maintaining a level of wellness consistent with the limitations imposed by the aging process and/or chronic illness. Gerontological nursing strives to identify and use the strengths of older adults and assists them to use those strengths to maximize independence. The older adult is actively involved to the fullest extent of his/her capabilities in the decision making which influences everyday living.‡

This description implicitly attends to concepts such as the right to health care and patient rights, which have gained acceptance in the past few years. Another concept that seems to be gaining support and that is implicit in this description is self-care. This concept involves attention to the teaching and learning aspects of health care. It is based on a sense of the personal responsibility of clients for promoting their health. The ANA description of gerontological nursing practice is reflected in consideration of the nursing process throughout this chapter.

These are the many definitions from which nurses may draw as they seek to define and interpret nursing in their own practice. Although the

*From Stone, V.: Gerontological nursing: student syllabus, Evanston, Ill., 1970, Video Nursing/American Journal of Nursing Co., p. 1a.
†From Schlotfeldt, R.M.: Nursing in the future, Nurs. Outlook **29**(5), 1981, p. 298.
‡From American Nurses' Association: Standards of gerontological nursing practice, Kansas City, Mo., 1976, ANA, p. 3.

ideas underlying these definitions are not necessarily new, they are expressed in new ways. Nurses should define nursing within the scope of professional nursing practice and the legal parameters established by the states in which they practice. Their definitions should also reflect their particular areas of nursing practice, such as gerontological nursing.

For other health care professionals these definitions can be used as a means of examining roles and functions of their particular discipline. Various components of the interpersonal process and holism are applicable whatever the discipline. Examination of the interpersonal process between client and minister, student, social worker, dietitian, client, and others is likely to help the caregiver acquire understanding and skills important to the relationship with older individuals. Substituting the appropriate term for "nurse" is a way for caregivers other than nurses to explore the roles and functions of their particular disciplines with older persons. Caregivers must be aware of the boundaries of their own disciplines and define their practice accordingly.

The Nursing Process

Nurses and other caregivers may use the framework of the nursing process for organizing their approach to practice, since the process is based on the scientific method. Since the scientific method is used by caregivers of various disciplines, it can serve as a mechanism for coordinating care for and communicating information to older persons.

The nursing process provides a conceptual framework for describing nursing actions (Chavasse, 1978). Nursing, as indicated previously, is care directed toward meeting the health needs of people. *Process* refers to a systematic ongoing course of action circumscribed by the needs of clients. The nursing process is universal in the sense that it can be used with individuals in various stages of development and by nurses throughout the world. Gerontological nursing process has this same conceptual framework, but activities vary according to the needs of older individuals.

Basically the nursing process consists of four phases that are described as discrete entities but that in actuality may overlap and occur in different sequences. These phases are (1) assessing, (2) planning, (3) implementing, and (4) evaluating. Certain activities are performed within each phase. For example, the first phase (assessing) involves collecting data and using these data in formulating nursing diagnoses. Equal consideration should be given to each phase of the nursing process; otherwise the process is incomplete, and the nursing action may be less effective.

Fig. 10-1 illustrates what may happen if emphasis is placed on assessing to the neglect of the other phases of the nursing process. A comprehensive and accurate health assessment is essential and may include data beyond

Fig. 10-1. **The nursing process.**

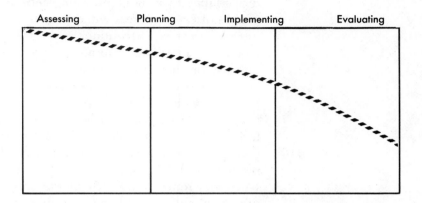

those needed for an adequate plan of care, but it is only one part of the nursing process. Justifying the collection of data that are not considered in the other phases of the nursing process may be challenged; planning and giving care without evaluating the outcomes is a questionable practice. Evaluating the outcomes of nursing action is necessary for determining its effectiveness, for determining if revision of the care plan is needed, and for documenting the nursing action (which has legal as well as practical aspects). Too often evaluation is the most neglected phase of the nursing process. The manner in which evaluation is carried out should be determined in the initial phases of assessing and planning. Unless attention is given to how evaluation will be managed from the beginning, it may be all but impossible to achieve an objective evaluation of the client's response to the nursing intervention. Evaluating outcomes of care is as essential as collecting data and making the nursing diagnosis; it should not be given short shrift or relegated to the "if I have time" category.

One of the reasons that evaluation of nursing actions results is neglected is that it is sometimes a difficult process. Nurses often are used to seeing rather dramatic responses from clients in acute care settings. However, the responses of older persons to nursing action may be varied and less dramatic. Involving older adults in the process of establishing goals and developing a mutually acceptable plan of action should be given high priority so that more realistic objectives and ways of evaluating outcomes may be established.

Teaching or learning needs are an example of the importance of evaluating outcomes of nursing action. Have you ever known a patient to administer an oral antibiotic for an ear infection into the ear because of a lack of understanding? Or an individual on a diet restricting fat who indicated that it was not a problem, since he never used butter—but that he could not eat his cereal without cream? Or an older patient who wore a nitroglycerine patch continuously for angina and talked about splitting wood for winter fuel? Information may not have been given to these individuals, or their ability to absorb it may have been compromised by anxiety, sensory changes, or slowed thought processes. Evaluating the outcome of the client's learning is important, especially if the individual lives alone and is responsible for self-care. Behavioral change can be facilitated by having older individuals repeat instructions, by exploring perceptions of older people on the need for changes in life-styles, and by providing a set of written instructions in large print for them to refer to when they return home. Whether teaching or learning has been effective is ultimately shown by whether individuals have modified their behavior. Older persons are resilient and can usually adapt to changes of aging if they understand what those changes are. To determine whether older persons understand what is happening and how they may help themselves is an important function of the health care provider. Evaluating client's response to teaching is essential in determining whether they understand the information essential for decision-making, self-care activities, and modification of behavior.

Implementing the nursing process requires a deliberate, systematic problem-solving approach. Nurses need knowledge and experience to make judgments about what is needed and how to proceed with ongoing activities. Nurses also need an affective dimension that motivates them to action and gives rise to the empathy and compassion important to care of the elderly. The nursing process is a means whereby nurses can organize their care of older persons and further develop skills important to the nurse-client relationship. Since information about approaches to nursing care of older adults is not as readily available as that for care of younger persons, information should be shared about ways of meeting their health care needs and problems.

Assessing

Assessing, the first phase of the nursing process, is the gathering of information to aid in the identification of health care needs and problems of clients. Assessing is a dynamic process achieved through the systematic collection, analysis, and interpretation of data. These data are essential for arriving at a nursing diagnosis and for initiating the subsequent phases of the nursing process.

Data are obtained from various sources, such as the client, client records, other persons having a significant relationship with the client, and observations of the nurse. These data provide clues to the health status of the client and the dimensions of the client situation (Yura and Walsh, 1978a,b).

Formulation of the nursing diagnosis marks the end of the assessment phase of the nursing process. Although elaboration on nursing diagnosis will appear later, a brief explanatory note is included here to illustrate the relationship between diagnosis and assessment. Diagnoses are judgments made regarding the health status of clients; they are the focus of nursing action. An example of a nursing diagnosis common among older clients is that of disturbed rest and sleep patterns (Gebbie and Lavin, 1974). This diagnosis should be made with caution, since the sleep-rest patterns of older persons differ from those of younger persons and among older individuals themselves. Sleep and rest are important to the person's state of well-being. A careful history of the sleep patterns of older persons is important for individualizing the care plan. Nurses are often in a key position to assist older persons adapt to changes in sleep patterns, since they know about aging changes affecting sleep patterns, medications that may disrupt sleep, and environmental factors affecting sleep.

Nursing diagnoses take into account actual or potential alterations in the health status of individuals, which are not necessarily disease related. The difference between nursing and medical diagnoses is important not only for the client's health but for legal reasons. Nursing diagnoses should identify needs or problems that nurses are prepared to treat and that fall within the scope of nursing practice. Nurses have the responsibility for making a referral when there is evidence of a need or problem that exceeds the scope of nursing practice as defined by state nurse practice acts (Fortin and Rabinow, 1979). Need for referral might arise when a screening procedure, such as for glaucoma, indicates the possibility of a pathological condition or when there is the possibility of a fracture. Documentation of the nursing process is one means of differentiating nursing from medical practice and of preventing legal problems.

As stated in the ANA *Standards of Gerontological Nursing Practice* (ANA, 1976) data collected in the assessment phase of the nursing process should be readily available. Documentation of the process of nursing is a means of ensuring continuity of care, of differentiating nursing from medical diagnoses, and most importantly of providing a data base essential to operationalizing the nursing process.

Assessment of older persons should include information about the various dimensions of the person, physical, psychological, sociological, and spiritual. It should also include information about the interaction of the person with the external environment. Just as the nursing process is incomplete unless each phase of the process is given equal consideration, assessment of older persons is incomplete unless attention is given to each of their dimensions. Of particular concern in older persons is the assessment of the spiritual dimension. A comprehensive assessment is particularly important for older persons, since many of their needs are psychological, sociological, and spiritual.

The spiritual dimension is intangible and subjective, and it permeates the entire being of the person. It affects the person's outlook on life and will to keep on being and becoming. Changes of aging, such as impairments of the sensory system and limitations of mobility, tend to limit the personal space of the older adult. Losses of various types, such as loss of work and loss of family and friends by death, also occur, diminishing the older person's social roles and functions. These losses also decrease the social support system at a time when older persons have greater need for social support. Life experiences and increasing awareness of mortality probably contribute toward the tendency for older persons to become more involved with development of the inner self (Jung, 1933; Neugarten and others, 1964) and spiritual concerns.

Gould (1972) presents evidence that a person's sense of time changes with age and with it the attitudes toward self and others in relation to time. He refers to the process that brings new beliefs about oneself and the world (Gould, 1975). Neugarten (1968) has also discussed differences in the way time is perceived by those in their middle years: the view of time left to live versus the time already lived. This developmental change may be evidenced by questions raised or comments made by older adults regarding the purpose of life and the relationship of the self to self, to others, to the universe, and to a deity, however defined (Smallwood and Stoll, 1975). Since the health status of older adults is influenced by their level of spiritual well-being as well as by their level of well-being in other dimensions, data should be gathered about their sense of time, attitudes, and beliefs—to indicate the level of their spiritual well-being.

Techniques. Assessing the older person's level of wellness requires certain tools and techniques. Tools for data collection include cognitive skills, interviewing skills, interpersonal skills, and observational skills. Techniques by which these skills may be adapted to meet the needs of older adults are critical to the interpersonal nurse-client relationship and the outcomes of the nursing process.

Interpersonal skills put older persons at ease and help establish a trusting relationship between them and health care providers, facilitating the data collection process. A sense of caring may be transmitted by the manner in which older persons are approached and sometimes through the use of touch. Care should be exercised to prevent a violation of trust and a diminishing of self-esteem in older persons. Acknowledging the right of older persons to participate in establishing a time for an assessment visit and to know that the nurse is arriving for the visit is an important part of the interpersonal process. Addressing older persons by title and name and giving them time to respond to a greeting are effective techniques in interpersonal skills.

Interviewing requires the ability to determine appropriate questions to ask for gathering essential data, language skills to facilitate the communication process (Edwards and Brilhart, 1981), and interpersonal skills to provide a psychological climate conducive to interview.

Observational skills are especially important in assessing the health status of older persons and need to be sharply honed. Observations should provide factual accounts of events in the physical world of the observer (Hein, 1980). Since observations are made through the senses and may be influenced by personal experiences and perceptions, the observer must guard against the subjective distortion of the older person's reality and interference with the caregiver-client relationship. An example is an older, bald gentleman who was lying in a hospital bed with his head in the sunlight streaming through the window. A nurse entering the room observed the bright sunlight, stepped over to the bedside, and adjusted the venetian blind, shutting out the sunlight. The gentleman rolled over and commented, "Oh, that felt so good on my head." The nurse failed to validate her interpretation of the observation with the older gentleman; her interpretation did not agree with his.

Sensitivity is also needed because of the reticence of older persons to discuss personal matters. Financial, sexual, and religious matters are sensitive areas for many older persons. Moreover, older persons often do not demonstrate the classic signs and symptoms of changes in health status that younger persons do. An increased pulse rate and a state of confusion rather than an elevated temperature may indicate an infection. Pain may not occur in the older person having a myocardial infarction; a change in skin color, moist skin, and a change in pulse rate may indicate the cardiac problem. Observation of changes in older persons is important.

Observations of older people also should include particular attention to nonverbal cues, which often reveal emotions not expressed in the caregiver-client verbal exchange. Older persons often tend to be stoic, and keep "a stiff upper lip" during periods of difficulty. Nonverbal cues need to be analyzed for congruence with the verbal cues, since contradictory messages may lead to inaccuracy in the nursing diagnosis (Hein, 1980; Edwards and Brilhart, 1981). Observations must be purposeful to be effective; data gathered through observation should supplement data collected by other means, such as interviewing.

Family dynamics and the client's social interaction with significant others should be observed closely for quality and quantity. Family relations may be strained because of lack of knowledge and understanding of the aging process and its behavioral response rather than because of a lack of caring. Since families and significant others are usually intimately involved with elderly individuals and their care, observation of their interactions can provide clues to their relationships. Accuracy of data on social roles and functions of these individuals is no less important than that of information gathered about other dimensions.

An example of the care that needs to be exercised in collecting data on the sociological dimension of older adults is reflected in the following incident. A resident of a high-rise apartment dwelling for the elderly commented that old age is a "no care" time of life. She complained that no one came around anymore, and that she was lonely. She related that she bought eggs from a farm woman who delivered them to her door—as much for having someone to talk to as for the produce itself. Further assessment of this resident's social interactions revealed that family members and friends visited frequently. Apparently this elderly woman felt neglected unless someone was with her most of the time. Without an in-depth assessment the caregiver might have been led to believe that the family of this lady neglected her. Although this woman's feelings of loneliness cannot be denied, her perception of the "no care" attitude in others must be questioned in view of the data. Her need for social interaction exceeded the coping ability of family and friends. Other options for meeting social needs had to be explored with this client.

Assessment tools. A number of tools are available for the assessment process, such as guides for history taking (LaMonica, 1979; Marriner, 1982) and for assessing the various dimensions and environments of older individuals (Yura and Walsh, 1978a,b; LaMonica, 1979; Murray, Huelskoelter, and O'Driscoll, 1980; Hogstel, 1981). Tools with demonstrated validity and reliability should be selected when available. Assessment tools are valuable, and caregivers need to examine them carefully when making a determination as to whether any adaptation of the tools is needed for their particular situations. Questionnaires should be scrutinized for items that may be superfluous, such as questions about family history—which may have little relevance for care of the elderly person. Since prolonged history taking can be fatiguing and may interfere with the accuracy of information on essential points, the aim of data collection should be to collect only data that influences the care of older persons. The trend is toward performing a health assessment that focuses on the strengths of the individual rather than on areas of weakness (Stokes, Rauckhorst, and Mezey, 1980).

Basic assessment tools may be organized around a systems framework model (Brown, 1981; Smith, 1981). These tools may be general in nature and useful for developing a systematic approach to the initial assessment (Mitchell, 1977). Consideration should also be given to the possible advantage of a multidimensional assessment tool. One such tool is the Older

Americans' Resources and Services Multidimensional Functional Assessment Questionnaire (OMFA) (Ebersole and Hess, 1981). This tool, originally developed to explore alternatives to institutionalization, is an outgrowth of work done at Duke University in Durham, North Carolina in response to a request from the Administration on Aging. Efforts have been directed toward developing a valid and reliable instrument that can be used in assessing functional ability and use of services. A comprehensive multidimensional tool can facilitate coordination of care and help to prevent duplication or gaps in services. Caregivers should be selective in deciding which assessment tools to use and what adaptations may be needed. One of the basic requirements for the assessment tool is to include items about each of the four dimensions of older persons.

A number of instruments are available for assessment of the person's various dimensions. Examples of these instruments, some of which have been cited previously, are (1) the physical assessment tool (Murray, Huelskoelter, and O'Driscoll, 1980), (2) the psychological assessment tool (Snyder and Wilson, 1977), (3) the social-psychological tool (Francis and Munjas, 1976), and (4) the spiritual assessment guide (Beland and Passos, 1981). Some of these instruments include information that facilitates the assessment process.

The Snyder and Wilson tool, for example, elaborates on the 10 elements to be explored and includes relevant questions to ask in each area. One element deals with the person's response to stress and coping and defense mechanisms. The tool affords a guide for exploring questions in an informal manner and at the same time provides an opportunity for older persons to talk to someone about their feelings and perceptions, which is often therapeutic in itself. At the close of the assessment period the caregiver can share the assessment with the client; they can then establish a set of goals for dealing with identified needs. A case in point is the elderly retired lady who expressed the need for additional activity outside the high-rise housing unit in which she lived. In discussing this need after the interview the client and the caregiver, a nursing student, set a goal directed toward resolving the client's need through volunteer work. The client soon found a position in the nearby city hall; she was especially pleased to learn that they would provide the necessary transportation. Both the client and the caregiver were gratified by the assessment and its results.

The assessment guide for the spiritual dimension (Beland and Passos, 1981) is organized around various subtopics, such as spiritual concern, spiritual despair, and the causes and defining characteristics of each. This organization should be emphasized because spiritual assessment is a sensitive area and is often limited to information about affiliation with an organized religion and its beliefs and practices. We believe along with others that every individual is a spiritual being and expresses spirituality in various ways. The guide for assessing the spiritual dimension identifies areas to be assessed regardless of the person's affiliation with an organized religion.

Other assessment tools are designed for making an in-depth assessment of specific areas such as the skin (Roach, 1977; Wells, 1978); geriatric behavior (Yesavage, Adey, and Werner, 1981); stress associated with life change events (Holmes and Rahe, 1967; Muhlenkamp, Gress, and Flood, 1975); and the feet (King, 1980; Livesey, 1981). These tools may be used for obtaining additional information when the basic assessment indicates the need for more specific information in certain areas. Judgment should be exercised regarding the need for a detailed assessment and the potential benefit to the client.

In addition to the tools just cited self-assessment tools are becoming available. One such tool is the Wellness Self-Assessment Tool (Clark, 1980). Although this tool is not directed specifically toward the elderly, it has relevance to some areas of their lives. A list of resources that might be useful in achieving a higher level of wellness is also available (Clark, 1980). Individual responsibility for well-being is becoming an increasingly important issue as the number and proportion of older adults increases and available resources dwindle. The older person's assumption of responsibility for self-assessment and for recording that data can be useful to caregivers when he or she requires assistance with health care needs or problems. Moreover, self-assessment can provide the older person with the sense of purpose and accomplishment important for integrity and self-esteem.

Other examples of instruments that older persons can use when the occasion demands are those cited by Butler and Lewis (1982). They include one to be used for insurance purposes and one for personal data. Having these records available in time of need facilitates the assessment process and is likely to speed up the process for obtaining needed health care service. Self-assessment is one way for older persons to retain some mastery over what happens when dependency needs arise.

Above all, an assessment of older persons by self or others should focus on strengths rather than weaknesses. Identifying strengths provides clues to the particular kind of support needed for promoting and maintaining the state of well-being. As a cane can be used to support the body's unaffected side, strengths of older persons enable them to enhance their independence. Too often older persons, because of "ageism" (Butler, 1969) or other factors, assume a more dependent role than is necessary and lose some of their cherished freedom. Hayter (1976) indicates that caregivers may unwillingly contribute to negative attitudes toward aging by the comments or questions they direct to the aged about physiologic functioning. Questions such as whether the person slept last night or when the person's bowels moved, according to Hayter, focus on physiological functioning and the likelihood of physiological decline. Hayter lists a number of positive aspects of aging, one of which is that older persons can be instead of do. Palmore (1979) also discusses what he considers to be the positive aspects of aging, including economic advantages and freedom from family responsibility, child rearing, and work. He classifies these aspects as individual or societal, according to the primary source of benefit. Palmore believes it is time to "accentuate the positive" and overcome fears about and prejudices against old age. Assessment of older persons' strengths should include attention to cultural beliefs and health practices and to their informal support network of family, friends, and neighbors.

Nursing diagnosis. Having reviewed many aspects of the assessment phase of the nursing process, pointing out various assessment tools and techniques that may be helpful in assessing older persons, it is appropriate to consider the nursing diagnosis, which concludes the assessment phase of the nursing process.

The nursing diagnosis is defined as a process of making inferences and coming to conclusions based on information obtained from individual clients (Aspinall, 1976). These conclusions provide the basis for individualized care plans. Client needs or problems that can be managed within the scope of nursing practice should be identified (Gebbie and Lavin, 1974).

Perhaps the definition of nursing diagnosis that comes closest to supporting the health-oriented approach is that of Dossey and Guzzetta (1981). They define signs and symptoms indicating actual or potential health problems that nurses are licensed for and capable of managing as the nursing diagnosis. They give actual problems priority over potential problems, but they use a health-oriented frame of reference.

According to Lash, there is general agreement that the nursing diagnosis:

- is made by the professional nurse
- is a summary statement
- is derived from patient data
- is about health problems
- is about therapeutic decisions amenable to nursing intervention
- is the necessary base for nursing care (Lash, 1978, p. 334)

The nursing diagnosis is needed for finalizing the assessment phase of the nursing process; it provides information essential for planning, the second phase of the nursing process.

Health care needs and strengths of older adults should be considered when arriving at a nursing diagnosis (Gleit and Tatro, 1981). Unmet needs, such as those for increased social interaction, tend to become problems, and existing strengths may be mobilized to support the older person's state of well-being. Seldom are older adults free of health problems—and seldom are they devoid of strengths. Older individuals are obviously survivors, yet the positive aspects of this status have rarely been systematically identified (Popkess, 1981). The nursing diagnosis should accentuate the positive. It should have a health-oriented approach to nursing intervention with older adults. For example, the older lady who identified the need for activity and interaction with other people outside the high-rise apartment in which she lived was quite capable of making the contacts necessary for getting into volunteer work. Having someone to help explore her needs and to encourage her to pursue her ideas was the only assistance required. This lady essentially met her own need for meaningful activity; she was both the source of her need and the resource for meeting her need. Exercising self-agency demonstrated strength, and the outcome of her efforts was rewarding to her.

An accurate nursing diagnosis is essential for planning and implementing effective care. This is certainly true for diagnosing the mental health needs of older people. Older persons are often depressed about life change events, and the challenge to caregivers is never greater than in this situation, since unmet needs may become problems leading to pathological depression. Helplessness often results in despair and suicide as a way out of an intolerable situation. Intervention directed toward promoting mental health is especially important for older people. Labeling persons is to be avoided, since labeling tends to contribute to depersonalization. "Mental incompetence," for example, is a label from which it is difficult if not impossible to recover. Nor is such a label useful in identifying strengths of individuals and in establishing goals of care.

Loss (and the subsequent grieving process) is one of the areas making accuracy in nursing diagnoses difficult to achieve. Questions arise, such as when does grieving become a pathological problem rather than a therapeutic adapting process? Does the normal grieving process take longer for the older adult than for the younger adult? Is a degree of depression normal for older adults? What criteria should be used for making an accurate nursing diagnosis of someone in a state of depression? Answers to these and other questions about the reaction of older persons to losses require additional research. The paucity of clear-cut norms contributes to the dilemma of gerontological nurses attempting to use a prescriptive approach to nursing intervention.

The Snyder and Wilson tool (1977), Elements of a Psychological Assessment, is useful for obtaining information about the older person's perceptions of personal experiences. The individual is asked to respond to questions in each of ten elements, to explain perceptions and ways of coping with various changes of aging. From this information and data collected from other sources the nurse may gain insight into the client's situation and arrive at a more accurate nursing diagnosis.

Arriving at a nursing diagnosis. Dossey and Guzzetta (1981) identify a three-step process for arriving at a nursing diagnosis. These steps are (1) observation of signs and symptoms that support the belief that there is a need or problem and the statement of that need or problem, (2) listing of possible causes of the problem, and (3) formulation of the diagnostic statement. The phrase "related to" should connect the statement of the problem and its probable cause, according to the authors of this approach. For example, potential dehydration is related to decreased fluid intake. This phrase is not likely to be misinterpreted as a medical diagnosis.

Dossey and Guzzetta suggest that nurses carry a list of the accepted nursing diagnoses and refer to it until they become more familiar. The list is published in *Proceedings of the 3rd and 4th National Conferences: Classification of Nursing Diagnoses* (Kim and Moritz, 1981).

Classifying nursing diagnoses. Classifying nursing diagnoses is a way of organizing data and promoting a more systematic approach to the nursing process. Identification of health care needs or problems amenable to nursing intervention is a means of describing the domain of nursing (Gebbie and Lavin, 1974). Developing universally acceptable nomenclature facilitates collaborative relationships between nurses and can be used to interpret nursing to other caregivers. Organizing data into useful blocks of related information is a precursor to prescriptive nursing interventions.

A list of 30 nursing diagnoses developed at the First National Conference on Classification of Nursing Diagnoses in 1973 and published in 1974 (Gebbie and Lavin) has continued to be used by a number of nurses. This list includes such diagnoses as alterations in faith and relationships with self and others. These diagnoses cover each of the four dimensions of the person, physical, psychological, sociological, and spiritual. Many nurses continue to use the list of diagnoses, probably because of its relative simplicity.

Tools for making a nursing diagnosis. According to Jasmin and Trygstad (1979), the tools of diagnosis are analysis and synthesis: analysis of the collected data and synthesis for developing a succinct statement of the client's needs or problems. Since the diagnosis guides nursing action and since many health care personnel are likely to share in the provision of health care services, a written diagnosis is preferable.

To analyze data means to separate pieces of information and to determine the ordering and categorizing needed to create a good data base.

Putting the material into a meaningful whole is part of the process of synthesis. Pieces of information from each of the person's dimensions (such as a blood pressure reading, a response to the Mental Status Questionnaire, a list of the older person's roles and functions, and information on how the individual perceives relationships to others) are not very useful in their singular form. When these pieces of information are put together, however, they begin to give a better idea about the individual as a whole person. The nursing diagnosis is a concise interpretation of data gathered about a given client. The diagnosis is based on scientific knowledge, experience, and the frame of reference of the nurse making the diagnosis. It gives direction to the planning phase of the nursing process.

Planning

Planning, the second phase of the nursing process, involves considering options for nursing intervention and establishing priorities for nursing action. The urgency of the need for resolution of the client's health care needs and problems determines the priority of actions to be taken (Marriner, 1982). Exploration of ways to deal with the needs and problems and knowledge of available resources is needed. Planning should be a collaborative process in which the older adult is involved to the fullest extent possible.

Standard III of the ANA *Standards of Gerontological Nursing Practice* (ANA, 1976) supports the right of the older adult and significant others to be involved in the planning process. The rationale accompanying the standard is that older adults are persons who both are and are becoming and who normally have the capacity to participate in planning what affects their state of well-being. Recognition of the older adult's right to participate in the planning of his or her own health care is one of the most important ways of acknowledging the personhood of the individual.

Care plans. Care plans are used for individualizing the approach to care and for ensuring its continuity. Determining who will carry out the various activities and when and how they should be carried out are important aspects of the planning process. The plan should have a rationale that helps the older person understand why the action is being proposed. The plan should be recorded so it becomes part of the communication system for the older individual and health care providers.

A written plan of care decreases the likelihood of omitting such components as the teaching of self-care, administration of medications, and attention to psychosocial needs. This formal plan of care becomes especially important when a number of health care personnel from various disciplines, such as dietitians, pharmacists, and physical therapists, are involved. Moreover, the written plan of care is useful in making changes in keeping with the changing conditions and circumstances of older adults.

Tebbitt (1981) cites the professional responsibility of health care providers for collaborating on the planning of continuity of care. This need should be emphasized with respect to older adults who frequently move from one level of care to another, from one health care institution to another, or from home to institution to home again. Not only is continuity of care critical for maintaining progress in such activities as bowel and bladder control and transfer skills but for supporting the motivation and morale of older persons. That the various health care providers know the plan of care is in itself reinforcing for the older person. The realization that various health care providers are using the plan of care reinforces the individual's feelings of self-worth and increases motivation for carrying out the plan.

Effective planning involves establishing goals mutually acceptable to the older person and the nurse or other health care providers. The nursing diagnosis suggests the desired outcomes of the intervention (Marriner, 1982). Behavioral objectives should be clearly stated to facilitate achieving specific objectives and evaluating their outcomes. This approach is useful for determining the need for revision of the plan and the direction such revision should take. Objectives should be realistic, that is, within the individual's ability to attain; otherwise the individual is likely to become discouraged and refuse to participate in them. The individual may be labeled *noncompliant*, for failing to meet the expectations of health care providers. This situation is likely to result in the client's decreased self-esteem and lack of adherence to the plan.

A number of guides are available for planning the nursing process. One guide deals with planning long-term care (Neal, Cohen, and Cooper, 1980). Its authors indicate that the guide is useful not only for planning care but for helping set criteria for evaluation that may be used for gerontological nursing. The specific guides in that book are presented in the nursing care plan format and are intended to be used as references from which to develop individualized plans of care. Guides are included for such need or problem areas as grief and mourning, mental status (which includes observable indicators of the individual's psychological functioning), and exercises for individuals over 65.

Yura and Walsh (1978b) describe the development and importance of a clearly written plan of care. According to them, the plan is an effective means of assuring the individual that his or her needs will be met and problems solved. Developing a plan of care with the client conveys the message that others are interested in him or her; so it tends to allay anxiety. Planning with the older person takes time, but it saves time in the long run.

Bower lists the purposes of nursing care plans as: ''(1) individualized and holistic care, (2) continuity of care, (3) communication of care, (4) evaluation of care, (5) comprehensive care, (6) coordination of care, and (7) team approach to nursing care."* These purposes are especially appropriate for older persons, who usually move in and out of the health care system more frequently than do younger persons. Benefits of nursing care plans may be lessened if they do not become a part of the client's permanent record or if the plans are not shared with health care providers when the client moves from one setting to another. For example, continuity of an older person's bowel and bladder training program may be disrupted by a short stay in a hospital if the hospital staff are unaware of it. When such disruptions occur, the quality of care of older persons is decreased, and the purposes of nursing care plans are thwarted.

The nursing care plan is the written summary of information gathered about the client during the assessment phase of the nursing process, according to Murray, Huelskoelter, and O'Driscoll (1980). It includes the individual's needs and problems, the plan for meeting these needs and resolving the problems, who is to carry out the planned action, and the priorities established for the proposed action.

A plan is the prescription for actions aimed at meeting the needs or resolving problems presented by clients. The planning should be comprehensive, no matter which dimension of the client is the source of the need or problem. Planning is the precursor of the third phase of the nursing process: implementing. The written plan of care signifies the end of planning and the beginning of implementing.

Implementing

Implementing is the action phase of the nursing process (Yurick and others, 1980). Implementation of the proposed plan of care may be direct, that is, carried out by the nurse, or indirect, that is, carried out by others under the direction of the nurse (Jasmin and Trygstad, 1979). The nurse is accountable for implementing the plan.

During the implementing phase of the nursing process, interpersonal aspects of the nurse-client relationship come into sharp focus. The plan of care mutually agreed on is activated, and the philosophies of the nurse and the client influence the action and its outcomes. If the nurse considers the client to be unique, the nursing action should reflect that by involving the client in the action and allowing ample time for the client to engage in activities of daily living. The client's philosophy becomes evident in his or her manner of attending to the various activities of the plan. If the nurse or other health care providers and the client believe in self-care, high priority will probably be given to instruction on self-care. Differences of opinion may arise between the nurse or health care provider and the client about the way the care plan is to be carried out. These differences should be

*From Bower, F.L.: The process of planning nursing care: a model for practice, ed. 3, St. Louis, 1982, The C.V. Mosby Co., p. 171.

resolved, often through compromise, to foster the kind of relationship necessary for accomplishing the goals of the plan.

An example of a dilemma for the nurse is the case of Mr. B., an 82-year-old bachelor, who has been having severe anginal attacks of increasing frequency and intensity. Mr. B. is a chain smoker and has decided that he cannot give up cigarette smoking entirely, in spite of the physician's advice. He asked the nurse whether four cigarettes a day would hurt him; he rationalized his position by saying that he had known many individuals who had heart attacks, who had never smoked a day in their lives. The dilemma for the nurse arises out of knowing the research findings on the effects of cigarette smoking and believing that the man has the right to participate in making decisions affecting his well-being and quality of life. For this man, who lived alone and had limited mobility, smoking was an important source of pleasure. For the therapeutic relationship to continue, the nurse had to compromise by accepting Mr. B's decision to reduce rather than stop smoking entirely. Respecting the older person's right to make decisions that are not congruent with research findings is hard. But respect for the person is essential to maintaining an effective relationship for the promotion of holistic well-being.

Another principle of care that is not always easily carried out is that of never doing for older persons what they can do for themselves. Care might be accomplished more quickly and effectively by the health care provider, but it may decrease the self-esteem of the older person and needlessly increase dependence. Judgment is needed in determining the self-care capabilities of older persons. If they lack the strength for total personal care, options should be discussed in keeping with their desires and capabilities. Knowing the consequences of actions is important during the implementing phase of the nursing process. Decisions should be based on their impact on the person's basic human needs. Disregarding the person and creating needless dependence are indefensible.

Implementing a care plan with older adults may require more time than would be required with younger adults, but this difference in time should be acknowledged as a necessary part of working with elderly persons. An unhurried manner and time allowed for response to a greeting or to questions are essential in establishing a relationship with older people. If older persons are pushed to respond too quickly, they may become confused (Wolanin and Phillips, 1981); the pressure to respond quickly may also interfere with the accuracy of their responses and cause them to withdraw. Time to communicate is as essential to the well-being of older persons as adequate time for participating in the activities of daily living and social activities and should be taken into account by health care providers.

Communication. Human beings have a great desire to share ideas and feelings, and an inability to do so can be highly frustrating and decrease their motivation to participate in various social activities. Impaired hearing reportedly has a greater psychological impact than decreased visual acuity. Information about new developments in devices that offset sensory impairment (such as the sound amplifier for the telephone and a light rather than a bell to signal incoming calls) should be shared with older individuals who need them. Manipulating the environment so as to compensate for sensory deficits should receive immediate attention. Examples of this manipulation are control of background noise and use of adequate lighting. Personhood is attained and maintained to a great extent through communication with others (Buscaglia, 1978), so lost or impaired ability to communicate has negative consequences for the elderly.

In some cases nonverbal means of communication may become the major means of communicating with an older person. Gestures, touch (Preston, 1973), and body posture may help convey a message of acceptance and caring. Providing opportunity for lip reading or signing may augment other aids and enhance the communication process. In any case it should be remembered that communication is a two-way exchange involving a sender and a receiver of a message. Each participant in the communication process should intermittently be a sender and a receiver. When the primary method of communication is nonverbal, thoughtful consideration should be given to the most effective way to use it.

Referrals. Since the health care needs and problems of older adults are complex and multiple in number, assistance may be needed from a number of health care providers other than nurses. Referral is a means of obtaining the needed assistance. Knowledge of available resources and how to tap them is essential to implementing the nursing process. An example is the referral to a teaching dietitian for questions about the client's nutritional status or the need for instruction on dietary modification. Another example is the referral to a podiatrist. Because of changes of aging that affect the feet and interfere with ambulation, such as loss of fat pads or splayfoot, older persons often require special services. Hard to cut toenails, ingrown toenails, calluses, and corns are conditions that can be extremely troublesome. For these types of conditions referral to appropriate and effective caregivers is an important part of nursing action.

The cost of health care services is sometimes raised with respect to referral. An important related question is the potential cost of not obtaining the additional services. This cost is not easily identified, since it falls within the preventive aspect of care; it should be considered in terms of human as well as economic factors. For example, what might be the cost of not obtaining the services of a podiatrist? The potential for infection from ingrown toenails is great among older individuals, whose circulation is often compromised and who often tend to have an elevated blood glucose level. The likelihood of limited mobility and decreased social interaction because of untreated bunions and corns is greater among older persons than young persons. It may not be a life or death issue, but it has implications for the quality of life of older individuals. It may have far-reaching implications in those with diabetes mellitus; the value of a lost limb, for example, is difficult to measure in strictly economic terms. Human factors, such as the change in body image and its impact on the person and loss of independence, should be considered. The nurse is in a position to be an advocate for the elderly and to use a holistic approach, which encompasses consideration of the person's total response to internal and external environmental changes.

Continuity of care. Continuity of care should be a part of implementing a care plan. It includes education of the client for self-care and may necessitate involvement of family members or significant others. It may involve more than one agency (Tebbitt, 1981). Although clients with chronic conditions such as diabetes mellitus and arthritis may be quite self-sufficient, a backup system should be available in case of emergency. Health care providers should be aware of the individual's kinship networks and their interrelationships (Strauss, 1975). Supporting the strengths of the client is important in the continuity of care; this may include pointing out that chronic conditions need not necessarily restrict ability to travel or to participate in other activities. Families may also need to be informed of resources, including those related to travel. Continuity of care should not be geographically limited; it can be arranged for individuals with various chronic conditions and in various settings.

Providing for continuity of care is especially important for older adults who move from one level of care to another in an institutional setting, from one institution to another, or from an institution to their homes. Telephone contacts help to arrange continuity of care, and so does the sharing of written care plans with agency staff members or families. Any type of ongoing program, such as bowel and bladder training or transfer training, should not be disrupted. Neglect of continuity of care has a price in human terms that exceeds monetary costs. Although continuing care depends many times on social policy legislation and the philosophy and efforts of health care providers and the agencies in which they work, it is not an impossible dream. To a great extent it depends on the standards of care of the various health care agencies.

Evaluating   Evaluating is the final phase of the four-step model of the nursing process. Its position within the nursing process framework does not, however, indicate its importance (Galton, 1981). Evaluating involves making a judgment about the effectiveness of the nursing action in terms of client response. Data are gathered, especially in the implementing phase, for evaluative purposes. Evaluation is an integral part of the whole nursing process.

The role of the older adult and significant others in the evaluation of progress is described in Standard VI of the *Standards of Gerontological Nursing Practice* (ANA, 1976). Standard VII states the need for an ongoing process of assessment and revision of plans and initiating new nursing action as indicated. Since the client is the focus of the nursing intervention, it is important to get input from the client regarding the outcomes when possible.

When client outcomes of the nursing intervention vary from what is anticipated, it may be the result of an incomplete or inaccurate assessment, or a change in the client's condition or situation; additional options may become available. Even a well-developed plan of care can go awry, since the plan is one thing and its implementation another. An example is the case of Mrs. B., an 84-year-old resident of a high-rise for the elderly, who was having difficulty taking her medications properly. To stay in the high-rise Mrs. B. had to be able to take care of herself. The nurse assessing the situation talked to the client and her neighbor across the hall about the possibility of the neighbor helping with the situation. Both Mrs. B. and the neighbor agreed on a plan to deal with the problem. All went well for a week, and the client's condition improved. For some unknown reason, both parties "disengaged" from responsibility for the administration of medications, and by the time of the nurse's next visit the plan had been scuttled. In evaluating the situation the nurse realized that Mrs. B. was an independent person who liked to control her schedule of activities (such as mealtimes, TV viewing, and time for taking medications) and that probably, once she felt better, she viewed the neighbor's help as intrusive and unnecessary. The neighbor probably also desired the freedom to pursue her interests without interruption. Although the client and the neighbor had been involved in the planning process and indicated their willingness to participate in implementation of the plan, they were unable to continue the arrangement for a prolonged period of time. This example points out the need for continuing evaluation and revision of a plan that for some reason fails to meet the need or resolve the client's problem. The fact that the plan of action, which was initially effective, had been discontinued does not negate the quality of the nursing intervention; it simply indicates the need for flexibility.

The following questions may be asked to facilitate the appraisal of the client's response to the plan of care. (1) Is the care effective? (2) What changes in the client's behavior indicate the effectiveness or ineffectiveness of care? In Mrs. B's case the care plan was effective for a short time;

however, she needed continual supervision with her medications. Therefore from a long-range perspective revision of the plan was indicated. In establishing criteria for evaluation it is necessary to consider whether the objective can be attained in a short time or whether long-term intervention is needed.

Little and Carnevali (1969) described evaluation as a three-step sequential process that includes the following: (1) establishing criteria to guide observations being made for evaluative purposes, (2) gathering information on client responses to nursing interventions with respect to established goals, and (3) comparing formative data to baseline data and to established criteria. In this third phase judgments are made about the client's behavioral change: its direction, stability, and realization. Evaluation is a complex process, but careful planning facilitates it and tends to ensure more systematic and objective results.

Various tools are available for use in evaluations. Olebaum (1974) cites benchmarks of adult wellness that can be used in assessing the older person's level of wellness and in establishing criteria against which to evaluate outcomes of care. Archer and others (1979) discuss the findings of a study aimed at identifying indicators for interventions facilitating the independence of older persons. Life-style indicators, including recreation and other semisocial activities, were assessed. Although the survey was conducted primarily to obtain data for program planning and implementation, some of the information on life-style indicators could be adopted for assessing the independence of older persons and evaluating outcomes of action taken to support or increase this independence, especially in the area of recreational activities. Other tools for evaluating the quality of care (Block, 1975; Yurick and others, 1980) include the Patient Appraisal and Care Evaluation (PACE) instrument from the former Department of Health, Education, and Welfare, Office of Long-Term Care. PACE is used for evaluating the quality of care actually given; it is client-centered and measures achievement of time-limited goals (Yurick and others). Hegyvary (1979) discusses nursing process as a basis for evaluating nursing care quality.

Evaluating outcomes of nursing intervention is important on a nurse-client level; it is also important for increasing older people's self-reliance in meeting their future health care needs. Self-care and self-help groups are ways older as well as younger persons may meet needs with minimal assistance from health care providers, thus conserving limited health care resources. Perhaps of greater importance is the self-respect and sense of mastery over their own lives and well-being that comes with more independence.

In summary the nursing process is an instrument used by nurses to help with making decisions about client care, predictions about the proposed nursing intervention's outcomes, and evaluations of the action's consequences. Concepts and theories from biophysiology, behavioral sciences, and the humanities are used to establish a rationale for the nursing process. Systematic use of the nursing process can be as useful for promoting and maintaining the well-being of older people as it is for younger persons.

Needs and Problems of Older Persons and the Nursing Process

Various aspects of the nursing process have been examined in terms of the needs and problems of older persons. The application of selected components of the nursing process is illustrated in Table 2. Although the material is limited in scope and depth, it is intended to focus attention on nursing diagnoses that may arise in the nurse's interaction with older adults. The cited examples are derived from actual nurses' interactions with older persons in noninstitutional settings. In some cases the same nursing diagnosis is used more than once, since it represents the diagnoses of two different clients, reflecting different approaches to care. These examples demonstrate the fact that although the structure of the nursing process is the same in each case, the nursing action varies because of the clients' individual differences. The variation in approach is also caused by individual differences among nurses who implement the nursing process.

The nursing diagnoses in Table 2 were drawn from the tentative list set forth by Gebbie and Lavin (1974) because their list is simplified and seems appropriate for illustrating use of the nursing process with older adults. Each of the four dimensions of older persons is represented, along with selected components of the nursing process.

In any case nurses need to formalize the process of nursing. Through the systematic and consistent use of the nursing process and documentation of the outcomes of nursing action, nurses can share information that should not only improve the care of individual clients but point out effective and ineffective approaches to care—which will contribute toward further development of gerontological nursing practice. Through use of the nursing process and the *Standards of Gerontological Nursing Practice*, nurses can meet the needs of older persons in our society.

Table 2. **Examples of Selected Nursing Diagnoses***	**Nursing diagnosis†**	**Nursing action**	**Evaluation of client outcomes**	**Comments**
	Biophysical			
	Impairment of urinary elimination (urgency, stress incontinence)	Encouraged 4 glasses of water daily (client taking diuretics for congestive heart failure); taught signs and symptoms of urinary tract infection; explained use of cranberry and orange juices to maintain acid flora	Client asymptomatic of tract infections	Client was interested in learning about her body changes and what might be done to offset the deficits; continued monitoring is indicated
		Encouraged use of Kegel's exercises to improve perineal and sphincter muscle tone; taught exercises	Client able to control stress incontinence, believes exercises are helping	Client was pleased with ability to perform the exercises and the outcomes of her efforts
		Discussed advantages and disadvantages of waterproof pants	Client able to control stress incontinence but wanted to consider pants for "emergencies"	Client who had limited social activities because of fear of incontinence may feel more secure in knowing that waterproof pants are available
		Discussed referral to a physician for evaluation of problem		

*Nursing action, evaluation of client outcomes, and comments based on clinical experiences of graduate students enrolled in the gerontological sequence of courses, Masters in Nursing Program, University of Kansas College of Health Sciences, School of Nursing, Spring 1982.

†Modified from Gebbie, K., and Lavin, M.A.: Classifying nursing diagnosis, **74**(2): February 1974. Copyrighted by the American Journal of Nursing Co.

Continued.

Table 2. Examples of Selected Nursing Diagnoses—cont'd	Nursing diagnosis	Nursing action	Evaluation of client outcomes	Comments
	Biophysical—cont'd			
	Respiratory disturbances and respiratory distress	Removed mucous plug	Client fatigued but appreciative of the fact that emergency was resolved	Laryngectomy had been performed following surgery for carcinoma of head and neck; nausea and pain interfere with fluid intake, resulting in thick, tenacious mucus; client was left alone during day except for visit from Visiting Nurses' Association nurse
		Attempted to increase fluid intake; recommended use of vaporizer	Nausea slightly decreased by medication; client using vaporizer	Fluid intake will probably not be sufficiently increased to handle the problem because of nausea
	Psychological			
	Grieving (older woman)	Encouraged reminiscence about loss of daughter	Client had difficulty initiating reminiscence of her life; however, she seemed appreciative of having someone to share her feelings with	Client was willing to reminisce, but it was a new experience to verbalize about relationship experiences
		Encouraged expression of feelings and crying as expression of regret	Tears were shed on several occasions; client verbalized anger over apparent senselessness of loss of daughter	
		Used touch—held her hand when talking about her feelings regarding her daughter's death	Client responded positively to touch	

Table 2. Examples of Selected Nursing Diagnoses—cont'd	Nursing diagnosis	Nursing action	Evaluation of client outcomes	Comments
	Psychological—cont'd			
	Grieving (older man)	Encouraged expression of feelings about death of sister	Client indicated that the nurse was the only one who cared about him	On previous visit client indicated he was making preparations to visit his sister; when he called to finalize plans, he learned that his sister had died and been buried a month before
		Asked how he had coped with the situation	Client able to talk freely about the event and support he received from neighbors and church friends	
	Sociological			
	Afraid of leaving floor of the high-rise building in which she resides	Explored client's feelings about socialization, history of social interaction, activities	Client shared information, uses walker following left hip replacement; arthritis in right hip further limits mobility; client lives on fifth floor of housing unit, is afraid to ride elevator (relative had been killed when elevator fell); niece, sister visit at least once a week; client uses telephone, listens to favorite radio station, is aware of current events	Will pursue situation further, but doubt that client will increase socialization that requires leaving the floor

Continued.

Table 2. Examples of Selected Nursing Diagnoses—cont'd	Nursing diagnosis	Nursing action	Evaluation of client outcomes	Comments
	Sociological—cont'd			
	Afraid of leaving home because of physical limitations	Performed sociological assessments, including one on social relationships	Client indicated she was not able to go places because of physical limitations; she agreed to try trip to grocery store	Physical assessment did not reveal problems preventing limited social activities; client expressed loneliness; nurse will pursue the possibility of increasing socialization
		Encouraged physical activity, such as walking to nearby grocery store, going to community center	Client walked to grocery store with a neighbor; seemed in better spirits	With continued encouragement, client may increase social activities and benefit from doing so
	Spiritual			
	Alterations with self and others (elderly woman with laryngectomy, in terminal phase of life—carcinoma of head and neck)	Explored her perceptions of the future	Through gestures, a device for aiding speech, and written messages client indicated that she expects to return to her hometown, first to a nursing home, then to her own home	Although conversation revealed a futuristic orientation, her plans for returning home seemed unreal—a form of denial

Table 2. Examples of Selected Nursing Diagnoses—cont'd	Nursing diagnosis	Nursing action	Evaluation of client outcomes	Comments
	Spiritual—cont'd			
	Altered self-concept (elderly woman who is legally blind)	Explored her feelings of despair and comments about taking her life if she could get the pills	Client talked freely about her feelings related to loss of vision, daughter's death, and another daughter's condition (Huntington's chorea) and subsequent admission to an out-of-town nursing home; she related that her son, with whom she lived, was recently diagnosed as also having Huntington's chorea; he was divorced and was trying to get custody of his young daughter who would come to live with the client and her son	Client cried during conversation but seemed relieved to be able to talk about her concerns; she acknowledged thoughts of suicide and that she would find it difficult to take her life; she spoke of bringing in some of her furniture from the farm and of planning in case the granddaughter would be joining the household; she will need further follow-up but the suicide crisis is probably over
		Gave positive feedback on her ability to help maintain home for son and to perform activities of daily living unassisted	Client smiled in response to the praise	

References

American Nurses' Association: Standards of gerontological nursing practice, Kansas City, Missouri, 1976, ANA.

Archer, S.E., and others: Life-style indicators for interventions to facilitate elderly persons' independence, Health Values 3(3):129-135, 1979.

Aspinall, M.J.: Nursing diagnosis—the weak link, Nurs. Outlook 24(7):433-436, 1976.

Beland, I.L., and Passos, J.Y.: Clinical nursing: pathophysiological and psychosocial approaches, ed. 4, New York, 1981, Macmillan, Inc.

Block, D.: Evaluation of nursing care in terms of process and outcome: issues in research and quality assurance, Nurs. Res. 24(4):256, 1975.

Bower, F.L.: The process of planning nursing care: nursing practice models, ed. 3, St. Louis, 1982, The C.V. Mosby Co.

Brown, D.J.: The nursing process system model, J. Nurs. Educ. 20(6):36-40, 1981.

Buscaglia, L.F.: Personhood: the art of being fully human, Thorofare, N.J., 1978, Charles B. Slack, Inc.

Butler, R.N.: The effects of medical and health progress on the social and economic aspects of the life cycle, Industrial Psychol. 1:1-9, 1969.

Butler, R.N., and Lewis, M.I.: Aging and mental health, ed. 3, St. Louis, 1982, The C.V. Mosby Co.

Chavasse, J.: The nursing process, World Irish Nurs. 7(1):1-2, 1978.

Clark, C.C.: Wellness self-assessment, Wellness Newsletter 1:1-4, 1980.

Clark, M.O.: The nursing process. II. For practical reasons, Nurs. Times 74(48):1986-1988, 1978.

Davis, B.A.: Gerontological nursing comes of age, J. Gerontol. Nurs. 1:6-7, 1975.

Dolan, J.A.: Nursing in a society: a historical perspective, ed. 14, Philadelphia, 1978, W.B. Saunders Co.

Dossey, B., and Guzzetta, C.E.: Nursing diagnosis, Nursing '81 11(6):34-38, 1981.

Ebersole, P., and Hess, P.: Toward healthy aging: human needs and nursing responses, St. Louis, 1981, The C.V. Mosby Co.

Edwards, B.J., and Brilhart, J.K.: Communication in nursing practice, St. Louis, 1981, The C.V. Mosby Co.

Fortin, J.D., and Rabinow, J.: Legal implications of nursing diagnoses, Nurs. Clin. North Am. 14(3):553-561, 1979.

Francis, G.M., and Munjas, B.A.: Manual of socialpsychologic assessment, New York, 1976, Appleton-Century-Crofts.

Galton, M.: The evaluation stage of the nursing process, Aust. Nurs. J. 10(10):50-52, 1981.

Gebbie, K., and Lavin, M.A.: Classifying nursing diagnosis, Am. J. Nurs. 74(2):250-253, 1974.

Gebbie, K.M., and Lavin, M.A., editors: Classification of nursing diagnosis: proceedings of the First National Conference, St. Louis, 1975, The C.V. Mosby Co.

Gleit, C.J., and Tatro, S.: Nursing diagnoses for healthy individuals, Nurs. Health Care 2(8):456-457, 1981.

Gould, R.L.: The phases of adult life: a study in developmental psychology, Am. J. Psychiatry 129(5):35, 1972.

Gould, R.: Adult life stages: growth toward self-tolerance, Psychol. Today 8(9):74-78, 1975.

Greenberg, B.M., and Zaranka, J.D.: Medical model–nursing model: a gerontological dilemma? J. Gerontol. Nurs. 1(4):6-14, 1975.

Hall, L.E.: Quality of nursing care. Address at meeting of the Department of Baccalaureate and Higher Degree Programs of the New Jersey League for Nursing, February 1955, Seton Hall University, Newark.

Harris, R.B.: A strong vote for the nursing process, Am. J. Nurs. 79(10):1999-2001, 1979.

Hayter, J.: Positive aspects of aging, J. Gerontol. Nurs. 2(1):19, 1976.

Hegyvary, S.T.: Nursing process: the basis for evaluating the quality of nursing care, Int. Nurs. Rev. 26(4):113-116, 1979.

Hein, E.C.: Communication in nursing practice, ed. 2, Boston, 1980, Little, Brown & Co.

Henderson, V.: The nature of nursing: a definition and its implications for practice, research, and education, New York, 1966, Macmillan, Inc.

Hogstel, M.O.: Communicating with the elderly. In Hogstel, M.O., editor: Nursing care of the older adult, New York, 1981, John Wiley & Sons, Inc.

Holmes, T., and Rahe, T.: The social readjustment rating scale, J. Psychosom. Res. 11(8):213-217, 1967.

Jasmin, S., and Trygstad, L.N.: Behavioral concepts and the nursing process, St. Louis, 1979, The C.V. Mosby Co.

Jung, C.G.: Modern man in search of a soul, New York, 1933, Harcourt Brace Jovanovich, Inc.

Karcher, C.J., and Linden, L.L.: Family rejection of the aged and nursing home utilization, Int. J. Aging Hum. Dev. 5:231-244, 1974.

Kim, M., and Moritz, D., editors: Classification of nursing diagnoses, Proceedings of the third and fourth National Conferences, New York, 1982, McGraw-Hill Book Co.

King, P.A.: Foot problems and assessment, Geriatr. Nurs. 1(3):182-186, 1980.

LaMonica, E.L., editor: The nursing process: a humanistic approach, Menlo Park, Calif., 1979, Addison-Wesley Publishing Co., Inc.

Lash, A.A.: A reexamination of nursing diagnosis, Nurs. Forum 17(4):332-43, 1978.

Lewis, L.: This I believe . . . about the nursing process—key to care, Nurs. Outlook 16:26-29, 1968.

Little, D., and Carnevali, D.: Nursing care planning, Philadelphia, 1969, J.B. Lippincott Co.

Livesey, C.W.: Happy feet, Can. Nurse 77(1):45-54, 1981.

Marriner, A.: The nursing process, ed. 3, St. Louis, 1982, The C.V. Mosby Co.

McGilloway, B.A.: The nursing process: a problem-solving approach to patient care, Int. J. Nurs. Stud. 17(2):79-80, 1980.

Mitchell, P.H.: Concepts basic to nursing, ed. 2, New York, 1977, McGraw-Hill Book Co.

Muhlenkamp, A., Gress, L.D., and Flood, M.A.: Perception of life change events by the elderly, Nurs. Res. 24(2):109-113, 1975.

Murray, R.B., Huelskoelter, M.M.W., and O'Driscoll, D.L.: The nursing process in later maturity, Englewood Cliffs, N.J., 1980, Prentice-Hall, Inc.

Neal, M.C., Cohen, P.F., and Cooper, P.G.: Nursing care planning guides for long-term care, Pacific Palisades, Calif., 1980, Nurseco.

Neilson, A.F.: Why do we need the nursing process? I. For legal reasons, Nurs. Times 74(48):1984-1985, 1978.

Neugarten, B., editor: Middle age and aging, Chicago, 1968, University of Chicago Press.

Neugarten, B., and others: Personality in middle and late life, New York, 1964, Atherton Press.

Olebaum, C.H.: Hallmarks of adult wellness, Am. J. Nurs. 74(9):1623-1625, 1974.

Palmore, E.: Advantages of aging, Gerontologist 19(2):220-222, 1979.

Peplau, H.: Specialization in professional nursing. In Riehl, J., and McVay, J., editors: The clinical nurse specialist interpretations, New York, 1973, Appleton-Century-Crofts.

Popkess, S.A.: Diagnosing your patient's strengths, Nursing '81 11(7):34-37, 1981.

Preston, T.: Caring for the aged: when words fail, Am. J. Nurs. 73:2064, 1973.

Roach, L.B.: Assessments: color changes in dark skin, Nursing '77 7:48-51, 1977.

Schlotfeldt, R.N.: Nursing in the future, Nurs. Outlook 29(5):295-301, 1981.

Smallwood, J., and Stoll, R.: Spiritual dimension of nursing practice. In Beland, I.T., and Passos, J.Y., editors, Clinical nursing: physiological and psychosocial approaches, ed. 3, New York, 1975, Macmillan, Inc.

Smith, B.: A systems model of the nursing process, Aust. Nurs. J. 11(4):33, 1981.

Snyder, J.C., and Wilson, M.F.: Elements of a psychological assessment, Am. J. Nurs. 77(2):235-239, 1977.

Stokes, S.A., Rauckhorst, L.M., and Mezey, M.D.: Health assessment—considerations for the older individual, J. Gerontol. Nurs. 6(6):328-336, 1980.

Stone, V.: Gerontological nursing: student syllabus, Evanston, Ill., 1971, Video Nursing.

Strauss, A.L.: Chronic illness and the quality of life, St. Louis, 1975, The C.V. Mosby Co.

Styles, M.M.: On nursing: toward a new endowment, St. Louis, 1982, The C.V. Mosby Co.

Tebbitt, B.V.: What's happening to continuity of care? Supervisor Nurse **12**(3):22-26, 1981.

Wells, T.J.: That minor skin problem could be trouble, RN Magazine **41**(7):41-46, 1978.

Wells, T.J.: Nursing committed to the elderly. In Reinhardt, A.M., and Quinn, M.D., editors: Current practice in gerontological nursing, vol. 1, St. Louis, 1979, The C.V. Mosby Co.

Wolanin, M.O., and Phillips, L.R.F.: Confusion: prevention and care, St. Louis, 1981, The C.V. Mosby Co.

Yesavage, J.A., Adey, M., and Werner, P.D.: Development of a geriatric behavioral self-assessment scale, J. Am. Geriatr. Soc. **29**(6):285-288, 1981.

Yura, H. and Walsh, M.B., editors: Human needs and the nursing process, New York, 1978a, Appleton-Century-Crofts.

Yura, H., and Walsh, M.B.: The nursing process: assessing, planning, implementing, evaluating, ed. 3, New York, 1978b, Appleton-Century-Crofts.

Yurick, A.G., and others: The aged person and the nursing process, New York, 1980, Appleton-Century-Crofts.

Chapter 11 **Support Systems Networks**

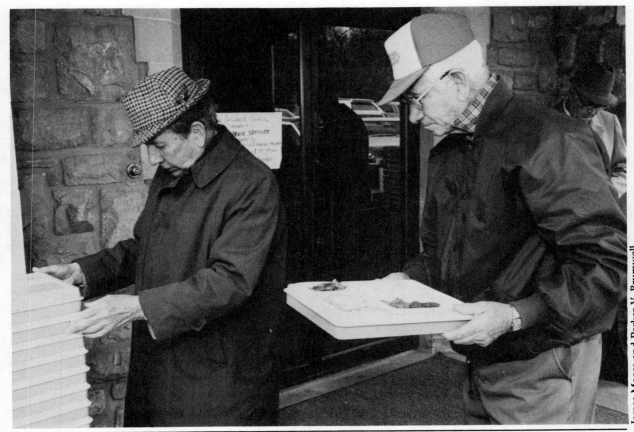

James Moore and Parker V. Brumwell

The survivor of 60 years or more is a person who has acquired the knowledge and skills essential for adapting to changes in the internal and external environments. Adaptation requires the individual to more effectively match abilities with environmental demands and to maintain a measure of independence. In adapting to changes of aging the person develops a resiliency that offsets many deficits. When challenges that arise from aging exceed the person's ability to cope independently, informal and formal support systems may be mobilized to assist the person to maintain integrity and continue the pursuit of personhood.

Systems Theory

The general systems theory presented by von Bertalanffy (1955) provides a theoretical framework for describing the total organization and its elements, such as the older adult and the networks systems. Although complexity occurs because of the dynamics among the various elements of a system (von Bertalanffy, 1955; Hazzard, 1971), the focus is on the whole organism or system and its purpose. Because of its holistic nature the systems theory is widely used by nurses and other health care providers concerned with older people.

The concept of the open living system exemplified by the older adult is based on the concepts of matter, energy, and information (von Bertalanffy). The older adult is able to exchange matter, energy, and information with the environment and may therefore be categorized as an open living system. Regulation of the older adult's system occurs in part through the dynamic interaction of elements, such as the thermoregulatory and neuroendocrine systems.

Hall and Fagan (1968) further defined the systems approach by differentiating systems from environment. This differentiation is based on factors (including the environment) affecting and affected by the system(s) of the object of study at a given time. Thus at the individual system level factors in the external environment, such as temperature and life space, should be taken into account along with those affecting the internal environment, mentioned previously.

In the systems approach the family may be viewed as an open system embedded in a social environment that influences family functioning (Unger and Powell, 1980). The family is an organized, functioning whole interacting interdependently with its environment. Input is received and output shared in an attempt by the family to maintain a steady state through self-regulation. New limits may be set from time to time because of the continuous interaction with other systems; the family system then attempts to regain and maintain a steady state within the newly established parameters.

Nursing also may be viewed within the systems framework. In the nurse-client dyad each individual is a nursing subsystem. The client becomes part of the nursing system when the health care needs exceed the individual's ability to cope independently. The nurse in turn becomes a part of the nursing system when implementing the nursing process in assisting the client to regain a steady state. The nurse and the client together determine a course of action and decide on who is to do what. Planning is preceded by a preliminary assessment of the client's needs and support systems network.

The informal and formal support systems network of the client can also be described within the systems theory framework. Each of these networks can be considered as either a separate system or a subsystem of the larger health care system. In many situations the informal support system composed of family, friends, and neighbors is sufficient to meet the needs of older clients. At other times additional assistance is needed and may be obtained from the formal support system composed of governmental and voluntary agencies. Whatever the situation, the nurse or other health care provider should know these support system resources and how to use them in assisting older people.

Sharing information with the client regarding needs assessment and available resources is an important function of the gerontological nurse. This function characterizes the interrelationship of open systems that can be used for satisfying unmet needs of older clients.

One of the major problems of older people is their increasing vulnerability related to deaths of family and friends and the ensuing losses to the support systems network. Older people are concerned not only with whether there will be anyone around who will care enough to assist with physical care, but also with whether others will respect their desire to exercise their basic human rights and to retain mastery over their affairs.

An example of this problem is Mr. B., the 82-year-old bachelor mentioned in Chapter 10, who lives alone on a small farm. He lets a neighboring family pasture their horses on his farm free of rent-because of the security he feels in knowing someone will be by every day. Recently Mr. B. was hospitalized for anginal pain and subsequently for a hernia repair. Although his recovery from the surgical procedure was remarkably uneventful and the nitroglycerine patches he wears are reasonably effective in controlling the anginal pain, Mr. B.'s convalescence has been disturbed by the fact that the neighbor who uses his pasture and another close neighbor have recently stopped by to express interest in purchasing his farm. Mr. B. is aware of his changing physical condition but desires to manage his affairs and remain on his farm for as long as possible. No matter how well intentioned, the approach of these neighbors about his property has caused Mr. B. to question the motives behind their neighborly acts, such as bringing in food. Since Mr. B. has tried to be a good neighbor and has paid well for help, such as transportation, he felt that he was maintaining his independence and good standing in the neighborhood. Being a kind person who finds it difficult to express feelings that might be construed as negative and who realizes the need for increasing social support, Mr. B. is distressed by this not-so-subtle reminder of his vulnerability. Whether or not the neighbors' interest in his well-being is sincere, the situation reinforces his insecurity and is a problem to be dealt with in future nurse-client interactions.

Mr. B.'s situation also illustrates the relationship between support systems. Because of the loss of some of his siblings by death, the declining capacities of his remaining siblings, and separation by geographical distance, Mr. B. is deprived of the measure of social support that ordinarily would have been provided by his family. In his situation the need for a relationship with extrafamilial support systems is apparent. Systems that are in keeping with the unique needs of older persons can function like family relationships in supporting them.

The Concept of Support

The concept of support essential to the well-being of the individual arises out of the person's early experiences within a family. It is operationalized in the dynamics occurring during the family's developmental process. The family tends to emphasize its independence rather than interdependence, especially with respect to extrafamilial support. This emphasis on independence sometimes inhibits acceptance of needed support by the older adult, even when the changes of aging result in various needs.

The idea of support is frequently referred to with respect to needs of the elderly, but a clear definition of it as it is used in clinical situations is lacking. Weiss (1976) speaks of the paucity of information on what to do during crisis episodes. He suggests that support is the most useful form of help. According to Weiss, support consists of communication and the apparent willingness of persons to help the dependent individual reestablish equilibrium. This communication may be verbal or nonverbal. Although consensus on the clinical definition of support is lacking, there is little if any disagreement on its value.

In an exploratory study of social networks, support, and coping Tolsdorf (1976) defines support as action that assists the dependent person to meet personal needs based on a particular situation. The nature of support varies according to the needs of individuals and the available resources. Support may include emotional, monetary, or other forms of support, such as goods and services. There is a variety of types of support that may be needed by older persons.

Support has sometimes been associated with strength. On occasion support is described as helping people to use their strength in adapting to life events (Hart and Reltweder, 1959; Weidenbach, 1964). Problem solving is also related to support. For example, Jones (1962) speaks of helping persons clarify problems; Hart and Reltweder mention the need to provide opportunity for individuals to express or solve problems; Gregg (1955) speaks of the need to assist the individual with problem solving. Others emphasize the need to teach, listen, and talk to the dependent individual (Gardner, 1979). These approaches point out the importance of communication skills in the provision of support (Preston, 1973; Gardner). Implicit in the concept of support is the importance of maintaining the strength of older individuals experiencing dependency needs.

Part of the difficulty in investigating the concept of support is related to the problem of measurement (Dean and Lin, 1977). Cobb (1976) offers a definition that seems to describe the essence of the concept as it is applied clinically. He speaks of social support as that which gives the individual the feeling of being loved, esteemed, and cared for. With this notion of support the dependent individual is viewed as a member of a network of mutual obligations. This suggests that outcomes of social support can be measured in terms of perception of information (Fuller and Larson, 1980). If this means of measurement were to be accepted, a consensus about the meaning of support would be more nearly realized.

Cobb indicates that theoretically the person's perception of social support should improve the ability to cope with life changes and related crises. Although interaction between life changes and social support has been supported by previous research (Cobb), Fuller and Larson cite the paucity of research on the predictability of life change events or crises that may occur among older people. Little is known, therefore, about the outcomes of support of older persons experiencing life change crises.

Fuller and Larson investigated one form of social support, emotional support, in an effort to determine whether it would help individuals cope with life change events. Cobb's definition of emotional support was used in this investigation; measurement criteria for the study included selected indices of physical and psychological health. Findings suggested that some type of support other than emotional might be helpful to persons during periods of stress or change. Fuller and Larson suggest that older persons might benefit more from knowing that they are needed than from passively receiving the concern of others.

Fuller and Larson's observation that the older person desires to be needed tends to agree with Cobb's definition of support, in which the individual perceives the self as a member of a network of mutual obligations. They cite the need for research on the effects of life events on the well-being of older people. They also cite the need for experimental research for discovering methods to counteract negative aspects of life changes. Since the influence of emotional and other forms of social support on the health of older persons is not clearly understood, further research is warranted. The concept of support held by elderly individuals is likely to influence not only their participation in the support network but their acceptance of support in case of need. The perceptions of older people are critical to their self-esteem, their desire to be needed, and the effective use of limited resources.

Support Systems

The notion of support has been explored as background for the idea of support systems. Just as the term *social* expands the concept of support to interaction among two or more individuals, the term *system* further expands it by reflecting an organization wherein an orderly way of providing supportive services is maintained. Support is activated within a basic social unit: someone needing assistance and someone willing to provide it. Needs of older persons sometimes exceed the capabilities of the basic social unit, and additional help must be sought from other support systems, informal and formal.

The concept of support systems, defined differently by different individuals, expands on that of social support. The basic support unit may have to be expanded into a support system when the needs of older people require additional assistance. Caplan defines support system as "an enduring pattern of continuous or intermittent ties that play a significant part in maintaining the psychological and physical integrity of the individual over time" (Caplan, 1974, p. 7). This definition reflects the continuity of support through its ongoing availability; it encompasses the spectrum of support services available through the informal and formal support systems.

Generally the concept of the social support system is viewed as helping older persons with three major needs: "socialization, the carrying out of tasks of daily living, and assistance during times of illness or crisis" (Gurian and Cantor, 1978, p. 186). The concept is further refined through use of the informal, semiformal, and formal systems, which is discussed in the following sections.

Briefly, the informal support system—family, friends, and neighbors—functions in a way that meets the instrumental and affective needs of individuals for such things as financial aid and emotional support. The informal system is given priority because it is the first line of support for most older persons (Gurian and Cantor).

The formal system is generally defined as composed of governmental agencies (such as Social Security) and voluntary agencies (such as the American Red Cross). This system functions primarily in an instrumental mode through programs that provide resources, such as income, transportation, and housing (Gurian and Cantor).

According to Gurian and Cantor, between the informal and formal support systems are individuals functioning in a semiformal helping role— for instance, mail carriers, storekeepers, and church members. These people often meet some of the socialization needs of older persons by taking time to exchange a few words with them when they meet. In addition these people often monitor the older person and report any unusual observations that might indicate a problem. This semiformal system is valuable to the welfare of older persons and the conservation of health care resources.

The various types of support systems are discussed in more detail later. Since support systems and networks are closely related and sometimes used interchangeably, the elements of both are discussed in the section on networks. One of the major differences between the two concepts is in the communication that links the support systems into a network. In a sense the network system is a dimension of the support system.

The Concept of Networks

The concept of networks is closely aligned with that of support and support systems. Support is aimed at meeting basic human needs, whereas a network is the interrelation of groups or systems. Older persons are often unaware that they are surrounded by multiple support systems until they need assistance.

Definitions of Networks and Functions

Networks are linkages of interrelated groups or systems that facilitate communication and mobilization of support when the need arises. The network's linkage of support systems provides a means of organizing a more comprehensive approach to satisfying the needs of older persons. Transportation, homemaker services, telephone reassurance, and health care are but a few of the services that can be mobilized through the support systems network.

The network is activated by such events as the illness of an older person or the death of a spouse. Various types of support may be mobilized: emotional support, food preparation, transportation, or running errands. The structure of the network is relatively invisible, but it is readily identified by its functions (Speck and Attneave, 1973).

The network's information exchange is put into operation by a number of persons who are not necessarily known to all the members of that particular network system. The network often extends beyond the boundaries of a particular group. An individual's network usually consists of significant human relationships that have lasting meaning to the individual (Speck and Attneave), but during periods of stress or crises many persons may participate in helping the affected person irrespective of any personal relationship. The network functions as a communication system, to facilitating the mobilization of needed support.

The importance of networks, according to Pilisuk (1980), is the extent to which their functions meet the essential needs of their members. These functions are summarized in the definition of supportive networks that refers to relationships and interpersonal contracts by which individuals maintain social identity and receive support, such as material aid, services, information, and new contacts (Walker, McBride, and Vachon, 1977). A reciprocating relationship is implied in this definition; its value cannot be denied.

Attributes of Social Support Networks

Pilisuk and Minkler (1980) suggest that the theory of social networks provides the most appropriate framework for study of the informal bonds of social support. A set of terms describes the interactions of individuals, or nodes, within a network, and each exchange provides a link among these nodes. Certain characteristics of social support networks provide a means of describing and analyzing these intentional systems of continuing support. They include (1) size, determined by the number of persons in social contact through a particular network, including contacts made only in times of need; (2) geographic location, which may range from those in a single dwelling site to those more widely scattered in a single neighborhood; and (3) similarity among members, in such areas as age, sex, income, education, marital status, or shared experiences such as bereavement, divorce, welfare status, or physical disability (Pilisuk and Minkler). These characteristics provide the basis for assessing the ability of networks to match the needs of individuals with appropriate services.

Types of Support Systems Networks

Informal Support Systems Network

Support systems networks of older adults, like support systems generally, tend to be categorized as informal and formal.

The informal support systems network is composed of family, friends, and neighbors. The family is the major resource of older persons (Shanas, 1979; Olsen and Cahn, 1980). Older persons tend to turn first to families, second to friends, and last to neighbors for assistance in times of adversity. Many services are available to older people through the auspices of the formal support systems network, but the informal support network is the resource of choice (Lindsey and Hughes, 1981; Sanders and Seelbach, 1981).

The family. The family is most often defined as a nuclear unit, composed of husband, wife, and their children, surrounded by a number of relatives

(Linton, 1936). Ball (1972) proposes a definition of family as a group of individuals living together in a social arrangement; this would include contemporary cohabiting relationships. These groups are characterized by relationships that provide gratification and emotional support similar to that provided by the more traditional family form. Ball's proposed definition acknowledges the existence of variant family forms within the informal support systems network.

The kinship group. The kinship group is a modified extended family composed of various nuclear families bonded together by affection and choice (Sussman and Burchinall, 1966). Members of this group share with each other in various ways, especially in providing emotional support.

Fictive kin. Fictive kin refers to a relationship between biologically unrelated individuals. Fictive kin are usually friends (Ball); they are comparable to family members who are related biologically or by marriage. Fictive kin are not necessarily adopted legally, but they are accepted into the family as regular members and often share family responsibilities.

An example of this type of relationship is a family that "adopts" an elderly neighbor and relates to that individual as to a grandparent. The individual is often invited to join the family for meals, trips to the grocery store, or family outings. Both the family and the older person benefit from this relationship.

According to Tibbitts (1977), most Americans live in a family or within a kinship system. In 1977 6.9 million families (14% of all families in the United States) were headed by a husband of 65 or over. These data reflect a significant change of this century: the longevity of the family after the children have left the parental home.

Although defining "living-together groups" as families allows for recognition of traditional and nontraditional family relationships, it raises questions about legitimization and the religious sanction of marriage, which are useful in defining status and functions. According to Sussman (1976), society needs a definition of family that allows for settling conflicts that may require extrafamilial protection of affected family members' rights. The nuclear family form is recognized as the definition best suited for this. The nuclear family is more easily identified and responsibilities for various kinds of support are more clearly delineated than is the case in nontraditional family groups. Nevertheless there are variant family forms; it behooves nurses to know these forms as they interact with older persons and their families.

The friendship network. Friendship is a relationship in which each person knows the other person well and shares a fondness and attachment for the other. Friendship usually arises out of common interests and similar backgrounds. Studies have led some to believe that the older person who has a friend as a confidant is better able to cope with the changes of aging than the one who lacks peer support (Lowenthal and Haven, 1968; Blau, 1973). Riley and Foner (1968), on the other hand, minimize the importance of friends next to that of family. They view friends and neighbors as being complements more than substitutes for kin. Blau and Rosow (1965) suggest that the relationship with the family may be negatively affected by its obligatory nature. Moreover, Blau suggests that social distancing occurs between generations because of differences in experience and interests and because children usually do not depend on their parents. After experiencing life events such as retirement and widowhood older persons need relationships with those who share their needs and interests (Ebersole and Hess, 1981).

Friends can share whatever resources they have—monetary resources, transportation, housing—without question. Also, according to Blau, the relationship with friends supports the individual's self-esteem and feelings of usefulness to a greater extent than family relationships do. Families often take older family members for granted and may not be sensitive to their self-esteem and need to feel needed. Friends also help maintain informal contact with persons outside the home (Riley and Foner). Contact between those who understand and appreciate one another provides for an exchange of ideas and expression of feelings, which may not be possible in the family circle. The quality of the relationship between friends is usually good, but it may not last as long as family relationships for various reasons. The nurse can help the older person to make contacts and establish new friendships when the loss of friends occurs.

Neighbors. The relationship among persons who live in close proximity varies. In rural areas neighbors may not live as close to each other as those in urban areas, but they may be close in terms of helping relationships. People living in rural areas usually know their neighbors, whereas those living in apartments may not know their neighbors. In most situations neighbors are not as likely to participate as independent resources in the informal support system network, but they can be an important component of it.

Neighbors can provide various types of support, usually for a limited period of time. Assistance with transportation, shopping, and food preparation during illnesses is the type of support usually provided by neighbors. Another help is monitoring. Neighbors often establish a means of determining that the older person is alright, such as observing that the window shades are raised in the morning or that the newspaper is picked up. In rural areas a sheet may be raised on a pole like a flag to signal that all is well. The telephone, when available, is another means of monitoring.

Neighbors tend to complement the other components of the informal support systems network.

Careful assessment of the informal support systems network of older clients is an important function of gerontological nurses. Older adults may have elderly children who are in a state of greater dependence than their parents. Changes in the composition of families brought about by divorce and consequent changes in family relationships have yet to be evaluated with respect to their effect on the older person's family support system. A family may or may not be a dependable source of support for older persons; the support system of older persons should be assessed on an individual basis.

Formal Support Systems Network

Formal support systems networks are another component of the total systems network. Formal support systems tend to provide broad-based programs in such areas as health, economy, transportation, and education (Gurian and Cantor, 1978). Various kinds of support have special techniques and technological treatments; they involve people prepared in various fields of endeavors.

Formal support systems are mechanisms that provide goods and services through organized programs of governmental and voluntary agencies. Goods such as food and clothing are often provided during crises such as fires or floods. Services such as transportation and educational programs may be provided. Formal support systems help many older persons to maintain their identity and integrity.

Although the elderly depend a great deal on the informal support system, they also rely to a great extent on formal support systems. Formal organizations are often impersonal, since they are organized to meet the needs of groups rather than individuals. They accomplish tasks by using technological advancements of the postindustrial society. Because of their nature formal systems tend to operate at an instrumental level rather than at an expressive level, which is characteristic of informal systems. In view of the many needs of older persons both the informal and formal support systems are necessary.

Formal support systems of maintenance and care began in the early twentieth century in the United States (Sussman, 1976). Programs of economic support such as welfare and social security are supported by taxation. Since older persons have contributed to these programs through taxation, they can consider their benefits as deserved. These programs exemplify the increasing use of formal support systems.

A communications network is necessary to help both the informal and formal support systems function effectively. Technology, which has become so much a part of the formal support systems in other areas, also contributes to the dissemination of information about the systems. However, in spite of the United States having one of the most extensive communication networks (Trager, 1976), people are often uninformed about available goods and services. This situation limits efforts to match the needs of older persons with appropriate service agencies. Dissemination of information about support services thus becomes one of the major challenges of those concerned with assisting the elderly. Little is gained by support services, no matter how necessary or effective they might be, if older people are unaware of them.

On the other hand, sometimes support services are not as accessible as they might be. This is more often the case in rural than in urban areas. Sometimes the support system itself may become a source of stress. Accessibility is not just a matter of geographical distance; lack of transportation may also limit access to goods and services. Either way, the formal support system becomes a stressor for the person who cannot reach it. Accessibility is an important factor in the evaluation of support services.

Furthermore, exploration of aging and supportive networks should consider the kinds of need that are common among older persons. These needs are often in individuals having one or more chronic conditions that affect their coping ability. Because many chronic conditions are progressive, the concept of long-term care has come into use. Initially this concept was defined with respect to institutions providing care (long-term care institutions). More recently, however, long-term care has come to be defined in terms of persons who have chronic conditions and require assistance for long periods of time in any setting. This shift in the definition of long-term care focuses attention onto the full spectrum of care meeting the needs of older persons.

Governmental and voluntary agencies compose the major part of the formal support system. Economic and social policies are implemented through various laws, including the Older Americans Act, the Social Security Act, Medicare, and Medicaid (Gurian and Cantor, 1978). Programs developed out of these legislative acts have for the most part been funded 50% or more by the federal government. State and local governments have made up the balance of funding in a partnership arrangement intended to decentralize the administration of various programs. Administration of the various services for older persons has been handled through state and area agencies on aging. Although these agencies generally do not provide direct services to the elderly, they contract for services on the basis of a needs assessment of given areas. This allows for provision of services according to the areas' specific needs.

Services provided through such acts as the Older Americans Act and the Social Security Act include nutrition, recreation, homemaker and home chore services, transportation, information and referral, and protective and legal services (Gurian and Cantor). These services are remarkable, but an increasing need for additional services in the home exists. A major thrust is being directed toward helping elderly persons remain in their customary places of residence for as long as possible.

Agencies of the formal support systems network are generally put into two groups: (1) governmental and (2) voluntary agencies. A brief description of each is presented in the following paragraphs.

Governmental agencies. Official governmental health agencies are created and given power through statutes enacted by elected lawmakers; they are financed by public taxes (Stewart, 1979). These official agencies are accountable to elected public officials. Generally federal and state agencies are involved in administering and coordinating programs, conducting research, establishing standards and qualifications, and analyzing statistics. Local agencies, county and city, carry out federal and state directives. They provide direct health services, such as health education, disease prevention, and health promotion. The formal support system is composed of a number of agencies designed to meet the instrumental needs of older persons in a rather impersonal manner; this manner is partly what distinguishes the formal support system from the informal system. Because of the nature of its programs and services and because they are planned for groups of people rather than for individuals, an impersonal approach can be expected; however, this is not always the case. In addition to governmental agencies a number of voluntary agencies in the formal support system contribute to the support of older persons.

Voluntary agencies. Voluntary agencies are described as having an "official" power; they are financed primarily by private and nontax monies. Examples of voluntary agencies are the American Cancer Society and the Visiting Nurses' Association, which have provided home health care services since 1885. These agencies provide services primarily for long-term care of the chronically ill or disabled. Since 1966 voluntary agencies have come to depend increasingly on federal and private, third-party insurers for pay for services to their clients (Stewart).

Perhaps one of the ways to improve service to older persons is to establish a closer working relationship between the informal and formal support systems networks. This relationship would involve developing an effective communication network to facilitate coordination and prevent overlap or duplication of services. A change in regulations might be needed so that older persons would not be penalized for availing themselves of services from both informal and formal support systems. Provision of services through these two systems would not necessarily be less expensive, but would be more humane. Blending the two support systems is particularly important in view of the rapidly increasing numbers of older persons and their predicted impact on health care systems.

The increasing number of persons who are 75 years of age and above, referred to as the frail elderly, require additional services as their health status changes. Many of these persons could remain in their own homes longer if appropriate supportive services were available. As their capacities and functional abilities decrease, the informal support system may be unequal to the task of meeting their health care needs. With assistance from the formal support system the informal system may continue to sustain older persons viably. An important function of gerontological nursing is not only knowing the resources of the informal and formal support systems but directing efforts toward achieving comprehensive care for the frail elderly through appropriate use of assistance from these two systems.

When a life change event occurs suddenly, resulting in a crisis in the informal support system, blending the two support systems could provide an additional sense of security. This possibility is pointed out in the following account of an event that quickly changed the pattern of the lives of several people. A 74-year-old woman died suddenly at home, leaving a number of older persons bereft of an important component of their informal support system. Her uncle of the same age, who lived with her, confronted the question of his future. Because of a cardiac condition he could hardly walk from one room to another. His comment to anyone listening was that he guessed he would have to go to a nursing home now. An older couple living in an upstairs apartment in the house also wondered about their future. Although they were not related to the deceased owner of the house, they had a close relationship with her that could be categorized as a fictive kinship. They assumed roles ordinarily performed by relatives and had enjoyed a family-like relationship for many years. They were struggling not only with the sudden loss of a close friend but with the likelihood of having to give up the apartment they had called home for 30 years. At the time of the crisis ownership of the home was undetermined; it was not known if a will transferred ownership to someone and if so to whom. What had been a viable kinship and friendship support system suddenly became incapable of functioning at the usual level, at least temporarily. Knowledge of the formal support network might have provided them with a sense of security and perhaps have alleviated some of their stress.

A number of the deceased lady's friends also experienced an acute sense of loss. Not only had she been a close friend with a number of her peers, but she had also been an important part of the social support system for several who were housebound by infirmities. She kept in frequent touch with them by telephone and shopped for them. This woman had undoubtedly been instrumental in keeping her friends out of an institution. Her sudden death gave rise to questions about how the needs of her friends would be met.

Assistance from the formal support system, such as Meals on Wheels and a homemaker service, could provide alternatives, but it is uncertain whether these older persons were aware of available services and how to tap them. The uncle of the deceased woman could continue living in that house for many years if he could have such services. The likelihood of this older man remaining in the house would also be enhanced if the older couple living in the upstairs apartment were willing to check periodically to see that he was all right. This arrangement would also be contingent on whether the couple would be able to continue living there. Perhaps more often than realized a need exists for mobilizing support from the formal system—perhaps on a temporary basis—when a break occurs in the informal support system.

In short, with the death of one person the situation of a number of frail elderly persons may suddenly be compromised. A mechanism is needed whereby their needs can be met and institutionalization prevented if possible. The kind of situation just described points out the need for a relationship between the informal and formal support systems that would provide continuity of care. Older persons may be able to return to managing within the informal support system once the crisis is over. A communication network is essential for coordinating support from the informal and formal systems and maximizing the benefits of these resources for the frail elderly.

A chart reflecting the components of the informal and formal systems is provided in Fig. 11-1 to help identify types of support. The chart also conceptualizes the resources of both systems and how they might be used to provide comprehensive care for older adults. In addition attention is directed toward the interrelationships among the communication networks that can make these systems more effective.

Models of Informal Support Systems

Two models of informal support systems currently in use are the family self-care model and the self-help model. Information on these models may be useful in assessing informal support systems and in helping families to plan care.

Family Self-care Model

The family self-care model is based on the concept that management of health care rests with the family itself (Pratt, 1977). It is an extension of the concept of individual self-care. Operationalizing family self-care requires answers to such questions as who performs the health care tasks, what forms of care are used, and how and where self-care is carried out.

Fig. 11-1. **Support systems.**

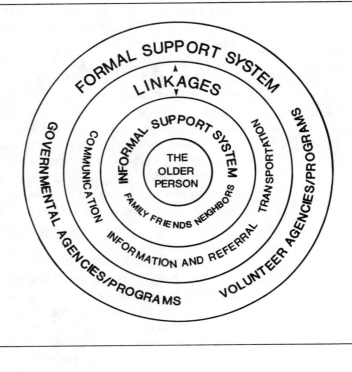

In the family self-care approach the family participates to a greater extent than in other forms of health care. It makes decisions about well-being and coordinates activities directed toward health promotion. A shift toward family self-care is evident in the kind of knowledge families seek regarding health care. An example of an issue they might face is whether to use extraordinary measures in the care of a seriously ill family member. In some cases the elderly couple elects to continue their particular life-style in spite of opposition from concerned adult children. The condition of the elderly couple may require concerted efforts by each spouse to keep body and soul together. This kind of relationship is sometimes called *symbiotic*. Adult children are often very anxious about their elderly parents; yet they may accept the parents' decision to remain in their own home and attempt to provide the help necessary to support their decision. This arrangement is not necessarily easier for the adult children, but in the family self-care model the family does not shirk what it considers to be its responsibility.

Self-help Model   Another model of an informal support system is the self-help model. Self-help is achieved through group efforts, which are usually organized around the needs of family members. These may be needs of either the individual family member requiring care or family members giving care. In either case self-help groups tend to be composed of those having concerns or problems in common, for instance families with a member who has had a stroke or who has Alzheimer's disease. Such families may meet to learn more about how to deal with the needs and problems of their family members, to obtain emotional support, and to have a social outlet. They may ventilate their feelings and learn how others are dealing with similar feelings and various aspects of care. Sometimes they give respite to each other: one might briefly take the other's charge, allowing the other an opportunity for shopping or a trip to the beauty shop. Relief afforded by someone who is experiencing a similar problem is supportive in and of itself. Whatever their makeup may be, self-help groups offer a great deal of support to families (who provide 80% to 90% of the care given to elderly family members).

Changing Relationships and the Informal Support Systems Network

Weiss (1969) speaks of the different kinds of relationships existing among individuals in the informal support systems network and their varied functions. Weiss believes that one relationship may serve several functions, such as nurturance and validation of worth. He suggests that relationships tend to become specialized in meeting certain needs and that individuals require a number of relationships to achieve and maintain a state of well-being. Rosow (1967) supports this theory of specialized functions in a relationship; he believes that friends cannot be functional substitutes for family or vice versa.

Relationship needs of older persons change during the later years. Progressive loss of relationships through death or other situations (such as geographical distance) and in some cases change in the nature of relationships contribute toward changing the relationship needs of older persons. Less demanding relationships may be needed because of declining physical strength and energy or decreased affluence. Customary activities that help maintain social contacts such as the exchange of gifts and letters may be discontinued. An important function of the informal support systems network is to assess the changing relationships of older adults and to provide appropriate support.

An excellent example of the manner in which relationships and functions of an older person may change and of the response of the informal support systems network is portrayed in the book *Gramp* (Jury and Jury, 1976). The story of the family's care for Gramp is beautifully illustrated in this true account of events occurring over a 3-year period. Although the circumstances that created the need for prolonged support of the ailing family member were unfortunate, the beautiful example of a caring family is unsurpassed. This family has made a remarkable contribution not only in carrying out the traditional function of caring for a dependent family member but in sharing the story of the process with those who may face similar circumstances. One can "learn a living" and learn about the worth and dignity of an older person by reading *Gramp*.

In the preceding paragraphs a brief description of the changing relationships among people and the informal support systems network has been presented. Although family structure and functions continue to change, research indicates that the family remains a major source of support for older adults. Friends and neighbors serve as an extension of the family and function in a complementary role in the informal support system. Effectiveness of the informal support systems network is evidenced to a great extent by the fact that 95% of the older adult population in the United States live in noninstitutional settings. While the formal systems network provides assistance, the preferred source of support is family, friends, and neighbors; this informal support system provides a greater amount of needed assistance. It remains to be seen how the advent of the family with two geriatric generations will affect the capabilities of the informal support systems. At this time the informal network is readily identifiable in urban and rural communities and continues to provide invaluable services to people.

Assessing Informal Support Systems

The following questions may be useful in gathering information about the informal support system of the older adult:

- How many persons live with you?
- What is your relationship to them?
- Whom would you call for help in time of need?
- Are there family members living close by?
- Are you in frequent contact with them?
- Is there anyone other than family that you could turn to for help?
- How do you manage household chores?

Answers to such questions provide information about the individual's ability to deal with the need for assistance should the occasion arise; they can also indicate whether additional resources from the formal support system might be needed in case of a change in health status.

Of more value in determining the family situation is specific information about the client's ethnic origin, cultural beliefs, and health practices. The need for health education should be assessed accordingly. Information may be needed about the formal support system, especially for families who have recently entered the country.

The importance of considering the family's cultural background is evident in a recent newspaper article entitled "The Later Years." Its author reports the experience of a family trying to meet the needs of an elderly parent (Haley, 1980). The mother, a Taiwanese, emigrated to the United States in 1968 to join her four children. Her life had been disrupted in 1947 by the Taiwanese uprising and the depletion of savings caused by the attempt to save her physician-husband's life. This elderly woman, on coming to the United States, visited each of her children and at first enjoyed being in a new country.

After about 7 years, however, this woman began to complain of various types of pain: arthritis and headaches. She became hypertensive and increasingly forgetful, demanding, and suspicious. In 3 more years she became very docile but needed to be reminded to carry out personal care activities, such as bathing and brushing her teeth. A thorough physical examination resulted in a diagnosis of senile dementia.

A daughter living in Kansas City had been sharing the responsibility of her mother's care with a sister and two brothers who lived in other states and another country. As the mother's condition worsened and care for her became more demanding, the arrangement whereby the mother spent a portion of the year with each child became impractical. Furthermore, it was felt that constant moving probably added to the mother's confusion.

The daughter in Kansas City, a medical/social worker, searched for a source of supportive care, such as a day-care program. She and her siblings were intent on finding a source of noninstitutional care. However, because of the severity of the mother's condition and the fact that she could speak only Japanese and Taiwanese the search for day-care proved unsuccessful; the attempt to find someone who could speak her language to stay with her also failed.

Finally the daughter found an intermediate-care facility in Los Angeles, the Japanese Retirement Home, which accepted her mother. In this setting the mother began talking with people in Japanese and participating in activities. Despite limitations the mother came to enjoy regular visits from a group of Taiwanese women and from one of her sons, who lived nearby. Being among people who speak her language and where the climate more nearly approximates that from which she came has made a great deal of difference in the quality of her life. Some of the concerns of the family, who reluctantly gave up part of its tradition of caring for an elderly parent, have been relieved.

This story points out the importance of obtaining support for the older person that respects his or her ethnic origins and cultural beliefs and practices. In this situation an appropriate ethnic resource was unavailable in Kansas City. Fortunately the family could avail itself of a resource located near one of its members.

Another way the informal support system functions is evident in the account of a family that for the most part cared for an elderly member in his own home for 2 years after a cerebral vascular accident. It is an example of how the kin network functions; it can be used for identifying important factors in assessing the family support system.

Mr. and Mrs. T., aged 88 and 84 years, respectively, at the time of the crisis, lived in their own urban home. Three of their daughters and one son lived nearby; the remaining son lived in a southeastern state. Immediately after suffering a cerebrovascular accident, Mr. T. was hospitalized; he was later transferred to a health care facility for a brief period of time; he was then taken home. His transfer to the health care facility would probably not have happened except for the fact that Mrs. T. had been home for only 2 days after surgery for a fractured hip when her husband became ill.

Mr. T.'s condition required a great deal of care. Because of right-sided hemiplegia and urinary and fecal incontinence constant attention was needed. During the 2 years prior to Mr. T.'s death, the adult children who shared the responsibility with their mother for his care never left her alone. The son who lived out of state was not immediately available, but he provided the emotional support important in long-term periods of illness. After Mr. T. died, the family expressed satisfaction in having kept him at home where he wanted to be and in having met his wishes and needs without undue delay.

In this situation the family was able to identify its needs for assistance and use various resources to meet them. A member of the extended family, who was a retired nurse, assisted in the physical care of Mr. T. on occasion and was a source of emotional support. A friend of the family, who could be categorized as fictive kin, provided a great deal of support in helping with food preparation, running errands, and emotional support. At times when the care was too taxing for the family, other persons were hired to help. On occasion the family physician made house calls and a podiatrist came to the home to treat Mr. T.'s ingrown toenails. During Mr. T.'s illness his family learned a great deal about basic nursing care and various health care resources. In spite of limitations following hip surgery, Mrs. T. participated in her husband's care. This story illustrates the strengths of a family and its ability to mobilize resources to care for its members during illness.

Assessing an older person should always include an assessment of the individual's informal support system. If this system is viable, it may prevent the institutionalization of an older person. Assistance through the informal system tends to support the self-esteem of the older individual because it helps him or her to maintain a sense of control over life events.

Assessing the support system of older adults involves recognizing differences among the various ethnic groups. For example, the strong kinship ties among black people may be the result of a greater cultural emphasis on kinship. Another hypothesis attributes it to the generally low socioeconomic level and need to share resources. According to Lee (1980), evidence supports both of these hypotheses. In view of the current information on kin ties, cultural factors are most often cited to explain black kin relationships. Cultural factors should be taken into account when assessing the needs or problems of older persons.

Examples of viable kin networks that continue over time are apparent among residents of a high-rise housing unit primarily lived in by black elderly people. Although the woman who described old age as a "no care" time of life had family members who kept in touch with her on a regular basis, she still felt lonely. This elderly lady, however, not only identified a need but initiated action to deal with it. Her problem-solving ability led her to buy eggs from a lady at the door; it was innovative and brought about some increase in socialization. Although a kin network existed in this situation, another resource was tapped in an attempt to satisfy a need of high intensity.

In still another situation in the high-rise, an elderly frail black woman moved her disabled older sister into her apartment so she could more easily give her the physical care she needed. The older sister's apartment was retained to provide storage for furniture and other possessions. Although keeping the apartment is a financial strain, the sacrifice is made because of the older sister's desire to keep her possessions. The adult daughter and grandchildren of the younger sister help care for the disabled sister. Strong kin networks are maintained in times of adversity; they are often useful even in unusual situations like this one.

Another example of cultural differences can be found in the informal support system of the American Indian. In this culture the support system is organized around the extended family rather than the nuclear family, as tends to be the case with the white family (Red Horse, 1980). Cultural beliefs and practices reinforce traditional family relationship patterns. Individual family members are integral members of a tribe; they gain identity and ego integrity through the harmonious balance between work and vital family functions (Red Horse, 1980). A responsibility for maintaining harmony with the environment is shared by all members of the tribe. This responsibility is discharged through interdependent functions.

Instead of retiring at some point in their later years, elders in the tribe are increasingly pulled into the mainstream of the tribe. Indians believe that they carry within them their ancestors' spirit. They are therefore concerned with preserving the unity and harmony that contributes to an ongoing sense of brotherhood and to the spirit of their ancestors. Elders in turn depend on the informal kin system for whatever support is necessary to maintain tribal relationships and to carry out tribal responsibilities.

It is interesting that the United States was founded by people supported by an informal network of family, friends, and neighbors, and that the needs of its people continue to be met in this way to a great extent in spite of societal changes brought about by the industrial revolution. The early settlers had varying ethnic origins, and those differences in cultural beliefs and practices persist. There is a blending of efforts to meet the needs of older people, but an attempt is often made to maintain their cultural and ethnic identities through the informal support systems. Maintaining the ethnic group identity does not negate the need for or the response to human needs of family, friends, and neighbors. Although the informal support systems of ethnic groups may be relatively invisible to outsiders, they are often viable and able to be activated in time of need.

The examples of client situations just cited point out the need for carefully assessing both the support systems of older adults from various ethnic groups and their particular needs. What might sometimes at first glance appear as indifference by the family is often an overwhelming need of the older person and an unrealistic expectation of the family. Older individuals may interpret a lack of response to their perceived needs as rejection, when the family may in fact be responding to the limits of its ability. An example is the need of older adults for social interaction. Relationships of older persons usually change in number and nature, contributing to a sense of loneliness. Because declining strength and energy limit their ability to participate in various activities and because economic factors prevent continuation of such customary activities as long-distance telephone calls, exchange of greeting cards and gifts, and entertaining, older adults may need less demanding types of relationships. This change in the nature of their relationships does not diminish their need for them. Because these needs may exceed the family's ability to cope with them, nurses should assess both these needs and the resources of the informal support system that may be mobilized to meet them.

Supporting the Support System

Mobilization of the informal support system to assist older persons often requires supporting the support system. Families may function well in the care of elderly members if they can have respite from time to time. Nurses are in a position to assess the situation and help meet the families' need for relief.

Northouse (1980) raises the question of who supports the support system. She points out that although a great deal of attention in recent literature focuses on persons in distress, little attention is given to the needs of the caregivers of distressed persons. She names factors affecting the family support system, such as the increased mobility of whole families and family members, the declining birthrate's impact on family resources, and increasing diversity with consequent changes in family structure. Northouse mentions the need for assessing the family as a support system and proposes nursing intervention for supporting the support system during periods of stress.

Northouse emphasizes the need for including the family as a component of health care. She indicates that since the family may have difficulty coping with the role of primary caregiver, its coping ability should be assessed and appropriate action taken.

In addition Northouse stresses the importance of helping the family to keep communication channels open. Maximizing the competence of the family includes teaching ways of dealing with the formal support system and of using its resources to supplement those of the informal support system. Families need an opportunity to express their feelings as they cope with changing situations. Families reeling under a sense of helplessness when the health status of one of its members changes can benefit from looking at their strengths and learning ways to use them effectively. According to Northouse, teaching families how to identify and use their resources may help the family regain a sense of control over situations and overcome feelings of helplessness.

In addition to learning their strengths families may need to recognize their weaknesses. Families often tend to cling to the desire to be independent and to see calling on others for assistance as a sign of weakness. In some cases the strength of the family is undermined by the inability to seek assistance such as respite care. If the family support system breaks down because of demands that exceed its strength, then care of its dependent member can be compromised. Lack of ability to recognize limitations may result in the family being forced to rely on outsiders for help; this situation might be prevented by recognition of limitations and acceptance of nonfamily resources.

Families should set realistic goals to build a sense of competence. Promoting the use of resources, such as the Visiting Nurses' Association and adult day-care services, is a means of supporting the family support system.

Helping families realize the importance of continuing extrafamilial activities is emphasized by Northouse. The need for an empathetic listener is pointed out along with the possibility that such a person might be discovered by family members while engaging in extrafamilial activities. If families have a person to whom they can turn to express their feelings and concerns, Northouse believes that they may feel supported and more able to cope with stress.

Although the article by Northouse is not directed specifically toward the elderly and their families, the suggestions she makes are applicable to them. Supporting the informal support system is likely to become increasingly important with the increasing longevity and numerical decline of family members who would ordinarily compose the family support system.

Recently interest in kinship relations has changed from studies describing kinship patterns to studies that attempt to explain them (Lee, 1980). More specific studies have focused on supportive aspects of elderly parent–adult child relationships. Less often is attention given to supportive relationships between elderly spouses. Furthermore, there is little in the literature about the interrelationships between elderly spouses and adult children in the informal support systems.

Kirkpatrick (1980) studied the elderly mother–adult daughter relationship and its effect on the length of the mother's hospital stay. Kirkpatrick became interested in the project because of recent research findings suggesting that the effects of stress were influenced by social support networks and that the health of an individual is affected by stress. The elderly mother's perception of her relationship with her adult daughter and its effect on her health were examined in this study. Kirkpatrick hypothesized that the better the relationship between mother and daughter, the shorter would be the length of the mother's hospitalization. Data failed to show any statistical significance in the relationship between the two variables, and the hypothesis was rejected.

Two factors pointed out by Kirkpatrick merit emphasis. One is the need for adult children to know available support systems they can use to help care for elderly mothers convalescing from episodes of illness that required hospitalization. The second is the finding that elderly married women tend to have on the average a longer hospital stay than women who are widowed. This is of particular interest. Since husbands tend to be older than wives, it may be that instead of being part of a viable support system, husbands contribute to the need for additional assistance. These factors indicate a need to assess the support system of older persons carefully.

Documentation of the nursing process carried out with older adults and their families is increasingly important. Documentation of actions and their outcomes is important, but of equal importance is that this information may be useful in other nurse-family interactions. Thoughtful nursing action is based on knowledge and experience validated by empirical experience and research. As this knowledge and experience is validated and formalized, it adds to the body of nursing knowledge, which in turn can be used to improve gerontological nursing practice.

Support Systems Networks and the Rural Elderly

Needs of the rural elderly are believed to differ from and be of greater magnitude than those of urban older persons. Of some 5 million Americans above 65 years of age, many are relatively isolated. Not only are rural older persons different from their urban counterparts in educational background, transportation, health, income, and housing, but there are differences in availability and accessibility of services to them, particularly of the formal support system.

Fewer studies have been conducted on the rural elderly than on the urban elderly (Luft, Hershey, and Morrell, 1976; Salber and others, 1976). One study reports on the attitudes of the rural elderly toward health and on their use of available community resources (Kersten, 1979). Findings revealed a significant relationship between their attitudes toward health and their use of community resources for health maintenance.

Kersten cites the need for home care in rural areas and for encouragement of self-care among the elderly. The need for home care is caused by the lack of readily available health care resources for the rural elderly and the relative inaccessibility of medical care. In addition, need is seen for educational programs that would provide the rural elderly with necessary self-care information. The investigator observed a paucity of support services in the rural area particularly of those services usually provided by the formal support system in urban areas.

Initially rural communities were organized around kinship groups, religious beliefs, or race (Conklin, 1980). Later other institutions developed, such as government, schools, and industry. In this relatively stable social structure informal community networks developed in response to needs or problems of the rural elderly and continue to be their major source of support.

In a sense triage is used in gaining access to services provided by the formal support system. Usually informal caregivers are the first to identify needs or problems and to give needed assistance. If the need or problem exceeds the ability of the informal caregivers, they often assist in locating appropriate resources in the formal support systems.

In many communities individuals referred to as gate-keepers are vital forces in the community. Knowledge of community attitudes and norms enables them to function in a unique manner; the gate-keepers often serve as a link between individuals and the community or between individuals and the formal support system. Whether or not gate-keepers have a close relationship with individual community members, they usually have face-to-face interactions with them facilitating the community members' acceptance of health care providers. Nurses initiating the nursing process with the rural elderly should be aware of the gate-keepers in the community and seek their assistance as circumstances indicate.

Examples of Support Systems and Services for Older Adults

Examples of support systems and services are numerous, yet many older adults have unmet needs because they do not know the available systems and services or how to tap them. A gap in the provision of services is created by not knowing them, since they cannot be considered in the planning of services for older adults. Anschutz (1982) found, however, some older adults who might have benefited from available resources who chose not to seek assistance. These persons either seemed not to perceive the need for help or expressed the desire to remain independent of extra-familial assistance. Different perceptions of need should be taken into account among older persons when assessing them.

Of critical importance in offering support is the concept of the whole person—body, mind, and spirit. Both the older person seeking health or wholeness and the nurse seeking to promote it are concerned with the process involved in attaining high-level wellness. The older person is a whole composed of many parts or subsystems. These parts normally work to maintain the individual's functioning. The whole person can thereby interact with the everchanging environment and while doing it find purpose in life. When change in either the internal or external environment interferes with the functioning of the whole person, support services may help offset the deficit and assist the person to regain a measure of well-being and wholeness. Knowledge of the needs or problems of the person and of support systems and available services is crucial to the nurse seeking to implement the nursing process within the holistic framework.

Sustaining the life force, or energy, of the older person requires a reverence for life and a caring expressed by nurse and client. In spite of adversity the older person often has a tremendous inner strength, which is an invaluable resource. Care should be taken to prevent depletion of the inner strength by erosion of the individual's fierce sense of independence. Establishing a relationship with the person and promoting interdependence should take priority; achieving this relationship takes sensitivity to the needs, wishes, and personhood of the older person.

A need for sensitivity to inner strength was occasioned by Mrs. K., a woman in her late 70s who had just learned that what initially had been diagnosed as a benign nasal polyp was believed to be malignant. Turning to her 88-year-old husband and her adult nurse/daughter, she said, "I don't want any tears. If you cry, I'll cry, and I don't want to. It's something I have to work through, but I can do it, if you let me do it my way."

**Multiple-service
Support Systems**

Commenting on the situation, the daughter said, "She's a very strong lady."

Although specific support systems and services exist for each of the four dimensions of the older person, there are support systems that provide multiple services capable of meeting a variety of needs. Shepherd's Center, in Kansas City, Missouri, is an example of a support system providing multiple services for older adults. Goals of the center are achieved through combining resources of the informal and formal support systems networks. The major part of the staff of the center is composed of volunteers; the formal component of the system comprises agencies, such as the Visiting Nurses' Association, that provide such services as health screening. The major function of the center is to provide alternatives to institutionalization for older persons. The program of the center is designed for and by older adults.

Shepherd's Center, created in the August of 1972, is defined as a concept rather than a place, although many of the programs and services are coordinated or conducted at one building. Shepherd's Center is an ecumenical project involving 25 church congregations, Catholic, Protestant, and Jewish (Cole, 1981). The center is incorporated, with a board of 24 representatives from the community, most of whom are above the age of 65. Programming is designed primarily to assist persons within an approximately 20-block target area to remain in their own homes and to be productive members of society. The uniqueness of Shepherd's Center arises out of the fact that for the most part it is older persons who meet the needs of older persons. Through such programs as life enrichment, health screening, and health education and services such as Meals on Wheels and handyman services, Shepherd's Center is a vital resource for many older persons. A purpose to life is realized by many older adults through the experience of giving and receiving support.

Program planning focused on the needs and interests of older adults is an annual event. A wide range of services and programs are provided, including transportation, companion aides, friendly visitors, security and protection services, adventures in learning, life enrichment, and health enrichment. These programs and services attend to the physical, psychological, sociological, and spiritual needs of older persons, reflecting the involvement of older persons in the planning process.

Changes in the programs occur from time to time according to the expressed needs and interests of the program participants. One of the newer programs is the hospice care program. A hospice provides care in a home-like environment for the terminally ill person and family. Supportive services are available on a 24-hour basis, 7 days a week, by qualified volunteers. These volunteers are selected and trained at the center for their roles in hospice care. Physical, emotional, and spiritual resources are available for meeting the needs of the terminally ill clients and their families.

The center, originally funded through the Missouri Department of Community Affairs, Office of Aging, under the provision of Title III, Older Americans Act of 1965, is currently supported by the community through contributions from churches, participants in the programs, clubs, foundations, and other community institutions. The Central United Methodist Church provides space and other support services needed for the various programs and activities, as do a number of other churches. The center thus reflects many community resources, which add to the quality of life of older persons. Moreover, older persons participating in the various activities are themselves important resources.

Since its inception the Shepherd's Center model has been emulated in many settings across the nation. Workshops are conducted for individuals interested in learning about the center and how the concept might be implemented in their home communities. Participants from various states and Canada gather to share in the learning experience. The sustained interest in Shepherd's Center by its older participants and by outside groups attests to its viability in meeting the basic needs of older adults.

The Four Dimensions of the Older Adult and Support Services

Overlap occurs among support services meeting the four dimensions of the older person. For example, day-care services may meet multiple needs, but the focus of a particular day-care program depends on the model upon which the program is established. Generally day-care services are organized around the medical model or the social model. This does not preclude the usefulness of either type of program in meeting needs in more than one dimension. Support services should be categorized according to the focus of each particular program. This approach requires analysis of the type of services provided but recognition that a given program may provide services that meet needs of older people in more than one dimension. Assessment of needs helps prevent gaps in services and promotes a more comprehensive approach to the needs of given individuals.

The following examples of services for older persons are by no means intended to represent the major services; nor are they mutually exclusive. The intent behind describing them is to show that a variety of services may be needed to meet the needs of the whole person.

The physical dimension. Day-care is a service provided at a place where older persons can spend part of a day or every day of the week if desired. The social model focuses on the social needs; the medical model as might be expected provides therapeutic services, such as physical therapy. Although day-care has not yet been widely accepted for care of older adults, it can be a vital service.

Day-care provides supervision of older persons, affording respite for the family. The medical model, which includes rehabilitative services, is a service supporting the physical dimension of older individuals. Not only the physical well-being of older persons but the well-being of the family support system may be maintained and promoted. Seeing gains made by the older family member and having an opportunity for shopping or other activities often gives the family a new lease on life. Day-care may halt a downward spiral and enable older persons and their families to gain a new perspective and hope.

With the increasing numbers of older persons and the thrust toward home care day-care centers are likely to become an important component of the formal support system. Cost of day-care is less than that of other types of institutional care. It is a means of sustaining the older person's support system, since it provides respite for the family. It is a service that can blend the informal and formal support systems into a continuum of services important to continuity of care and to the family support system.

The psychological dimension. One of the resources available for meeting the psychological needs of older persons is the elderhostel (College at my age? 1980). This resource is based on the assumption that the older person is never too old to learn.

The elderhostel is a nationwide program that encourages older individuals to participate in curricular and extracurricular activities on college and university campuses. Participants live in student dormitories, eat in the school cafeterias, attend classes of various types, and enjoy such extracurricular activities as watermelon feasts and plays offered in the school theaters. The older persons have an opportunity to make new friends not only with people their own age but with younger college students (University of Kansas, 1980).

Course offerings include such subjects as the psychology of communication and underground space. Participants often take courses for credit; some are interested in pursuing degrees, but others use the credit to see how they "measure up" in the academic world. Older persons often seize the opportunity for the education that was unavailable earlier in life; they tend to take more solid courses.

Although the elderhostel program began only 5 years ago with five participating colleges, some 300 colleges and universities participated in the 1981 summer programs (College at my age? 1980). The concept of lifelong learning is being realized by pioneering older adults on college and university campuses across the nation.

The sociological dimension. Various programs and activities that meet the social needs of older adults are available. These include captioned films for the deaf offered at libraries and colleges and ballroom dance classes offered at community centers. Creative workshops for developing skills such as writing, sculpting, painting, and working with ceramics are available in many centers for older adults. Great books clubs and Toastmasters' Clubs offer additional opportunities for making new friends, discussing ideas, learning new skills, and trying out new roles.

The spiritual dimension. Support for the spiritual dimension of older persons may be found through established synagogues and churches of various religious denominations. Increasing numbers of churches have programs and services of interest to older adults: Bible study groups and a variety of other group activities.

A number of churches are using a holistic approach to the aged, for instance, the Lutheran Church of America (LCA). Its "layered" organizational structure, starting with the LCA and followed by the Lutheran Social Service, Inc. (LSS), the Synod (composed of four states), the Metropolitan Lutheran Ministries, and the local churches, has task forces on older adults and facilitates program planning, coordination of services, and implementation of programs. A needs assessment provides data for planning the program. Needs documented by a 1982 LSS report include inadequate income, health problems, and lack of church-related groups for older people, especially in rural areas. Other needs include lack of in-home religious counseling and tape ministry, lack of transportation, loneliness, scarcity of information on protective services, and lack of screening programs for vision and hearing, particularly in rural areas (Stoulil, 1981).

The media are used to announce available services and how to make contact with them. Talking Books, a service provided through libraries, can help the visually impaired and the isolated to keep thinking; it is a means of affirming the older person's self-image as a thinking, feeling human being. There is need for resources that can be used for groups and for those who may have recently become isolated or who have tended to be private persons all their lives. Among the materials available to older visually impaired persons are audiotapes, including tapes of the Bible. There are numerous resources for supporting the spiritual dimension of the older person.

Another community-based program designed to help people live independently is Lifeline. Lifeline is an emergency call system, which the individual can activate by pushing a small wireless button attached to the clothing. Response to the call for help is available 24 hours a day; it is especially useful for the frail elderly. The Department of Health and Human Services is exploring potential reimbursement for this service for certain populations (for instance, those who are bedfast or wheelchair bound) as a result of the findings of their 3-year study of the Lifeline system (Lifeline Systems, 1982).

Additional Resources   Not the least of the resources are printed materials on various topics of interest to older persons and their families. Books listing resources are often available in local communities (Where to turn, 1977); they often give the name of the agency providing the service, the type of service it offers, and its address and telephone number. References on specific topics are available, such as those from the American Heart Association and the Arthritis Foundation. There is a book entitled *Special Devices for Hard of Hearing, Deaf, and Deaf-Blind Persons* (Hurvitz and Carmen, 1981). This reference lists numerous devices, their purposes, descriptions, prices, and makers.

A manual, *Your Health and Aging* (Glickman and Lipshutz, 1981), offers education and support to older adults and their caregivers; it is a compilation of information based on input of community residents 60 years of age or above. This manual is also a resource for professionals who are involved with educational programs and group activities for older adults. It is an outgrowth of a 2-year model project funded through the Administration on Aging and is available from the Division of Gerontology, Office of Urban Health Affairs, New York Medical Center. Content of the report is organized around three major topics: (1) living a healthy life, (2) specific disease conditions such as arthritis and diabetes mellitus, and (3) social services (including a description of various services that may be useful to older persons). The material is set in large type and includes a bibliography. The concepts of self-care are discussed in this material. This reference may be used by individuals who want to learn about themselves and by those who are responsible for group activities and programs.

Listings of programs and services are available through news media and public libraries. An example is the column "The Later Years," published in the *Kansas City Times;* it contains information about programs and services, such as free tax assistance, legal assistance, health clinics, diet, and program schedules for activities sponsored by the Parks and Recreation District. These informational resources are available in many areas of the nation; they are an important part of the support systems network.

Summary   The older person is likely to need support from the informal and formal support networks to maintain integrity and personhood in the later years. An important function of the gerontological nurse is assisting older persons to identify unmet needs and appropriate resources for meeting those needs. The nurse initiating the nursing process is in a position to help an older client learn information that the client may subsequently be able to use in adapting a life-style to allow him or her a greater sense of mastery in the face of life change events.

Supporting the strengths of older persons requires knowing them and their support systems network, both informal and formal. It may necessitate teaching older persons the importance of interdependence when changes of aging decrease their independence. Assisting older persons requires an appreciation of them as thinking, acting, feeling human beings whose integrity and personhood are worthy of support.

References

Anschutz, M.G.: The relationship between needs and utilization of informal support resources and formal community resources by elderly homeowners for maintenance of independent living, master's thesis, Lawrence, Kan., 1982, University of Kansas.

Ball, D.W.: The family as a sociological problem: conceptualization of the taken-for-granted as prologue to social problem analysis, Soc. Problems 19:295-307, 1972.

Blau, Z.S.: Old age in a changing society, New York, 1973, New Viewpoints.

Caplan, G.: Support systems and community mental health: lectures on concept development, New York, 1974, Behavioral Publications.

Cobb, S.: Social support as a moderator of life stress, Psychosom. Med. 38(5):300-314, 1976.

Cole, E.D.: The Shepherd Center. In Berghorn, F.J., Schafer, D.E., and others, editors: The dynamics of aging: original essays on the processes and experiences of growing old, Boulder, Colo., 1981, Westview Press, Inc.

College at my age? UMKC Magazine 11(2):15, 1980.

Conklin, C.: Rural community care givers, Soc. Work 25(6):495-496, 1980.

Dean, A., and Lin, N.: The stress buffering role of social support: problems on prospects for systematic investigation, J. Nerv. Ment. Dis. 165:403-417, 1977.

Ebersole, P., and Hess, P.: Toward healthy aging: human needs and nursing response, St. Louis, 1981, The C.V. Mosby Co.

Elderhostel, University of Kansas, Gerontol. Rev. 3(2):1, 1980.

Fuller, S.S., and Larson, S.B.: Life events, emotional support, and health of older people, Res. Nurs. Health 3(2):81-89, 1980.

Gardner, K.G.: Supportive nursing: a critical review of the literature, J. Psychiatr. Nurs. 17(10):10-16, 1979.

Glickman, S., and Lipshutz, J.: Your health and aging, New York, 1981, Division of Gerontology, Office of Urban Health Affairs, New York University Medical Center.

Gregg, D.: Reassurance, Am. J. Nurs. 55:171-174, 1955.

Gurian, B.S., and Cantor, M.H.: Mental health and community support systems for the elderly. In Usdin, G., and Hofling, C.K., editors: Aging: the process and the people, New York, 1978, Brunner/Mazel, Inc.

Haley, J.: The later years: Taiwanese daughter overcame obstacles to find help for her sick mother, The Kansas City Star, December 31, 1980.

Hall, A.D., and Fagan, R.E.: Definition of a system. In Buckley, W., editor: Modern systems research for the behavioral scientist, Chicago, 1968, Aldine Publishing Co.

Hart, B., and Reltweder, A.: Support in nursing, Am. J. Nurs. 59:1398-1401, 1959.

Hazzard, M.E.: An overview of systems theory, Nurs. Clin. North Am. 6(3):385-393, 1971.

Hurvitz, J. and Carmen, R.: Special devices for hard of hearing, deaf, and deaf-blind persons, Boston, 1981, Little Brown & Co.

Jones, E.M.: Who supports the nurses? Nurs. Outlook 10:476-478, 1962.

Jury, M., and Jury, D.: Gramp, New York, 1976, Grossman Publishers.

Kersten, J.: Attitudes of the rural elderly toward health and their use of available community health resources, master's thesis, Lawrence, Kan., 1979, University of Kansas.

Kirkpatrick, S.L.: Study of the association between elderly-mother/adult-daughter relationship and length of hospitalization of mother, masters thesis, Lawrence, Kan. 1980, University of Kansas.

Lee, G.R.: Kinship in the seventies: a decade review of research and theory, J. Marriage Family 42(4):923-934, 1980.

Lifeline Systems: Results of HEW-funded study of lifeline, Noblesville, Ind., 1982, Lifeline Systems, Inc.

Lindsey, A.M., and Hughes, E.M.: Social support and alternatives to institutionalization for the at-risk elderly, J. Am. Geriatr. Soc. 29(7):308-315, 1981.

Linton, R.B.: The study of man, New York, 1936, Appleton-Century-Crofts.

Lowenthal, M.F., and Haven, C.: Interaction and adaptation: intimacy as a critical variable, Am. Sociol. Rev. 33:20-30, 1968.

Luft, H.S., Hershey, J.C., and Morrell, J.: Factors affecting the use of physician's services in a rural community, Am. J. Pub. Health 66(9):865-871, 1976.

Northouse, L.L.: Who supports the support system? J. Psychiatr. Nurs. 18(5):11-15, 1980.

Olsen, J.K., and Cahn, B.W.: Helping families cope, J. Gerontol. Nurs. 6(3):152-154, 1980.

Pilisuk, M.: Supportive networks: life ties for the elderly, J. Soc. Issues 36(2):95-115, 1980.

Pilisuk, M., and Minkler, M.: Supportive networks: life ties for the elderly, J. Soc. Issues 36(2):95-116, 1980.

Pratt, L.: Changes in health care ideology in relation to self-care by families, Health Educ. Monogr. 5(2):121-135, 1977.

Preston, T.: Caring for the aged: when words fail, Am. J. Nurs. 73:2064, 1973.

Red Horse, J.G.: American Indian elders: unifiers of Indian families, Social Casework 61(8):490-493, 1980.

Riley, M.W., and Foner, A.: Aging and society, vol. 1. An inventory of research findings, New York, 1968, The Russell Sage Foundation.

Rosow, I.: Forms and functions of adult socialization, Soc. Forces 44(1):35-45, 1965.

Rosow, I.: Social integration of the aged, New York, 1967, The Free Press.

Salber, E.G., and others: Access to health care in a southern rural community, Med. Care 14(12):971-986, 1976.

Sanders, L.T., and Seelbach, W.C.: Variations in preferred care alternatives for the elderly: family versus nonfamily sources, Fam. Relations 30(3):447-451, 1981.

Shanas, E.: The family as a social support system in old age, Gerontologist 19(2):169-174, 1979.

Speck, R.V., and Attneave, C.L.: Family networks, New York, 1973, Pantheon Books, Inc.

Stallwood, J., and Stoll, R.: Spiritual dimensions of nursing practice. In Beland, I.R., and Passos, J.Y., editors: Clinical nursing: pathophysiological and psychosocial approaches, ed. 3, New York, 1975, Macmillan Pub. Co., Inc.

Stewart, J.E.: Home health care, St. Louis, 1979, The C.V. Mosby Co.

Stoulil, C.A.: Lutheran Social Service aging report, Wichita, Kan., 1982, Lutheran Social Service.

Sussman, M.B.: The family life of old people. In Binstock, R.H., and Shanas, E., editors: Handbook of aging and the social sciences, New York, 1976, Van Nostrand Reinhold Co.

Sussman, M.B., and Burchinall, L.G.: Kin family network: unheralded structure in current conceptualizations of family functioning. In Farber, B., editor: Kinship and family organization, New York, 1966, John Wiley & Sons, Inc.

Tibbitts, C.: Older Americans in the family context, Aging 270-271:6-11, 1977.

Tolsdorf, C.: Social networks, support, and coping: an exploratory study, Fam. Process 15(4):407, 1976.

Trager, N.P.: Available communication networks for the aged in the community. In Oyer, H.J., and Oyer, E.D., editors: Aging and communication, Baltimore, 1976, University Park Press.

Unger, D.G., and Powell, D.R.: Supporting families under stress: the role of social networks, Fam. Relations **29**(4):566-574, 1980.

Von Bertalanffy, L.: General systems theory, Main Currents Modern Thought **11**:75-83, 1955.

Walker, K.N., McBride, A.I., and Vachon, M.L.S.: Social support networks and the crisis of bereavement, Soc. Sci. Med. **11**:35-41, 1977.

Weidenbach, E.: Clinical nursing: a helping act, New York, 1964, Springer Publishing Co., Inc.

Weiss, R.S.: The fund of sociability, Trans-action **6**:36-43, 1969.

Weiss, R.S.: Transition states and other stressful situations. In Caplan, G., and Killelea, M., editors: Support systems and mutual help—multidisciplinary explorations, New York, 1976, Greene and Stratton.

Where to turn: a directory of health, welfare, recreation, and educational resources in the metropolitan Kansas City area, Kansas City, Mo., 1977, Voluntary Action Center.

Epilogue

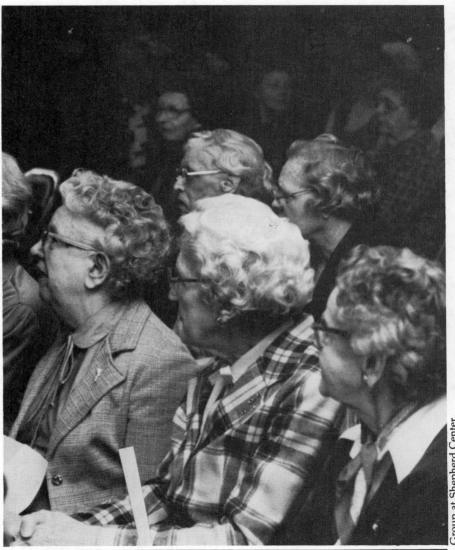

Since the beginning of time, aging has been viewed as a universal human experience in the natural order of things that takes place within the context of social change. With the passage of time and the advance of science, health care has improved, increasing longevity for many individuals. In 1900 the life expectancy in the United States was 47 years. The average life expectancy is now 74 years, with an increment expected in each future census. A life expectancy of approximately 84 years is projected for the end of the century. Currently 15,000 persons are known to be over 100 years of age (AARP, 1983).

Historically changes have affected the societal view of the individual. Currently society has entered what is referred to as the era of information and communication, and it is scrutinizing the role and functions of its older members. Never before has there been such a large population of older people throughout the world nor so many resources of information on "learning a living." During the industrial era people were viewed as expendable, especially those over the age of 55. Little attention was given to individuals leaving the world of work or to their need for socialization into what has often been referred to as "roleless roles." With increasing longevity and the consequent increasing number of older persons, attention is now being given to the contribution older persons can make to society.

Perspectives of Aging Past and Present

Social movements reflecting varying views of individuals are evident in the pages of history, beginning with the pagan orientation, in which individuals were used for the benefit of the state. The Christian era gave rise to the view of the individual as a person worthy of being accorded dignity and respect. This era was followed by the industrial period when the worth of the individual tended to be discounted, especially if the individual became nonproductive in the economic system.

With the transition into the information and communication era, the societal view of the individual fluctuates like an ECG needle on paper tape between depersonalization and repersonalization. This fluctuation makes it difficult to determine the extent of the trend toward personalization. The goal of gerontologists is that the personhood of each older individual be recognized.

Questions are now being raised as to who should make decisions about who should live and who should die, and the questions touch on such factors as economic and medical resources and the value of human life. A case in point, occurring on December 2, 1982, brings this issue sharply into focus. A retired, 61-year-old dentist with a heart disease and suffering a sudden, rapid deterioration of his condition became the first recipient of a mechanical heart. In this case there was little time to consider this act's ethical ramifications; ethical issues regarding the use of mechanical replacement of vital organs are likely to be raised increasingly over time. Scientists are already discussing possibilities of other bionic devices for prolonging biological life, raising questions about humanness, personhood, and the acceptance of aging and death. Can dependence on mechanical devices such as the air compressor that keeps the artificial heart functional be humanistic when the locus of control over a vital life function is outside the body? The impact of this type of procedure on the quality of the older person's life is staggering to contemplate when the moral and religious ramifications are analyzed.

From a nursing perspective the older person is worthy of care on the basis of humanness and certain needs. Although the nursing profession and some of its individual members were affected by the negative societal attitude toward aging and the aged, within recent years special attention has been directed toward the unique health care needs of the older segment of society. In 1966 the ANA established what is now called the Division of Gerontological Nursing Practice. This division, designed to meet the health needs of the elderly, became an integral part of the total ANA organizational structure and has steadily increased its membership.

The *Standards of Gerontological Nursing Practice* have been developed and implemented by the ANA Division of Gerontological Nursing Practice. These standards are used by the nursing profession and by individual nurses for evaluating the outcomes of gerontological nursing care and practice. In addition, they are used by outside agencies for the evaluation of care and by the legal profession for questions regarding gerontological nursing practice.

Furthermore, efforts have been directed toward the recognition and education of gerontological nurses. Inclusion of instruction on gerontological nursing has been successfully encouraged in undergraduate and graduate curricula. Nurses who have directed their energies toward learning about care of older persons and practicing in the field of gerontological nursing have been recognized partly because of the ANA certification program for gerontological nurses and degree-granting educational programs.

These developments in gerontological nursing have been initiated in response to societal needs. Demand for further developments of this nature is increasing with the rapidly increasing population of older people and the growing awareness of their needs. The nursing profession continues to provide health care for older adults. This epilogue, touching the historical evolution of society and the concomitant development of gerontological nursing, provides a foundation from which projections for the future can be made for nursing and other disciplines.

Perspectives of the Future and Challenges of Aging

There is a need to explore the transitional phase between past and present developments and the anticipated changes and challenges of the future. A large population segment of the future will be older people; they will experience major changes in life-style, work, leisure activities, and interpersonal relationships. An overview of potential change is necessary, even though projections for the future may vary in accuracy. Such a philosophical analysis is essential for placing older human beings in perspective within the dynamic sociocultural milieu of the global village.

In the emerging era of information and communication a bright future depends on the judgment and wisdom of human beings. If older persons are recognized and appreciated as fully human beings, their wisdom may be brought to bear on the concerns of society. The wisdom of all people is needed to prevent the destruction of humankind and the physical world and to achieve world brotherhood. This concept of brotherhood encompasses the tenets of the Judeo-Christian belief system. Our philosophical stance bases the concept of world brotherhood on the worth and dignity of human beings as exemplified by the life of Christ and the values he es-

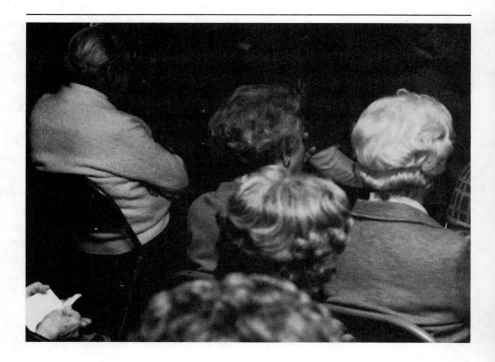

poused. This brotherhood would value each human being and all mankind. Respect for life should bring about a better quality of life, which is a right of all human beings, including the older members of society.

"Learning a living," an experience of older people, means developing the art and science of life to achieve full humanness. This requires developing a philosophy of life that encompasses the entirety of life and its experiences, including the spiritual dimension. Some may view the spiritual dimension as continuing beyond the realm of physical existence. Many believe that the concept of life after death forms the foundation on which the worth of the human being is established and which is the basis for a fuller appreciation of the gift of life. In any case, the spiritual dimension is the essence of hope, giving meaning to life and encouraging the will to live.

A human being stands on the shifting sands of change but may be rooted in unchanging convictions based on eternal values that provide stability and contribute toward the attainment of life's goals. By choosing life, such an individual is motivated by a sense of social responsibility and concern for the well-being of others to better the human condition according to his or her value system. This philosophical stance is ageless and timeless in its implications. Our expectation is that human beings will ascribe more fully in the future to this major element of the eternal value system, the brotherhood of man.

If brotherhood were achieved, the global village would become a community of caring family, friends, and neighbors intensely interested in promoting health and well-being among all of the villagers. In such an event, the sharing of resources would be based on this concept: to each according to his or her needs and from each according to his or her abilities. For example, it would be important that food distribution not become a weapon in the hands of politicians. The potential for living life fully would be realized through the concern of one human being for another.

It appears to us that the denial of the aging process continues to interfere with the development of human potential. Research efforts tend to be directed toward extending physical life through artificial means such as the mechanical heart, whereas less attention is given to the quality of such a life. The question can be raised as to when a human being's qualities are lessened by dependence on an external mechanical device. A device may disrupt spiritual development and the acceptance of life and death as naturally occurring events. Is it possible to attend to both the finiteness of physical being and the quality of life concurrently? Should we continue to pursue extraordinary means of extending life and almost ignore the issue of how one can live and die as a fully integrated human being?

Furthermore, cloning and genetic engineering raise another set of questions about humanness and the right to self-determination. In the natural order of things individuality has tended to be favored over consideration of the group. Cloning and gene splicing could alter the natural cycle of human life and development. What does scientific advancement mean to the individual and to future human brotherhood?

The effects of scientific advancement on individual rights and responsibilities to the social group is a major issue. Where should the line be drawn between extending life and accepting death? What is the value of human life, and who should decide it? What are the qualitative aspects of an extended life? Can self-determination and the exercise of individual rights be realized without compromising the social group?

From our perspective respect for and appreciation of the individual's unique qualities and possible contributions to humankind is the keystone to a bright new world. Assisting each older person to realize the fullness of life is a meaningful goal, which must exist along with the goal of increasing longevity.

The challenge of the future is the qualitative development of human beings over the mere quantitative extension of life. Regardless of the length of life, the individual comes to an end point of physical being. Assisting persons to a greater realization of their potential has an effect on the quality of their lives and in turn on that of the social group. Failure to confront death may deprive the person of some of the finer experiences of life and human relationships: when life seems endless, time for appreciation of the beauty and fragrance of a rose may be put off, and meaningful relationships with other persons may be neglected. Attention should be focused on improving the quality of life even as it ebbs. Helping each person to share in the lifelong process of giving and receiving recognizes the worth and dignity of every person; respect for personhood will lead to a bright new world of human brotherhood.

Reference

AARP: Centenarians send message via their active lifestyles: 15,000 are 100 or older, Am. Assoc. of Retired Persons News Bull. **24**(5):15, 1983.

Index

Social Security, 174
Social Security Act, 238-239
Social support networks, 234
Society, attitude of, to older person, 28, 31
Sociological aging, 37, 80-82
  theories of, 47
Sociological definition of human person, 19
Sociological development in later years, 45-47
Sociological dimension, support services for, 256
Sociological nursing diagnoses, 221-222
Sordes, 67
Special Devices for Hard of Hearing, Deaf, and Deaf-Blind Persons, 257
Speech discrimination, loss of, 75
Speech perception, 75
Spirit, definition of, 82-83, 106
Spirit-titre, 86, 106
Spiritual aging, 37, 48
Spiritual changes of aging, 83-89
  in later years, 48-49
Spiritual dimension of personality, 23
  assessment of, 201-202, 205-206
  compared with biopsychosocial dimensions, 84
  motivation through, 106-107
  support services for, 256-257
Spiritual nursing diagnoses, 222-223
Staff, attitude of, 188-189
Staffing in health care centers, 182
Standards of gerontological nursing practice, 7, 176-180
Standards of Gerontological Nursing Practice, 7, 218, 263
  and availability of data, 201
  and evaluation, 216
  and participation of older person in planning, 186, 210
  for positive attitude, 189
Statement on the Scope and Practice of Gerontological Nursing, 185, 189
Stimulus persistence, 73
Stimulus-response psychology, 96
Striving, 99
Subordinate systems, 2
Superordinate systems, 2

Support services, accessibility of, 238
Support, concept of, 230-232
Support systems, 232-233
  blending of, 240-241
  definition of, 232
Support systems network, 227-260
  concept of networks, 233-234
  concept of support, 230-232
  formal, 229, 233, 237-241
  four dimensions of older adult and
    physical, 254-255
    psychological, 255
    sociological, 256
    spiritual, 256-257
  informal; *see* Informal support systems networks
  losses in, 229-230
  multiple-service, 253-254
  and rural elderly, 251-252
  and services for older adults, 252-257
  social, 234
  supporting, 248-250
  and systems theory, 228-230
  types of, 234-241
Supporting support system network, 248-250
Symbiotic relationship, 242
Synthesis
  of data, 209-210
  as mode of inquiry, 39
Systematic data collection, 177
Systems differentiated from environment, 228
Systems framework
  assessment tools organized around, 204-205
  nursing in, 229
Systems, theory, 228-230

T

Tabula rasa, 96
Talking Books, 256
Task performance, research on, 117-118
Team nursing, 193-194
Tension states and motivation, 100, 104
Terminal drop, 75
Tests
  cognitive ability, interpretation of, 76
  for perception, 73-74